T0358930

Pediatric Emergency Medicine

Editors

SEAN M. FOX
DALE P. WOOLRIDGE

EMERGENCY MEDICINE CLINICS OF NORTH AMERICA

www.emed.theclinics.com

Consulting Editor
AMAL MATTU

May 2018 • Volume 36 • Number 2

ELSEVIER

1600 John F. Kennedy Boulevard • Suite 1800 • Philadelphia, Pennsylvania, 19103-2899

http://www.theclinics.com

EMERGENCY MEDICINE CLINICS OF NORTH AMERICA Volume 36, Number 2
May 2018 ISSN 0733-8627, ISBN-13: 978-0-323-58350-3

Editor: Colleen Dietzler
Developmental Editor: Casey Potter

Emergency Medicine Clinics of North America (ISSN 0733-8627) is published quarterly by Elsevier Inc., 360 Park Avenue South, New York, NY, 10010-1710. Months of issue are February, May, August, and November. Business and Editorial Offices: 1600 John F. Kennedy Boulevard, Suite 1800, Philadelphia, PA 19103-2899. Customer Service Office: 6277 Sea Harbor Drive, Orlando, FL 32887-4800. Periodicals postage paid at New York, NY, and additional mailing offices. Subscription prices are $100.00 per year (US students), $336.00 per year (US individuals), $644.00 per year (US institutions), $220.00 per year (international students), $455.00 per year (international individuals), $791.00 per year (international institutions), $220.00 per year (Canadian students), $405.00 per year (Canadian individuals), and $791.00 per year (Canadian institutions). International air speed delivery is included in all *Clinics'* subscription prices. All prices are subject to change without notice. **POSTMASTER:** Send address changes to *Emergency Medicine Clinics of North America*, Elsevier Periodicals Customer Service, 11830 Westline Industrial Drive, St. Louis, MO 63146. Customer Service (orders, claims, online, change of address): Elsevier Periodicals **Customer Service, 11830 Westline Industrial Drive, St. Louis, MO 63146. Tel: 1-800-654-2452 (U.S. and Canada); 314-453-7041 (outside U.S. and Canada). Fax: 314-453-5170. E-mail: journalscustomerservice-usa@elsevier.com (for print support)**; **journalsonlinesupport-usa@elsevier.com (for online support)**.

Reprints. For copies of 100 or more of articles in this publication, please contact the Commercial Reprints Department, Elsevier Inc., 360 Park Avenue South, New York, NY 10010-1710. Tel.: 212-633-3874; Fax: 212-633-3820; E-mail: reprints@elsevier.com.

Emergency Medicine Clinics of North America is covered in *MEDLINE/PubMed (Index Medicus), Current Contents/Clinical Medicine, EMBASE/Excerpta Medica, BIOSIS, SciSearch, CINAHL, ISI/BIOMED,* and *Research Alert.*

Contributors

CONSULTING EDITOR

AMAL MATTU, MD, FAAEM, FACEP
Professor and Vice Chair, Department of Emergency Medicine, University of Maryland School of Medicine, Baltimore, Maryland

EDITORS

SEAN M. FOX, MD, FACEP, FAAP
Associate Program Director, Emergency Medicine Residency Program, Department of Emergency Medicine, Carolinas Medical Center, Charlotte, North Carolina

DALE P. WOOLRIDGE, MD, PhD, FAAEM, FAAP, FACEP
Associate Director Pediatric-Emergency Medicine Combined Residency Program, Professor of Emergency Medicine and Pediatrics, Department of Emergency Medicine, The University of Arizona, Tucson, Arizona

AUTHORS

RYAN FEY, MD
Assistant Professor of Surgery, University of Minnesota Medical School, Burn Center Director, Hennepin County Medical Center, Department of Surgery, Minneapolis, Minnesota

AARTI GAGLANI, MD
Division of Emergency Medicine, Phoenix Children's Hospital, Phoenix, Arizona

MARY GASPERS, MD
Associate Professor, Department of Pediatrics, Pediatric Critical Care Medicine, University of Arizona College of Medicine–Tucson, Banner–University Medical Center Tucson, Tucson, Arizona

TONI GROSS, MD, MPH
Division of Emergency Medicine Phoenix Children's Hospital, Department of Child Health, The University of Arizona College of Medicine–Phoenix, Phoenix, Arizona

JAMES (JIM) L. HOMME, MD
Assistant Professor of Pediatrics and Emergency Medicine, Associate Program Director, Pediatric and Adolescent Medicine Residency, Department of Emergency Medicine, Division of Pediatric Emergency Medicine, Mayo Clinic, Rochester, Minnesota

VIVIAN HWANG, MD, FACEP, FAAP
Associate Program Director, The Altieri PEM Fellowship, Assistant Clinical Professor of Emergency Medicine, The George Washington University School of Medicine & Health Sciences, Assistant Professor of Emergency Medicine and Pediatrics, Virginia Commonwealth University School of Medicine, Inova Fairfax Medical Campus, Falls Church, Virginia

MAYBELLE KOU, MD, FACEP, FAAP
Program Director, The Altieri PEM Fellowship, Associate Clinical Professor of Emergency Medicine, The George Washington University School of Medicine & Health Sciences, Assistant Professor of Emergency Medicine and Pediatrics, Virginia Commonwealth University School of Medicine, Inova Fairfax Medical Campus, Falls Church, Virginia

AARON N. LEETCH, MD
Assistant Professor, Departments of Emergency Medicine and Pediatrics, The University of Arizona, Tucson, Arizona

EMILY C. MACNEILL, MD
Associate Professor, Emergency Medicine, Carolinas HealthCare System, Charlotte, North Carolina

CHRISTYN MAGILL, MD
Attending Physician, Department of Emergency Medicine, Division of Pediatric Emergency Medicine, Carolinas Medical Center, Levine Children's Hospital, Charlotte, North Carolina

ANNA McFARLIN, MD, FAAP
Assistant Professor of Emergency Medicine and Pediatrics, Program Director, Combined Emergency Medicine-Pediatrics Residency, Children's Hospital of New Orleans, Louisiana State University Health Sciences Center, New Orleans, Louisiana

JENNY MENDELSON, MD
Assistant Professor, Department of Emergency Medicine and Pediatrics, Division of Pediatric Critical Care Medicine, University of Arizona College of Medicine–Tucson, Banner–University Medical Center Tucson, Tucson, Arizona

GARRETT S. PACHECO, MD
Assistant Professor, Departments of Emergency Medicine and Pediatrics, University of Arizona College of Medicine–Tucson, Banner–University Medical Center Tucson, Tucson, Arizona

AMY L. PUCHALSKI, MD
Attending Physician, Department of Emergency Medicine, Division of Pediatric Emergency Medicine, Carolinas Medical Center, Levine Children's Hospital, Charlotte, North Carolina

NADIRA RAMKELLAWAN, MD
Pediatric Emergency Medicine Fellow, The Altieri PEM Fellowship, Inova Fairfax Medical Campus, Falls Church, Virginia

STACY L. REYNOLDS, MD
Associate Professor, Department of Emergency Medicine, Division of Pediatric Emergency Medicine, Carolinas Medical Center, Charlotte, North Carolina

EMILY ROSE, MD, FAAP, FAAEM, FACEP
Director for Pre-Health Undergraduate Studies, Director of the Minor in Health Care Studies, Assistant Professor of Clinical Emergency Medicine, Keck School of Medicine of USC, University of Southern California, LAC + USC Medical Center, Los Angeles, California

TIM RUTTAN, MD
Department of Pediatric Emergency Medicine, Dell Children's Medical Center of Central Texas, Austin, Texas

GENEVIEVE SANTILLANES, MD
Associate Professor, Department of Emergency Medicine, Keck School of Medicine of USC, University of Southern California, Los Angeles, California

PAUL C. SCHUNK, MD
Department of Pediatric Emergency Medicine, Dell Children's Medical Center of Central Texas, Austin, Texas

ASHLEY M. STROBEL, MD
Assistant Professor of Emergency Medicine, University of Minnesota Medical School, Hennepin County Medical Center, University of Minnesota Masonic Children's Hospital, Minneapolis, Minnesota

KHOON-YEN TAY, MD
Assistant Professor of Clinical Pediatrics, Division of Emergency Medicine, Children's Hospital of Philadelphia, Philadelphia, Pennsylvania

CHAD D. VISCUSI, MD
Assistant Professor, Departments of Emergency Medicine and Pediatrics, University of Arizona College of Medicine–Tucson, Tucson, Arizona

CHANTEL P. WALKER, MD
Fellow, Pediatric Emergence Medicine, Carolinas HealthCare System, Charlotte, North Carolina

JESSICA J. WALL, MD, MPH
Clinical Associate Emergency Medicine Faculty, Department of Emergency Medicine, Penn Presbyterian Medical Center, Philadelphia, Pennsylvania

BRYAN WILSON, MD
Chief Resident, Departments of Emergency Medicine and Pediatrics, The University of Arizona, Tucson, Arizona

Contents

Section 1: Common

fractures, deterioration and neurosurgical intervention are rare and hospital admission can be avoided.

Paul C. Schunk and Tim Ruttan

Syncope is a common presentation to the emergency room. Unlike in the adult population, most pediatric syncope has non-life-threatening causes, and minimal evaluation in the emergency department is appropriate with parental reassurance. Despite this benign prognosis, care must be taken to find uncommon and potentially fatal causes. The primary purpose of evaluation of the patient with syncope is to determine whether the patient is at increased risk for death and needs either admission to the hospital or an expedited outpatient evaluation. This article reviews some of the most dangerous causes of syncope in the pediatric patient.

Aarti Gaglani and Toni Gross

Nearly 20 years ago, standards were established for hospitals to assess and treat pain in all patients. Research continues to demonstrate evolving trends in the measurement and effective treatment of pain in children. Behavioral research demonstrating long-lasting effects of inadequate pain control during childhood supports the concepts of early and adequate pain control for children with painful conditions in the acute care setting. The authors discuss pain concepts, highlighting factors specific to the emergency department, and include a review of evidence for pharmacologic and nonpharmacologic treatments.

Anna McFarlin

The term "brief resolved unexplained event" was created to replace "apparent life-threatening event," narrowing the definition and providing evidence-based guidelines for management. The emphasis is placed on using clinical clues to classify patients as low risk or exclude them from the categorization altogether. Infants who meet low-risk classification can be briefly observed in the emergency department and be discharged home. Infants who demonstrate elements suggestive of a specific etiology should be evaluated and treated accordingly. Patients who demonstrate no specific findings yet who are high risk should be evaluated for the most common etiologies of apneic events and be admitted.

Amy L. Puchalski and Christyn Magill

Advances in medical imaging are invaluable in the care of pediatric patients in the emergent setting. The diagnostic accuracy offered by studies using ionizing radiation, such as plain radiography, computed tomography, and fluoroscopy, are not without inherent risks. This article reviews the evidence supporting the risk of ionizing radiation from medical imaging as well as discusses clinical scenarios in which clinicians play an important role in supporting the judicious use of imaging studies.

Emily C. MacNeill and Chantel P. Walker

An inborn error of metabolism should be considered in any neonate who presents to the emergency department in extremis and in any young child who presents with altered mental status and vomiting. In children with un-known diagnoses, it is crucial to draw the appropriate laboratory studies before the institution of therapy, although treatment needs rapid institution to mitigate neurologic damage and avoid worsening metabolic crisis. Although there are hundreds of individual genetic disorders, they are roughly placed into groups that present similarly. This article reviews the approach to the patient with unknown metabolic diagnosis and up-to-date management pearls for children with known disorders.

Section 2: Critical

Chad D. Viscusi and Garrett S. Pacheco

Noninvasive ventilation (NIV) has emerged as a powerful tool for the pedi-atric emergency management of acute respiratory failure (ARF). This ther-apy is safe and well tolerated and seems to frequently prevent both the need for invasive mechanical ventilation and the associated risks/compli-cations. Although NIV can be the primary treatment of ARF resulting from multiple respiratory disease states, it must be meticulously monitored and, when unsuccessful, may aid in preoxygenation for prompt endotracheal intubation and invasive mechanical ventilation. The following article re-views the physiologic effects of NIV and its role in common respiratory dis-eases encountered in pediatric emergency medicine.

Garrett S. Pacheco, Jenny Mendelson, and Mary Gaspers

Pediatric mechanical ventilation is first initiated by emergency physicians (EPs) when performing active airway management in a critically ill or injured child. When initiating and adjusting mechanical ventilation, the child has unique anatomy and physiology to consider. The EP is the first to respond to ventilator alarm triggers and the initial medical provider to resuscitate the ventilated pediatric patient who is deteriorating while in the emergency department. This article uses cases to provide a framework to initiate and troubleshoot mechanical ventilation of pediatric patients in the emergency department.

Jessica J. Wall and Khoon-Yen Tay

Posttonsillectomy hemorrhage represents a potentially life-threatening condition that occurs in up to 5% of pediatric patients. Minor bleeding often precedes severe hemorrhage. Patients with minor or self-resolving bleeding should be observed in the emergency department or admitted for monitoring. Patients with severe bleeding should be immediately assessed for airway and hemodynamic stability. Management of severe bleeding includes immediate surgical consultation or initiation of the transfer process to a center with surgical capabilities, direct pressure to the site of hemorrhage with or without the addition of a hemostatic agent, possible rapid sequence intubation, and management of hemodynamic instability with volume resuscitation.

Shock, a state of inadequate oxygen delivery to tissues resulting in anaerobic metabolism, lactate accumulation, and end-organ dysfunction, is common in children in the emergency department. Shock can be divided into 4 categories: hypovolemic, distributive, cardiogenic, and obstructive. Early recognition of shock can be made with close attention to historical clues, physical examination, and vital sign abnormalities. Early and aggressive treatment can prevent or reverse organ dysfunction and improve morbidity and mortality.

Although the overall incidence of and mortality rate associated with burn injury have decreased in recent decades, burns remain a significant source of morbidity and mortality in children. Children with major burns require emergent resuscitation. Resuscitation is similar to that for adults, including pain control, airway management, and administration of intravenous fluid. However, in pediatrics, fluid resuscitation is needed for burns greater than or equal to 15% of total body surface area (TBSA) compared with burns greater than or equal to 20% TBSA for adults. Unique to pediatrics is the additional assessment for nonaccidental injury and accurate calculation of the percentage of total burned surface area in children with changing body proportions, which are crucial to determine resuscitation parameters, prognosis, and disposition.

Traumatic brain injury is a highly prevalent and devastating cause of morbidity and mortality in children. A rapid, stepwise approach to the traumatized child should proceed, addressing life-threatening problems first. Management focuses on preventing secondary injury from physiologic extremes such as hypoxemia, hypotension, prolonged hyperventilation, temperature extremes, and rapid changes in cerebral blood flow. Initial Glasgow Coma Score, hyperglycemia, and imaging are often prognostic of outcome. Surgically amenable lesions should be evacuated promptly. Reduction of intracranial pressure through hyperosmolar therapy, decompressive craniotomy, and seizure prophylaxis may be considered after stabilization. Nonaccidental trauma should be considered when evaluating pediatric trauma patients.

Stacy L. Reynolds

Thoracic injuries account for less than one-tenth of all pediatric trauma-related injuries but comprise 14% of pediatric trauma-related deaths. Thoracic trauma includes injuries to the lungs, heart, aorta and great vessels, esophagus, tracheobronchial tree, and structures of the chest wall. Children have unique anatomic features that change the patterns of observed injury compared with adults. This review article outlines the clinical presentation, diagnostic testing, and management principles required to successfully manage injured children with thoracic trauma.

EMERGENCY MEDICINE
CLINICS OF NORTH AMERICA

THE CLINICS ARE NOW AVAILABLE ONLINE!
Access your subscription at:
www.theclinics.com

PROGRAM OBJECTIVE

The goal of *Emergency Medicine Clinics of North America* is to keep practicing emergency medicine physicians and emergency medicine residents up to date with current clinical practice in emergency medicine by providing timely articles reviewing the state of the art in patient care.

LEARNING OBJECTIVES

Upon completion of this activity, participants will be able to:
1. Review treatment approaches for pedatric respiratory conditions
2. Recognize and manage pediatric pain, thoratic trauma, and head injury
3. Discuss emergency management and care of pediatric shock and burns

ACCREDITATION

The Elsevier Office of Continuing Medical Education (EOCME) is accredited by the Accreditation Council for Continuing Medical Education (ACCME) to provide continuing medical education for physicians.

The EOCME designates this enduring material for a maximum of 15 *AMA PRA Category 1 Credit*(s)™. Physicians should claim only the credit commensurate with the extent of their participation in the activity.

All other healthcare professionals requesting continuing education credit for this enduring material will be issued a certificate of participation.

DISCLOSURE OF CONFLICTS OF INTEREST

The EOCME assesses conflict of interest with its instructors, faculty, planners, and other individuals who are in a position to control the content of CME activities. All relevant conflicts of interest that are identified are thoroughly vetted by EOCME for fair balance, scientific objectivity, and patient care recommendations. EOCME is committed to providing its learners with CME activities that promote improvements or quality in healthcare and not a specific proprietary business or a commercial interest.

The planning committee, staff, authors and editors listed below have identified no financial relationships or relationships to products or devices they or their spouse/life partner have with commercial interest related to the content of this CME activity:
Colleen Dietzler; Ryan Fey, MD; Sean M. Fox, MD; Aarti Gaglani, MD; Mary Gaspers, MD; Toni Gross, MD, MPH; James(Jim) L. Homme, MD; Vivian Hwang, MD, FACEP, FAAP; Alison Kemp; Maybelle Kou, MD, FACEP, FAAP; Aaron N. Leetch, MD; Emily C. MacNeill, MD; Christyn Magill, MD; Amal Mattu, MD; Anna McFarlin, MD, FAEM, FAAP; Jenny Mendelson, MD; Garrett S. Pacheco, MD; Amy L. Puchalski, MD; Nadira Ramkellawan, MD; Stacy L. Reynolds, MD; Emily Rose, MD, FAAP, FAAEM, FACEP; Tim Ruttan, MD; Genevieve Santillanes, MD; Paul C. Schunk, MD; Ashley M. Strobel, MD; Khoon-Yen Tay, MD; Chad D. Viscusi, MD; Vignesh Viswanathan; Chantel P. Walker, MD; Jessica J. Wall, MD, MPH; Bryan Wilson, MD; Dale Woolridge, MD, PhD, FAAEM, FAAP, FACEP.

UNAPPROVED/OFF-LABEL USE DISCLOSURE

The EOCME requires CME faculty to disclose to the participants:
1. When products or procedures being discussed are off-label, unlabelled, experimental, and/or investigational (not US Food and Drug Administration [FDA] approved); and
2. Any limitations on the information presented, such as data that are preliminary or that represent ongoing research, interim analyses, and/or unsupported opinions. Faculty may discuss information about pharmaceutical agents that is outside of FDA-approved labelling. This information is intended solely for CME and is not intended to promote off-label use of these medications. If you have any questions, contact the medical affairs department of the manufacturer for the most recent prescribing information.

TO ENROLL

To enroll in the *Emergency Medicine Clinics* Continuing Medical Education program, call customer service at 1-800-654-2452 or sign up online at http://www.theclinics.com/home/cme. The CME program is available to subscribers for an additional annual fee of $244.40 USD.

METHOD OF PARTICIPATION

In order to claim credit, participants must complete the following:
1. Complete enrolment as indicated above.
2. Read the activity.

3. Complete the CME Test and Evaluation. Participants must achieve a score of 70% on the test. All CME Tests and Evaluations must be completed online.

CME INQUIRIES/SPECIAL NEEDS

For all CME inquiries or special needs, please contact elsevierCME@elsevier.com.

Foreword

Pediatric Emergencies

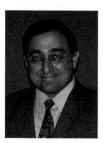

Amal Mattu, MD
Consulting Editor

There are few presentations that strike more fear in the hearts of emergency physicians than the presentation of a sick child. Why is that? Perhaps it is because a child is supposed to be happy and playful, a source of bubbly energy with decades of future productive life and joy, and therefore, there is far more to lose if things go south. Or perhaps it is because devastating illness is so unexpected in children…it is simply not supposed to happen. Or perhaps it is simply because we fear what we do not understand. After all, we have all heard countless times the mantra that "kids are not just small adults." We are often made to believe that children are a different creature with different presentations and different diseases. We are often made to believe that general emergency physicians are poorly equipped to fight the battle against childhood maladies.

Fortunately, if knowledge is power, you hold in your hands a powerful weapon in this battle. In this issue of *Emergency Medicine Clinics of North America*, Guest Editors Drs Sean Fox and Dale Woolridge, both dual-trained emergency physicians-pediatricians, have assembled a team of amazing educators in emergency medicine to give you powerful skills in caring for sick children. They have divided this issue into two sections: the first section addresses common conditions, and the second section addresses critical conditions.

In the first section on common conditions, the authors address apnea and the new "BRUE." Other common conditions, such as minor head trauma, pain management, dehydration, syncope, and bronchiolitis, are addressed. You will find that the authors have taken extra care to address the quandary of when to obtain radiographic or CT imaging in children. This first section largely addresses typical "urgent care" presentations and will be invaluable to those providers working in fast-tracks and ambulatory centers.

The second section, on the other hand, addresses higher acuity and critical illnesses of importance in most emergency departments. The authors here discuss airway emergencies and ventilator management, shock, burns, and major trauma. These articles

Emerg Med Clin N Am 36 (2018) xv–xvi
https://doi.org/10.1016/j.emc.2018.02.002
0733-8627/18/© 2018 Published by Elsevier Inc.

emed.theclinics.com

address areas of confusion by presenting evidence-based approaches to these very challenging patient presentations.

The Guest Editors and authors are to be commended for their work. Though this is not intended to be a comprehensive review of pediatric emergency medicine, the contents of this issue of *Emergency Medicine Clinics of North America* brings significant clarity to the management of often confusing and controversial topics. Regardless of your current level of training and comfort in managing pediatric patients in the acute setting, this issue is certain to help you feel well armed in your next battle to save the life of a sick child.

Amal Mattu, MD
Department of Emergency Medicine
University of Maryland School of Medicine
Baltimore, MD 21201, USA

E-mail address:
amalmattu@comcast.net

Preface

Pediatric Emergencies: The Common and the Critical

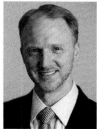
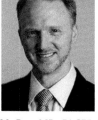

Sean M. Fox, MD, FACEP, FAAP   Dale P. Woolridge, MD, PhD, FAAEM, FAAP, FACEP

Editors

Caring for children in the emergency department (ED) is both rewarding and challenging. Children have a tremendous ability to remind us about the importance of our role in the medical care environment. They provide us the opportunity to make critical interventions when they are the most impactful. They also remind us of the humanitarian aspects of our vocation, and they, often, make us smile even during the most difficult of shifts, proving to be a redemptive resource even amid chaos.

While caring for children brings many of us significant satisfaction, it is certainly not without its challenges. The utterance of "kids aren't little adults" is typically invoked when caring for children in the ED. While this statement is meant to remind providers of the fact that pediatric patients represent a unique population, it can also engender trepidation in care providers. Unquestionably, children represent a special patient population that deserves specific attention to the variances in their anatomy and physiology, but these are aspects of medical management that need to be accounted for in all special populations and should not engender fear. Our goal in presenting this compilation of topics is to empower emergency medicine providers by helping them stay abreast of the common as well as the critical conditions that children will present with to our EDs.

We have several individuals who deserve our appreciation. We would like to thank our team of pediatric emergency medicine experts who have helped us present the most current evidenced-based approach to these common and critical conditions. We would also like to thank you, the reader, who has dedicated yourself to providing excellent care for all of your patients—even those who belong to this special population. In addition, we would like to thank all of our patients and their families, as they continually give us the amazing opportunities to help them all the while teaching us

Emerg Med Clin N Am 36 (2018) xvii–xviii
https://doi.org/10.1016/j.emc.2018.02.001
0733-8627/18/© 2018 Published by Elsevier Inc.

emed.theclinics.com

so much. Last, we would be remiss if we did not recognize those who sacrifice on our behalf: our wives, children, and families. Thank you all!

Sean M. Fox, MD, FACEP, FAAP
Emergency Medicine Residency Program
Department of Emergency Medicine
Carolinas Medical Center
Medical Education Building, Third Floor
1000 Blythe Boulevard
Charlotte, NC 28203, USA

Dale P. Woolridge, MD, PhD, FAAEM, FAAP, FACEP
Department of Emergency Medicine
University of Arizona
1501 North Campbell Avenue
PO Box 5057
Tucson, AZ 85724-5057, USA

E-mail addresses:
smfoxmd@gmail.com (S.M. Fox)
dale@aemrc.arizona.edu (D.P. Woolridge)

Section 1: Common

Evaluation and Management of Dehydration in Children

Genevieve Santillanes, MD, Emily Rose, MD*

KEYWORDS

- Dehydration • Oral rehydration • Subcutaneous rehydration • Intravenous fluid
- Fluid bolus • Hyponatremia • Hypernatremia

KEY POINTS

- The degree of pediatric dehydration may be difficult to clinically quantify.
- Dehydration may be treated with oral, subcutaneous, or intravenous fluids.
- Most children with mild to moderate dehydration can be successfully rehydrated with oral rehydration.
- When intravenous fluids are chosen for rehydration, isotonic solutions should be used to avoid iatrogenic hyponatremia.

DIAGNOSIS

This article discusses evidence-based treatment of dehydration due to acute gastro-enteritis in children. Many other common childhood illnesses, such as bronchiolitis, influenza, gingivostomatitis, and urinary tract infections, may cause dehydration as well. Although some of these other illnesses require specific therapy, the approach to associated dehydration is generally the same as presented in this article. Although diarrhea and dehydration are major causes of morbidity and mortality in low-income countries, this review focuses on treatment in high-income countries. Treatment considerations vary based on health care resources, incidence of preexisting poor nutrition, and common pathogens.

Children with dehydration are commonly divided into severity subgroups by percent of weight lost during the illness. Minimal or no dehydration is commonly defined as a loss of less than 3% of body weight, mild dehydration is a 3% to 5% loss, moderate dehydration is a 6% to 9% loss, and severe dehydration is a loss of 10% or more of the preillness weight, although severity subgroupings vary somewhat in different

The authors received no funding for the preparation of this article and have no relevant financial disclosures.

Department of Emergency Medicine, Keck School of Medicine, University of Southern California, 1200 North State Street, GH Room 1011, Los Angeles, CA 90033, USA

* Corresponding author.

E-mail address: emilyrose010@gmail.com

published guidelines (**Tables 1** and **2**). If a reliable preillness weight is available, the degree of dehydration can be calculated (Equation 1). A weight just prior to the illness, however, is not generally available and severity of dehydration must be estimated based on clinical signs and symptoms.

The formula for calculating fluid deficit is as follows:

$$\text{Fluid deficit (mL)} = \% \text{ dehydration} \times \text{weight (kg)} \times 10$$

$$\% \text{ dehydration determined clinically OR weight change}$$

$$-\left(\frac{(\text{previous weight} - \text{current weight})}{\text{previous weight}}\right) \times 100 \qquad (1)$$

The ability to recognize dehydration has important clinical implications. Untreated dehydration may lead to electrolyte disturbances, acidosis, and end-organ damage due to hypoperfusion, including renal insufficiency and cardiovascular instability. An accurate assessment of the severity of dehydration, however, can be challenging. Historical features, including duration of illness, frequency and characterization of vomiting and diarrhea, urine output, preillness weight, and recent oral intake should be ascertained.[1,2] Guidelines recommend checking vital signs, general appearance, appearance of oral mucosa, and respiratory pattern.[2] Eyes should be examined for a sunken appearance and presence or absence of tears should be

Table 1
Commonly taught clinical symptoms/signs associated with dehydration

Symptom	Minimal Dehydration (<3% Loss of Body Weight)	Mild–Moderate Dehydration (3%–9% Loss of Body Weight)	Severe Dehydration (≥10% Loss of Body Weight)
Mental status	Normal	Normal, fatigued, restless or irritable	Apathetic, lethargic, unconscious
Heart rate	Normal	Normal–increased	Tachycardia (bradycardia possible if severe)
Breathing	Normal	Normal, fast	Deep
Pulse quality	Normal	Normal–decreased	Weak, thread, or difficult to palpate
Systolic blood pressure	Normal	Normal or low	Low
Anterior fontanelle	Normal	Sunken	Very sunken
Mucous membranes	Moist	Dry	Parched
Eyes	Normal	Slightly sunken	Deeply sunken
Tears	Present	Decreased	Absent
Skin fold elasticity	Pinch with instant recoil	Recoil in <2 s	Recoil in >2 s
Capillary refill	Normal	Prolonged	Prolonged, minimal
Extremities	Warm	Cool	Cold, mottled, cyanotic
Urinary output	Normal–decreased	Decreased	Minimal
Estimated fluid deficit	30–50 mL/kg	100 mL/kg	>100 mL/kg

Data from Colletti JE, Brown KM, Sharieff GQ, et al. The management of children with gastroenteritis and dehydration in the emergency department. J Emerg Med 2010;38(5):686–98; and Steiner MJ, DeWalt DA, Byerley JS. Is this child dehydrated? JAMA 2004;291(22):2746–54.

Table 2
Succinct clinical signs indicating the degree of dehydration

Degree	Percentage	Clinical Signs
Mild/none	<4	No clinical signs
Moderate	4–6	Some physical signs Individual signs mildly or moderately abnormal
Severe	>7	Multiple physical signs Individual signs markedly abnormal May develop hypotension or acidosis

From Children's Health Queensland Hospital and Health Services. Intravenous fluid guidelines—paediatric and neonatal. Available at: c-foam.com/au/wp-content/uploads/2016/04/Paeds-fluids-guidelines.pdf. Accessed April 17, 2017.

noted. Skin findings may include prolonged capillary refill time and tenting (**Table 3**).[2]

Unfortunately, some of these traditionally taught signs and symptoms are neither particularly sensitive nor specific. A 2004 *JAMA* systematic review of the literature on the physical examination in dehydration found 3 clinical signs clinically helpful in detecting 5% or greater dehydration: prolonged capillary refill time, abnormal skin turgor, and an abnormal respiratory pattern.[3] That systematic review also found that cool extremities, weak pulse, and lack of tears were possibly, but less clearly, helpful tests for detecting 5% or greater dehydration.[3] Increased heart rate, sunken fontanelle, and poor overall appearance were found not clinically useful.[3] Three physical examination findings found clinically useful in decreasing the likelihood of 5% dehydration were absence of dry mucous membranes, normal overall appearance, and absence of sunken eyes. The traditionally taught physical examination findings for dehydration should be checked and documented but their presence

Table 3
Clinical examination methods for diagnosing dehydration

Finding	Method	Normal Value	Examination Pitfalls
Skin turgor	Pinch a small skin fold on lateral abdominal wall (at level of umbilicus)	Immediate	Excess subcutaneous fat or hypernatremia may falsely normalize turgor in dehydrated children; malnutrition and primary skin disorders may falsely prolong turgor
Capillary refill	Compress palmar surface of distal fingertip with child's arm at the level of the heart in a warm environment, gradually increase pressure and release immediately; estimate time to restoration of color	1.5–2 s	Ambient temperature, location, lighting, medications and autonomic dysfunction (primary: complex regional pain syndrome or secondary: cardiogenic shock) may impact results

Data from Steiner MJ, DeWalt DA, Byerley JS. Is this child dehydrated? JAMA 2004;291(22):2746–54; and King CK, Glass R, Bresee JS, et al, Centers for Disease Control and Prevention. Managing acute gastroenteritis among children: oral rehydration, maintenance, and nutritional therapy. MMWR Recomm Rep 2003;52(RR-16):1–16.

does not necessarily indicate severe dehydration and does not preclude oral rehydration.

PROGNOSIS

Although dehydration is not a major cause of mortality in the United States, it is one of the most common reasons for unscheduled hospital admissions in children of all ages in the United States.[4] In North American countries where life-threatening complications and death due to dehydration are rare, quality improvement focuses on decreased admission rates, decreased emergency department (ED) length of stay, and decreased unplanned return visits.

Ideally, the least invasive treatment plan is used in EDs while avoiding treatment failures with resultant in prolonged stays, return visits, and potentially avoidable admissions. Oral rehydration is recommended for most children with mild to moderate dehydration. A Cochrane review found that only 1 of every 25 children receiving intravenous (IV) fluids for dehydration failed oral rehydration therapy (ORT) and required IV fluids.[5]

IV fluid administration does not seem to decrease ED repeat visits in children with mild to moderate dehydration.[6] Serum bicarbonate values also were not associated with ED revisits.[7,8] Increased frequency of vomiting before initial visit and a higher heart rate at discharge were, however, predictors of return visits.[9]

CLINICAL MANAGEMENT

The goal of clinical management is to replace fluid deficits and ongoing losses in the least invasive yet effective manner. Effective circulating volume has an impact on distal tissue perfusion and untreated hypovolemia may result in ischemic end-organ damage. Emergent correction of severe dehydration should occur; treatment of severe dehydration is typically with IV therapy but can be successful by alternative means, such as with ORT, via nasogastric tube (NGT), and by subcutaneous administration. In moderate hypovolemia, ORT, IV, or subcutaneous fluid may be used.

ORT is recommended for children with mild-moderate dehydration. This recommendation is included in multiple guidelines for treatment of gastroenteritis or diarrhea, including the guidelines published by the American Academy of Pediatrics; the Centers for Disease Control and Prevention; the Canadian Paediatric Society; the European Society for Pediatric Gastroenterology, Hepatology, and Nutrition; and European Society for Pediatric Infectious Diseases; and the World Health Organization.[2,10–13] See **Table 4** for relevant guidelines. Oral rehydration is not appropriate in patients with altered levels of consciousness, paralytic ileus, severe dehydration, or shock. Patients may also present with other contraindications to oral rehydration, such as severe respiratory distress or possible surgical process.

Despite the recommendations of multiple professional societies, oral rehydration seems underused in the United States.

A reported concern regarding ORT is prolonged ED length of stay because ORT administration over 2 hours to 4 hours is recommended.[2] ORT, however, has been shown to require less staff time and result in a shorter ED length of stay compared with IV hydration.[14] One randomized controlled study found that equal percentages of patients receiving oral and IV hydration were rehydrated at 4 hours.[15] Another study found that the mean ED length of stay of children receiving IV hydration exceeded 4 hours.[16] Length of stay is also shorter in hospitalized patients receiving oral rehydration.[5,17] Another concern is that initial use of oral rather than IV hydration results in increased failure of ED rehydration; however, randomized controlled trials have found that oral rehydration results in a lower rate of admission than IV hydration.[14,15]

Table 4
Relevant guidelines regarding oral rehydration therapy

Professional Society and Practice Parameter	Year of Publication	Patient Population
American Academy of Pediatrics Practice parameter: the management of acute gastroenteritis in young children	1996	Previously healthy children aged 1 mo–5 y living in developed countries with acute gastroenteritis
Centers for Disease Control and Prevention Managing acute gastroenteritis among children: oral rehydration, maintenance, and nutritional therapy	2003	Infants and children with acute diarrhea
European Society for Pediatric Gastroenterology, Hepatology, and Nutrition/ European Society for Pediatric Infectious Diseases Evidence-based guidelines for the management of acute gastroenteritis in children in europe: update 2014	2014	Previously healthy children aged 5 and under living in Europe with acute gastroenteritis
Canadian Paediatric Society Oral rehydration therapy and early refeeding in the management of children with gastroenteritis	2006 Reaffirmed 2016	Children with gastroenteritis
Canadian Paediatric Society Emergency department use of oral ondansetron for acute gastroenteritis-related vomiting in young children	2011 Reaffirmed 2016	Children 6 mo–12 y with vomiting due to gastroenteritis
World Health Organization Department of Child and Adolescent Health and Development Clinical management of acute diarrhea: WHO/UNICEF joint statement	2004	Children in developing nations with diarrheal diseases

Oral Rehydration Technique

Patients with mild to moderate dehydration should receive 50 mL/kg to 100 mL/kg of oral rehydration solution (ORS) over 2 hours to 4 hours to correct the fluid deficit.[2] In addition, ongoing fluid losses from vomiting or diarrhea should be replaced.[2] For children with significant vomiting, ORS should initially be administered in 5-mL aliquots every 1 minute to 2 minutes.[11] Administration of fluid with a teaspoon, syringe, or dropper may facilitate initial fluid resuscitation. Fluid volumes can be increased as tolerated. Repletion for ongoing fluid losses may be estimated at 5 mL/kg to 10 mL/kg (5 mL/kg for each emesis and 10 mL/kg for each diarrheal episode).[2]

Multiple ORSs are commercially available. Ideal ORSs have been developed to improve water absorption across the intestinal mucosa (**Table 5**). The ideal glucose-based ORS has a 1:1 glucose-to-sodium ratio to take advantage of glucose and sodium cotransport across the intestinal mucosa, improving water absorption. For this reason, commercially available ORSs are preferable to other clear liquids, such as sports drinks and other fluids, which have a high osmolality and inappropriate carbohydrate-to-sodium ratio. Furthermore, hyperosmolar solutions, such as soda, may cause an osmotic diarrhea in children with gastroenteritis, worsening fluid losses. Polymer-based ORSs, including rice-based, wheat-based, and maize-based solutions, have been developed with the goal of slowly releasing glucose into the gut as the polymer is broken down.[18] The evidence for use of polymer-based solutions is

Table 5
Composition of appropriate and inappropriate rehydration solutions

	Carbohydrate, g/L	Sodium, mmol/L	Potassium, mmol/L	Base, mmol/L	Osmolality, mmol/L
WHO (current recommendations)	13.5	75	20	30	245
WHO (original formula)	20	90	20	30	311
Pedialyte[a]	25	45	20	30	250
Enfalyte[b]	30	50	25	34	200
Rehydralyte[a]	25	75	20	30	305
Sports drink	45	20	3	3	330
Coca-Cola Classic[c]	112	2	0	13	750
Apple juice (full-strength)	120	3	32	0	730
Chicken broth	0	250	8	0	500

[a] Ross Laboratories (Abbott Laboratories) (Colombus, OH).
[b] Mead-Johnson Laboratories (Princeton, NJ).
[c] Coca-Cola Corporation (Atlanta, GA).
Adapted from Practice parameter: the management of acute gastroenteritis in young children. American Academy of Pediatrics, Provisional Committee on Quality Improvement, Subcommittee on Acute Gastroenteritis. Pediatrics 1996;97(3):426–7; with permission; and *Data from* Shapiro HL. Standard rehydration fluid. Lancet 1977;2:407; and King CK, Glass R, Bresee JS, et al, Centers for Disease Control and Prevention. Managing acute gastroenteritis among children: oral rehydration, maintenance, and nutritional therapy. MMWR Recomm Rep 2003;52(RR-16):1–16.

poor and performed in populations with a high incidence of cholera. Plain water alone is inappropriate and may lead to hyponatremia and hypoglycemia. Multiple recipes for homemade ORS have been published, but homemade solutions carry the risk of mixing errors, which could lead to solutions with inappropriately high sodium levels. Frozen ORS has been shown to be better tolerated by children and may increase the success of oral rehydration.[19]

Ondansetron (Zofran)

Many children with dehydration due to gastroenteritis also present with vomiting, which can be a barrier to ORT. Oral ondansetron has been shown effective in increasing the proportion of children who cease vomiting in EDs.[20] It also reduces the need for IV fluids and decreases immediate hospitalization.[20] Its effect, however, may be less in clinical practice.[21,22] One large retrospective study found that although ondansetron use increased over a 10-year period, the rate of IV hydration did not decrease.[21] More than 85% of children receiving IV hydration did not receive oral ondansetron, which could indicate that ondansetron was not used in children at the highest risk of failed ORT or that IV hydration was used in children who might have tolerated ORT.[21]

An American Academy of Pediatrics practice parameter did not specifically evaluate use of antiemetics but stated that consensus opinion was that antiemetic drugs were not needed in the treatment of gastroenteritis. Importantly, these guidelines were published in 1996 before the availability of generic ondansetron and have not been updated.[11] Since that time, multiple studies have been published on the use of ondansetron for pediatric gastroenteritis and its use has become more common. The

Canadian Paediatric Society recommends that a single dose of oral ondansetron be considered in children presenting to an ED with mild to moderate dehydration due to gastroenteritis-related vomiting.[23] ORT should be initiated 15 minutes to 30 minutes later. Diarrhea is a common side effect of ondansetron, so ondansetron is not routinely recommended for children with the predominant symptom of moderate to severe diarrhea.[23]

Early use of oral ondanseton is reasonable in children presenting with dehydration and vomiting to facilitate successful oral rehydration. The pediatric dose of ondansetron is 0.15 mg/kg per dose. A commonly used simplified dosing regimen is presented in **Table 6**.

Refeeding

Breastfed infants and toddlers should continue to breastfeed throughout rehydration process.[2,10,12] Children and formula-fed infants should be fed an age-appropriate diet once the initial rehydration process is completed. Full-strength milk or formula can be given at this point; avoiding lactose is generally not necessary.[2,11,12] Although fatty foods and foods high in simple sugars should initially be avoided,[11] overly restrictive diets are not necessary. The classic bananas, rice, applesauce, and toast diet is low in energy density, protein, and fat and is no longer recommended.[11]

Nasogastric Rehydration

Nasogastric hydration is an option for infants and children who cannot or will not take sufficient oral fluids. Nasogastric fluids may be a particularly good option for infants who are unable to ingest sufficient oral fluids due to respiratory distress. Nasogastric hydration is suggested as an option in the American Academy of Pediatrics clinical practice guideline on bronchiolitis.[24] If nasogastric rehydration is chosen, local anesthesia can be used before insertion of the NGT. Options include nebulized lidocaine, application of viscous lidocaine jelly, and atomized lidocaine. Once the NGT is placed, a commercial ORS can be administered.

Intravenous Fluid Rehydration

IV fluid administration is clinically indicated in severe dehydration or with failure of alternative rehydration techniques described previously for mild to moderate dehydration. The recommended pediatric bolus dose is 10 mL/kg to 20 mL/kg, which may be repeated as needed. The rate of bolus administration is typically over an hour but the ideal administration time is not clearly defined.[25,26] Hypovolemic shock mandates rapid repletion.

There is great practice variation in fluid administration.[27,28] Variation occurs in use of IV fluids (vs alternative techniques), rate of administration, and type of fluid used. Isotonic fluid is recommended to restore circulatory volume because hypertonic or hypotonic solutions may lead to cerebral edema and alter electrolyte composition. The risk of hyponatremia with low sodium content fluids in children has been demonstrated and recently highlighted in the medical literature.[29–34] The most commonly

Table 6 Ondansetron dosing	
Weight	**Dose**
8–15 kg	2 mg
15–30 kg	4 mg
>30 kg	6–8 mg

used isotonic fluid is 0.9% sodium chloride (normal saline [NS]). There is also emerging evidence for balanced salt solutions to avoid hyperchloremia.[35] Balanced solutions used in children include Plasma-Lyte 148 (also known as Plasma-Lyte A) and Lactated Ringer solution (also known as Hartmann solution) (**Table 7**).[36] These solutions have additional organic anion (eg, acetate, gluconate, and citrate) and so have lower concentration of chloride than NS.

There are no large, randomized controlled trials comparing NS with any of the balanced solutions in either adults or children. Most of the literature evaluating outcomes associated with fluid type has been in animal models. A prospective multicenter trial of 100 children with dehydration secondary to acute gastroenteritis demonstrated that Plasma-Lyte A was superior to NS in improvement of metabolic acidosis (as determined by serum bicarbonate levels).[37]

NS was originally invented for the management of cholera epidemics in the early 1800s. It has been the most commonly used fluid since that time and is less expensive than available balanced solutions. NS, however, does not match plasma's physiologic composition (see **Table 7**). NS infusion consistently induces or worsens metabolic acidosis and contains a chloride level approximately 40% higher than the plasma concentration. Supraphysiologic chloride levels increase systemic inflammation and can cause renal vasoconstriction and decrease glomerular filtration rate.[38,39] Better outcomes have been demonstrated in adults treated with balanced solutions in conditions, such as diabetic ketoacidosis and surgical and infectious etiologies of

Table 7
Composition of common crystalloid solutions

	Plasma	0.9% Sodium Chloride	0.9% Socium Chloride with 5% Glucose	Plasma-Lyte 148 (Plasma-Lyte A)	Lactated Ringer Solution (Compound Sodium Lactate or Hartmann Solution)
Sodium (mmol/L)	136–145	154	154	140	130
Potassium (mmol/L)	3.5–5.0	0	0	5	4
Magnesium (mmol/L)	0.8–1.0	0	0	1.5	0
Calcium (mmol/L)	2.2–2.6	0	0	0	3
Chloride (mmol/L)	98–106	154	154	98	109
Acetate (mmol/L)	0	0	0	27	0
Gluconate (mmol/L)	0	0	0	23	0
Lactate (mmol/L)	0	0	0	0	28
Osmolality (mOsmol/kg H_2O)	287	286	578	271	256
pH	7.35–7.45	4.5–7	4.5–7	4–8	5–7

From Reddy S, Weinberg L, Young P. Crystalloid fluid therapy. Crit Care 2016;20:59; and Children's Health Queensland Hospital and Health Services. Intravenous fluid guidelines—paediatric and neonatal. Available at: c-foam.com/au/wp-content/uploads/2016/04/Paeds-fluids-guidelines.pdf.

illness.[40-45] The impact on these conditions in children is yet unknown and NS continues to be the isotonic crystalloid most commonly used in the acute management of dehydration.

The ideal rate of rehydration is not clearly established. Rapid rehydration (60 mL/kg) has not been demonstrated to improve clinical signs of rehydration faster than standard (20 mL/kg) bolus fluid administration.[25] A rapid rehydration protocol (1 hour vs 3 or more hours) does seem safe and decreases ED length of stay.[26]

Maintenance Fluids

There are 2 methods used for calculation of maintenance fluids after rehydration therapy:

1. Hourly rate (4, 2, 1 rule):
    4 mL/kg for the first 10 kg, 2 mL/kg for the second 10 kg, and 1 mL/kg for additional weight over 20 kg
2. Maintenance for a 24-hour period:
    less than 10 kg: 100 mL/kg
    10 kg or greater: 1000 mL for first 10 kg plus 50 mL/kg for any increment of weight over 10 kg

The second method results in slightly more fluid but the difference between the 2 methods does not seem clinically significant. The kidney compensates by concentrating or diluting urine to meet physiologic needs.

Dextrose

Dextrose should be given to hypoglycemic patients. The addition of dextrose to IV fluids is commonly used at a concentration of 5% to 10% solution. This concentration is typically rapidly absorbed by cells and does not remain in the intravascular space. It does not significantly contribute to the tonicity of IV fluids compared with sodium but does increase osmolarity (see **Table 7**). Dextrose is frequently added to maintenance fluid but may also be given with IV fluid boluses. The addition of dextrose to IV fluid boluses results in reduced ketone levels but has not been demonstrated to impact hospitalization rates or rate of metabolic acidosis.[46] Dextrose exacerbates hypokalemia (secondary to the stimulation of insulin release) so hypokalemia must be concomitantly treated if dextrose is administered.

Subcutaneous Rehydration

An alternative but less frequently used method for rehydration is the use of subcutaneous infusion of fluids. Subcutaneous rehydration was commonly used in the first half of the last century but fell out of favor when improved supplies and techniques for IV rehydration became available.[47] One barrier to subcutaneous hydration is that hyaluronan present in subcutaneous tissues resists the spread of fluid through the subcutaneous tissues.[47] In the past, animal-derived hyaluronidase was used to temporarily hydrolyze hyaluronan, facilitating absorption of fluids from the subcutaneous space, but use was limited by high rates of allergic reactions and anaphylaxis.[47] Recombinant human hyaluronidase (Hylenex; Halozyme Theraputics, San Diego, California) is now available, which makes subcutaneous rehydration a more useful option.

Subcutaneous rehydration may be useful in cases of failed ORT in children with anticipated difficult or failed IV access. One study of subcutaneous rehydration in children found that the subcutaneous catheter was inserted on the first attempt in 90% of children and on the second attempt in the remainder of children, with a median of

19 mL/kg of fluid given in the first hour.[48] Health care providers in another study found subcutaneous fluid administration less difficult than IV fluid administration.[49]

The technique for subcutaneous fluid administration is simple. The chosen site, usually the upper back, is cleansed, as it would be for an IV line placement. The skin is pinched and a 22-gauge to 24-gauge angiocatheter or butterfly needle is inserted into the subcutaneous tissue at a 30° to 45° angle. A folded 2-in × 2-in gauze can be placed under the needle before securing the line to maintain the angle. 150 units (1 mL) of recombinant human hyaluronidase is injected and fluid administration with NS or lactated Ringer solution can be initiated.[47]

DISEASE COMPLICATIONS
Hyponatremia/Hypernatremia

Most cases of hypovolemia caused by acute gastroenteritis are isonatremic, but either hyponatremia or hypernatremia may occur. The serum sodium concentration is the best estimate of water balance in relation to solute. A normal value implies balance, but it does not reveal volume status. When the sodium is abnormal, there must be caution in the administration of fluids with attention given to the rate of change in sodium. Overly rapid correction of hyponatremia or hypernatremia may result in osmotic demyelination syndrome, cerebral edema, or seizures.

Hyponatremia in hypovolemic children is usually caused by the intake of hypotonic solutions. A diminished ability to excrete free water occurs with antidiuretic hormone (ADH) secretion. Hypovolemia triggers ADH secretion, but other stimuli not uncommon in acute gastroenteritis, such as pain, nausea, vomiting, stress, and hypoglycemia, also induce ADH secretion and can exacerbate hyponatremia.[50]

In hyponatremia due to hypovolemia and increased free water retention, isotonic saline both corrects the volume depletion and raises serum sodium. This occurs because isotonic saline has a higher concentration of sodium (154 mEq/L) and correction of hypovolemia decreases ADH secretion, which allows urinary excretion of excess water. Hypokalemia should be treated if concomitant with hyponatremia because the addition of potassium increases the tonicity of the solution and raises the serum sodium more rapidly. IV potassium should be avoided in patients with decreased kidney function or oliguria.

Symptomatic hyponatremia (altered mental status or seizure) should be immediately treated with a hypertonic saline bolus at 3 mL/kg to 5 mL/kg of 3% sodium chloride.[51] The sodium concentration of 3% hypertonic saline is 513 mEq/L. In an emergency, sodium bicarbonate from the crash cart can be used to increase plasma sodium levels if there is a delay in obtaining hypertonic saline from the pharmacy. Sodium bicarbonate has a sodium level of 595 mEq/L and a dose of 1 mEq/kg to 2 mEq/kg is appropriate. Once acute central nervous system symptoms have resolved, the remaining sodium correction should occur at a rate less than 8 mEq/L to 12 mEq/L in 24 hours. Correction should occur initially rapidly because the pathophysiology of symptomatic hyponatremia involves worsening cerebral edema. The risk of morbidity from delayed therapy is greater than the risk of complication from overly rapid correction and osmotic demyelination. A commonly cited goal is a correction of serum sodium at a rate of 2 mEq/L per hour with a goal of raising serum sodium by 5 mEq/L in the first several hours.[52] The rate at which the sodium shift initially occurred also correlates with risk of complications. If the water deficit developed slowly (over days), complication rates from rapid correction are higher. Hypernatremia should be corrected at a rate of less than or equal to 0.5 mEq/L per hour (10–12 mEq/L/d) to avoid neurologic sequelae.[53,54]

Indications and Interpretation of Laboratory Values

A finger-stick glucose or serum electrolyte panel is indicated in patients with altered mental status, severe dehydration, or other clinical concern for abnormalities. Electrolytes are commonly obtained in moderate to severe dehydration and when IV fluids are administered. No laboratory value, however, is either sensitive or specific for the prediction of dehydration in children.[7,55] Sodium levels correlate with water balance but are not helpful in determining degree of dehydration. Typically, predicative laboratory values are clinically apparent—the well-appearing child has normal laboratory test results and the ill-appearing child has abnormal values. The only laboratory measurement that seems valuable in decreasing the likelihood of 5% dehydration is serum bicarbonate concentration of greater than 15 mEq/L to 17 mEq/L with a likelihood ratio range of 0.18 to 0.22.[3,56,57] Vega and Avner[56] found that an absolute bicarbonate concentration of less than 17 mEq/L was consistent with dehydration of 5%. Patients with bicarbonate levels of greater than 15 mmol/L were unlikely to have severe dehydration.[57] Urea is impacted by renal blood flow and elevated levels frequently correlates with dehydration.[55] In a group of hospitalized children with acute gastroenteritis, a serum urea nitrogen level greater than 45 mg/dL was specific for at least 5% dehydration.[57]

CONTROVERSIES

One study examined the use of dilute apple juice followed by a patient's preferred oral fluids rather than flavored, commercially available ORS.[58] This study of children with mild gastroenteritis who were either minimally dehydrated or not dehydrated found that the group randomized to dilute apple juice was less likely to require IV rehydration in the next week.[58] Children with more significant degrees of dehydration were not included in the study, so it is unclear if results can be extrapolated to children with more than minimal dehydration. This study was performed in previously healthy children in Canada and the results likely do not extrapolate to children in countries where poor preillness nutrition is more prevalent and where different etiologies of diarrhea are common.

SPECIAL CIRCUMSTANCES

Nonphysiologic ADH release (also known as syndrome of inappropriate antidiuretic hormone secretion) may occur in ill children and result in decreased free water excretion and potential hyponatremia. Lack of appropriate release of ADH (central diabetes insipidus) results in polyuria and potential hypernatremia. Additionally, infants have immature renal function and are more prone to electrolyte abnormalities. Increased insensible water losses from the skin may occur in premature/young infants as well as those treated with phototherapy or radiant heaters. Fever, burns, and mechanical ventilation as well as gastrointestinal losses also increase water loss. Oliguric patients have decreased urinary water loss.

Probiotics, specifically *Lactobacillus rhamnosus* GG and *Saccharomyces boulardii*, have been shown to reduce the duration and intensity of symptoms of acute gastroenteritis.[10] Probiotics have also been demonstrated to decrease length of stay by over 24 hours in hospitalized patients with dehydration due to acute gastroenteritis.[59] The exact clinical indications, frequency, and dose remain unknown. Zinc supplementation is recommended in children over 2 months old in the developing world for the treatment of dehydration associated acute gastroenteritis.[2]

SUMMARY

Pediatric dehydration occurs frequently and is most commonly secondary to acute gastroenteritis. The degree of fluid deficit may be difficult to clinically quantify and there is no laboratory value that is either sensitive or specific to estimate the degree of dehydration in children. Rehydration may occur via oral, subcutaneous, or IV routes. Oral rehydration is underused in the United States. IV fluids should be isotonic to avoid iatrogenic hyponatremia and its potentially devastating neurologic sequelae. NS is the most commonly used fluid in pediatrics, but there is emerging evidence for the use of balanced solutions, such as plasmalyte.

REFERENCES

1. Colletti JE, Brown KM, Sharieff GQ, et al. The management of children with gastroenteritis and dehydration in the emergency department. J Emerg Med 2010;38(5):686–98.
2. King CK, Glass R, Bresee JS, et al, Centers for Disease Control and Prevention. Managing acute gastroenteritis among children: oral rehydration, maintenance, and nutritional therapy. MMWR Recomm Rep 2003;52(RR-16):1–16.
3. Steiner MJ, DeWalt DA, Byerley JS. Is this child dehydrated? JAMA 2004;291(22): 2746–54.
4. Wier LM, Hao Y, Owens P, et al. Overview of children in the emergency department, 2010. 2013. Available at: https://www.hcup-us.ahrq.gov/reports/statbriefs/ sb157.pdf. Accessed April 24, 2017.
5. Hartling L, Bellemare S, Wiebe N, et al. Oral versus intravenous rehydration for treating dehydration due to gastroenteritis in children. Cochrane Database Syst Rev 2006;(3):CD004390.
6. Freedman SB, Thull-Freedman JD, Rumantir M, et al. Emergency department revisits in children with gastroenteritis. J Pediatr Gastroenterol Nutr 2013;57(5): 612–8.
7. Wathen JE, MacKenzie T, Bothner JP. Usefulness of the serum electrolyte panel in the management of pediatric dehydration treated with intravenously administered fluids. Pediatrics 2004;114(5):1227–34.
8. Freedman SB, DeGroot JM, Parkin PC. Successful discharge of children with gastroenteritis requiring intravenous rehydration. J Emerg Med 2014;46(1):9–20.
9. Freedman SB, Powell E, Seshadri R. Predictors of outcomes in pediatric enteritis: a prospective cohort study. Pediatrics 2009;123(1):e9–16.
10. Guarino A, Ashkenazi S, Gendrel D, et al. European Society for Pediatric Gastroenterology, Hepatology, and Nutrition/European Society for Pediatric Infectious Diseases evidence-based guidelines for the management of acute gastroenteritis in children in Europe: update 2014. J Pediatr Gastroenterol Nutr 2014;59(1): 132–52.
11. Practice parameter: the management of acute gastroenteritis in young children. American Academy of Pediatrics, Provisional Committee on Quality Improvement, Subcommittee on Acute Gastroenteritis. Pediatrics 1996;97(3):424–35.
12. Leung A, Prince T, Canadian Paediatric Society, Nutrition and Gastroenterology Committee. Oralrehydration therapy and early refeeding in the management of childhoodgastroenteritis. Paediatr Child Health 2006;11(8):527–31.
13. World Health Organization Department of Child and Adolescent Health and Development. Clinical management of acute diarrhoea: WHO/UNICEF joint statement [WHO/FCH/CAH/04.7]. Geneva (Switzerland): World Health Organization; 2004.

14. Atherly-John YC, Cunningham SJ, Crain EF. A randomized trial of oral vs intravenous rehydration in a pediatric emergency department. Arch Pediatr Adolesc Med 2002;156(12):1240–3.

15. Spandorfer PR, Alessandrini EA, Joffe MD, et al. Oral versus intravenous rehydration of moderately dehydrated children: a randomized, controlled trial. Pediatrics 2005;115(2):295–301.

16. Bender BJ, Ozuah PO. Intravenous rehydration for gastroenteritis: how long does it really take? Pediatr Emerg Care 2004;20(4):215–8.

17. Fonseca BK, Holdgate A, Craig JC. Enteral vs intravenous rehydration therapy for children with gastroenteritis: a meta-analysis of randomized controlled trials. Arch Pediatr Adolesc Med 2004;158(5):483–90.

18. Gregorio GV, Gonzales ML, Dans LF, et al. Polymer-based oral rehydration solution for treating acute watery diarrhoea. Cochrane Database Syst Rev 2016;(12):CD006519.

19. Santucci KA, Anderson AC, Lewander WJ, et al. Frozen oral hydration as an alternative to conventional enteral fluids. Arch Pediatr Adolesc Med 1998;152(2): 142–6.

20. Fedorowicz Z, Jagannath VA, Carter B. Antiemetics for reducing vomiting related to acute gastroenteritis in children and adolescents. Cochrane Database Syst Rev 2011;(9):CD005506.

21. Freedman SB, Hall M, Shah SS, et al. Impact of increasing ondansetron use on clinical outcomes in children with gastroenteritis. JAMA Pediatr 2014;168(4): 321–9.

22. Keren R. Ondansetron for acute gastroenteritis: a failure of knowledge translation. JAMA Pediatr 2014;168(4):308–9.

23. Cheng A. Emergency department use of oral ondansetron for acute gastroenteritis-related vomiting in infants and children. Paediatr Child Health 2011;16(3):177–82.

24. Ralston SL, Lieberthal AS, Meissner HC. Ralston SL, Lieberthal AS, Meissner HC, et al. Clinical practice guideline: the diagnosis, management, and prevention of bronchiolitis. Pediatrics. 2014;134(5):e1474–e1502. Pediatrics 2015;136(4):782.

25. Freedman SB, Parkin PC, Willan AR, et al. Rapid versus standard intravenous rehydration in paediatric gastroenteritis: pragmatic blinded randomised clinical trial. BMJ 2011;343:d6976.

26. Nager AL, Wang VJ. Comparison of ultrarapid and rapid intravenous hydration in pediatric patients with dehydration. Am J Emerg Med 2010;28(2):123–9.

27. Freedman SB, Sivabalasundaram V, Bohn V, et al. The treatment of pediatric gastroenteritis: a comparative analysis of pediatric emergency physicians' practice patterns. Acad Emerg Med 2011;18(1):38–45.

28. Janet S, Molina JC, Maranon R, et al. Effects of rapid intravenous rehydration in children with mild-to-moderate dehydration. Pediatr Emerg Care 2015;31(8): 564–7.

29. Hanna M, Saberi MS. Incidence of hyponatremia in children with gastroenteritis treated with hypotonic intravenous fluids. Pediatr Nephrol 2010;25(8):1471–5.

30. Moritz ML, Ayus JC. Improving intravenous fluid therapy in children with gastroenteritis. Pediatr Nephrol 2010;25(8):1383–4.

31. Neville KA, Sandeman DJ, Rubinstein A, et al. Prevention of hyponatremia during maintenance intravenous fluid administration: a prospective randomized study of fluid type versus fluid rate. J Pediatr 2010;156(2):313–9.e1-2.

32. Neville KA, Verge CF, Rosenberg AR, et al. Isotonic is better than hypotonic saline for intravenous rehydration of children with gastroenteritis: a prospective randomised study. Arch Dis Child 2006;91(3):226–32.
33. Choong K, Kho ME, Menon K, et al. Hypotonic versus isotonic saline in hospitalised children: a systematic review. Arch Dis Child 2006;91(10):828–35.
34. Montañana PA, Modesto i Alapont V, Ocón AP, et al. The use of isotonic fluid as maintenance therapy prevents iatrogenic hyponatremia in pediatrics: a randomized, controlled open study. Pediatr Crit Care Med 2008;9(6):589–97.
35. Weinberg L, Collins N, Van Mourik K, et al. Plasma-Lyte 148: a clinical review. World J Crit Care Med 2016;5(4):235–50.
36. Myburgh JA, Mythen MG. Resuscitation fluids. N Engl J Med 2013;369(25): 2462–3.
37. Allen CH, Goldman RD, Bhatt S, et al. A randomized trial of Plasma-Lyte A and 0.9 % sodium chloride in acute pediatric gastroenteritis. BMC Pediatr 2016;16:117.
38. Zhang Z, Xu X, Fan H, et al. Higher serum chloride concentrations are associated with acute kidney injury in unselected critically ill patients. BMC Nephrol 2013;14:235.
39. Chowdhury AH, Cox EF, Francis ST, et al. A randomized, controlled, double-blind crossover study on the effects of 2-L infusions of 0.9% saline and plasma-lyte® 148 on renal blood flow velocity and renal cortical tissue perfusion in healthy volunteers. Ann Surg 2012;256(1):18–24.
40. Yunos NM, Bellomo R, Hegarty C, et al. Association between a chloride-liberal vs chloride-restrictive intravenous fluid administration strategy and kidney injury in critically ill adults. JAMA 2012;308(15):1566–72.
41. Shaw AD, Bagshaw SM, Goldstein SL, et al. Major complications, mortality, and resource utilization after open abdominal surgery: 0.9% saline compared to Plasma-Lyte. Ann Surg 2012;255(5):821–9.
42. Mahler SA, Conrad SA, Wang H, et al. Resuscitation with balanced electrolyte solution prevents hyperchloremic metabolic acidosis in patients with diabetic ketoacidosis. Am J Emerg Med 2011;29(6):670–4.
43. Raghunathan K, Shaw A, Nathanson B, et al. Association between the choice of IV crystalloid and in-hospital mortality among critically ill adults with sepsis*. Crit Care Med 2014;42(7):1585–91.
44. Rochwerg B, Alhazzani W, Gibson A, et al. Fluid type and the use of renal replacement therapy in sepsis: a systematic review and network meta-analysis. Intensive Care Med 2015;41(9):1561–71.
45. Rochwerg B, Alhazzani W, Sindi A, et al. Fluid resuscitation in sepsis: a systematic review and network meta-analysis. Ann Intern Med 2014;161(5):347–55.
46. Levy JA, Bachur RG, Monuteaux MC, et al. Intravenous dextrose for children with gastroenteritis and dehydration: a double-blind randomized controlled trial. Ann Emerg Med 2013;61(3):281–8.
47. Spandorfer PR. Subcutaneous rehydration: updating a traditional technique. Pediatr Emerg Care 2011;27(3):230–6.
48. Allen CH, Etzwiler LS, Miller MK, et al. Recombinant human hyaluronidase-enabled subcutaneous pediatric rehydration. Pediatrics 2009;124(5):e858–67.
49. Spandorfer PR, Mace SE, Okada PJ, et al. A randomized clinical trial of recombinant human hyaluronidase-facilitated subcutaneous versus intravenous rehydration in mild to moderately dehydrated children in the emergency department. Clin Ther 2012;34(11):2232–45.

50. Neville KA, Verge CF, O'Meara MW, et al. High antidiuretic hormone levels and hyponatremia in children with gastroenteritis. Pediatrics 2005;116(6):1401–7.
51. Brenkert TE, Estrada CM, McMorrow SP, et al. Intravenous hypertonic saline use in the pediatric emergency department. Pediatr Emerg Care 2013;29(1):71–3.
52. Verbalis JG, Goldsmith SR, Greenberg A, et al. Diagnosis, evaluation, and treatment of hyponatremia: expert panel recommendations. Am J Med 2013;126(10 Suppl 1):S1–42.
53. Bolat F, Oflaz MB, Guven AS, et al. What is the safe approach for neonatal hypernatremic dehydration? A retrospective study from a neonatal intensive care unit. Pediatr Emerg Care 2013;29(7):808–13.
54. Sterns RH. Disorders of plasma sodium–causes, consequences, and correction. N Engl J Med 2015;372(1):55–65.
55. Shaoul R, Okev N, Tamir A, et al. Value of laboratory studies in assessment of dehydration in children. Ann Clin Biochem 2004;41(Pt 3):192–6.
56. Vega RM, Avner JR. A prospective study of the usefulness of clinical and laboratory parameters for predicting percentage of dehydration in children. Pediatr Emerg Care 1997;13(3):179–82.
57. Yilmaz K, Karabocuoglu M, Citak A, et al. Evaluation of laboratory tests in dehydrated children with acute gastroenteritis. J Paediatr Child Health 2002;38(3):226–8.
58. Freedman SB, Willan AR, Boutis K, et al. Effect of dilute apple juice and preferred fluids vs electrolyte maintenance solution on treatment failure among children with mild gastroenteritis: a randomized clinical trial. JAMA 2016;315(18):1966–74.
59. Freedman SB, Ali S, Oleszczuk M, et al. Treatment of acute gastroenteritis in children: an overview of systematic reviews of interventions commonly used in developed countries. Evid Based Child Health 2013;8(4):1123–37.

Bronchiolitis
From Practice Guideline to Clinical Practice

Maybelle Kou, MD[a],*, Vivian Hwang, MD[a], Nadira Ramkellawan, MD[b]

KEYWORDS

- Bronchiolitis • ED management • Guidelines pediatric respiratory emergency
- Respiratory distress • AAP CPG • RSV • Therapy • Diagnosis

KEY POINTS

- Bronchiolitis is a common but challenging cause of respiratory distress in infants and children presenting to an emergency department.
- Emergency physicians must be able to stabilize those patients with escalating illness, distinguish patients with impending respiratory failure, and determine who may be discharged safely home.
- Emergency practitioner must be familiar with the American Academy of Pediatrics' clinical practice guideline for bronchiolitis in order to apply best practices appropriately.

This article discusses recent literature to inform the implementation of the American Academy of Pediatrics' (AAP's) bronchiolitis clinical practice guideline (CPG) into the emergency department (ED) management of bronchiolitis in children aged 1 month to 23 months. Recommendations on general resuscitation or inpatient management of bronchiolitis are not discussed.

BRONCHIOLITIS: FROM GUIDELINES TO CLINICAL PRACTICE: AN EMERGENCY DEPARTMENT PERSPECTIVE
The Guidelines

The 2014 update of the AAP's 2006 bronchiolitis CPG reflects a minimalist approach to bronchiolitis and addresses the care of previously healthy infants and children, most of whom do not need major intervention.[1] Before the 2006 CPG, widespread practice

Disclosure Statement: The authors do not have a direct financial interest in subject matter or materials discussed in the article or with a company making a competing product.
[a] The Altieri PEM Fellowship, Inova Fairfax Medical Campus, The George Washington University School of Medicine, Virginia Commonwealth University School of Medicine, Inova Fairfax Campus, 3300 Gallows Road, Falls Church, VA 22042, USA; [b] Pediatric Emergency Medicine Fellow, The Altieri PEM Fellowship, Inova Fairfax Medical Campus, 3300 Gallows Road, Falls Church, VA 22042, USA
* Corresponding author. % J. Eichorn, Emergency Department, 3300 Gallows Road, Falls Church, VA 22042.
E-mail address: maybelle.kou@inova.org

variation existed.[2] Despite increasing evidence that many bronchiolitis therapies lack effect, several recent studies describe the unnecessary resource and treatment utilization that still occurs globally.[3] Many infants still routinely receive medications with no proven benefit.[2] Although the 2014 guidelines have not yet had a major impact on all physician behavior, recent quality initiatives are promising in the reduction of unnecessary treatments in the inpatient setting.[4]

Disparity in treatment and evaluation

A comparison of general versus pediatric emergency physician (EP) treatment of bronchiolitis revealed poor adherence to the CPG and greater use of non–evidence-based therapies or testing in general EDs (GEDs) 77% of this large pediatric cohort received their care in GEDs[5] which suggests a lack of awareness of published CPGs and/or challenges in implementation of the guidelines in GEDs that might have contributed to these findings. With advances in knowledge diffusion via collaborative media sites targeting general EPs, synopses of evidence-based guidelines are increasingly available.[6]

Bronchiolitis: The Disease

Bronchiolitis is a disease of the lower respiratory tract most prevalent in children less than two years of age. Respiratory syncytial virus is a common cause, although other viruses such as human metapneumovirus and human rhinovirus have also been implicated.[7] The clinical respiratory effects stem from damage of epithelial cells in the terminal bronchi leading to edema, inflammation, excessive mucous production, and epithelial cell sloughing.[8] This cascade causes widespread obstruction of bronchioles from mucous plugging and causes atelectasis resulting in varying levels of respiratory distress. Symptoms may range from mild nasal congestion, to copious secretions, wheezing, and/or rales (crackles). Ventilation-perfusion mismatch due to obstruction causes hypoxia, rather than the smooth-muscle contraction of airways seen in reactive airway disease.

Epidemiology

Bronchiolitis outbreaks span the winter months into spring, with peaks in January and February. Boys and girls are equally affected. Worldwide, 3.4 million hospitalizations occur annually.[9] In the United States, 1.4 million outpatient and ED visits per year result in 150,000 admissions of patients less than 5 years old.[10] Risk factors that increase the likelihood of developing bronchiolitis include having an older sibling, exposure to cigarette smoke, daycare attendance, and birth within 2 months of the peak season.

Diagnosis

Bronchiolitis remains a clinical diagnosis with a wide spectrum of illness. Many patients with mild symptoms can be discharged with minimal to no ED intervention as recommended by the CPG.[11]

To Intervene or Not to Intervene

The CPG targets children with mild to moderate symptoms of bronchiolitis.[1] Findings such as a history of poor feeding, severe retractions, oxygen saturation of 92% or less, and a respiratory rate of 60/min or more were found to be predictive of major interventions and possible hospitalization in one study.[12] However, any child in shock (frank or impending), hypoxemia, and/or respiratory failure needs urgent stabilization and treatment (**Fig. 1**).

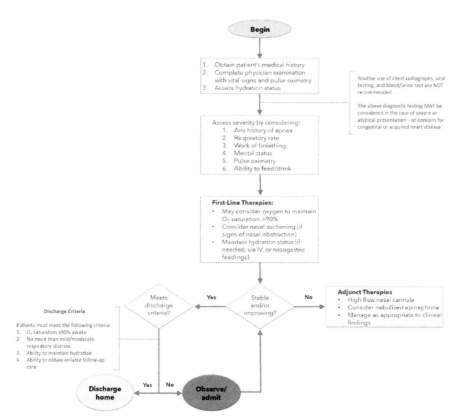

Fig. 1. Algorithm for acute bronchiolitis management. IV, intravenous; O_2, oxygen. (*From* Jain S. PV Card: Algorithm for acute bronchiolitis management. ALiem; November 7th, 2016. Available at https://www.aliem.com/2016/11/pv-card-algorithm-acute-bronchiolitis-management/.)

Risk Assessment and Predictors of Severe Illness

Bronchiolitis can lead to a wide spectrum of illness that may worsen during an ED stay. A retrospective study of previously healthy RSV-infected patients that subsequently developed respiratory failure (and mechanical ventilation) had lethargy, grunting, and a $PaCO_2$ of 65 mm, Hg or greater at initial ED presentation.[13] Past medical conditions, such as uncorrected or undiagnosed congenital heart disease, neuromuscular disease, immunodeficiency, or lung disease due to prematurity, also contribute to higher risks for progression of illness and need for hospitalization.

Respiratory Syncytial Virus Prophylaxis

Palivizumab for RSV immunoprophylaxis decreases hospitalizations in high-risk groups with an estimated population-weighted efficacy to reduce hospitalizations of 70%.[10] Only high-risk infants and those born at less than 32 weeks' gestational age, however, are eligible to receive prophylaxis and only during the peak of the RSV season in the first year of life. Many patients eligible to receive prophylaxis do not receive it.

Consideration of Apnea in Young Infants with Respiratory Syncytial Virus

The association of apnea and bronchiolitis in infants is important. Apnea may manifest with reported cessation of or irregular breathing. A prospective study reported 5% of hospitalized patients with bronchiolitis had apneic events.[14] Historical risk factors included a postconception age of less than 48 weeks, low birth weight, low or high respiratory rates, and low room air oxygen saturation. No increased risk was attributed to any particular viral pathogen. Increased morbidity was found when children were premature, had mothers with asthma, or had parents who smoked.[15]

Thresholds for Hospitalization

Poor feeding, severe retractions, oxygen saturation of 92% or less, and a respiratory rate of 60/min or more are general thresholds for hospitalization. A severity scale can be helpful to distinguish patients in need of an intervention[16] (**Table 1**). Decisions to hospitalize are subjective and can be due to social factors including parental reliability and home environment.[17] The validity of clinical scoring tools to predict thresholds for bronchiolitis severity or hospitalization is unproven.[18] A recent study describes a modified respiratory index score[19] that predicts hospitalizations based on the need for respiratory support or intravenous hydration; however, in this non-US study, the criterion for admission included oxygen saturations less than 95%.

Utility of Testing

Viral testing

Viral testing does not predict outcomes in otherwise healthy patients with symptoms of bronchiolitis and is not recommended even with a concern for viral coinfection.[7] Testing may be considered to guide management of illness in high-risk patients with comorbidities (and if influenza is suspected).[20,21] Testing for the purpose of cohorting admitted patients is common practice but increases resource utilization.[22] A recent study of hospitalized children implicated human rhinovirus (HRV) coinfection with increased hospital stay due to pneumonia. This suggests testing of hospitalized children with severe bronchiolitis may be helpful in the instance of HRV bronchiolitis.[23]

Urinalysis

It is well described that urinary tract infections occur concomitantly with RSV bronchiolitis in infants, and a recent study demonstrates coinfection also occurs in children 2 to 23 months of age.[24]

Serology

Bloodwork is not routinely recommended. Evaluation for serious bacterial infection (SBI) other than UTI has been shown to increase antibiotic use, ED length of stay (LOS), and/or inpatient admissions in patients with bronchiolitis.[25]

Table 1
Bronchiolitis assessment for infants younger than 12 months

	Mild	Moderate	Severe
Interest in feeding	Normal	Slightly decreased	Not interested or able
Respiratory rate	<2 mo >60/min; >2 mo >50/min	>60/min	>70/min
Chest retractions	Mild	Moderate	Severe
Nasal flare or grunting	Absent	Absent	Present
Pulse oximetry	>92%	88%–92%	<88%
General behavior	Normal	Irritable	Lethargic

Adapted from Ravaglia C, Poletti V. Recent advances in the management of acute bronchiolitis. F1000Prime Rep 2014;6:103. Available at: http://www.ncbi.nlm.nih.gov/pubmed/25580257. Based on SIGN, 2005 Based on SIGN (2005) and PREDICT (NZ); with permission.

Advances in genomic research may hold future promise in prognosis. Recent (preliminary) studies correlate greater RSV disease severity with viral load, and a weakened or delayed host response early in infection via measurements of RSV gene copy numbers.[26]

Diagnostic Imaging

Chest radiography

Well-appearing children do not need diagnostic imaging and are more likely to receive antibiotics if performed.[27] Studies document only modest decreases in chest radiography since publication of the CPG, however.[28] The clinical criteria to warrant chest radiography in children with bronchiolitis are ill defined. A 2015 meta-analysis to investigate clinical predictors of airspace disease (infiltrate or atelectasis) could not determine a correlation between physical examination findings and positive chest radiograph in a pooled analysis.[29] Bronchiolitis mimics, such as myocarditis, congestive heart failure, and complications from pneumonia, may justify the imaging of children with moderate to severe or lingering illness.

Bedside or point-of-care ultrasound

Studies of point-of-care ultrasound (POCUS) in the evaluation of pediatric patients with pulmonary disease are limited. A meta-analysis of ultrasound diagnosis of pediatric pneumonia described lung ultrasound (LUS) as a reliable test, especially in younger children whereby visualization is easier because of the smaller thoracic diameter and lung volumes.[30] A study of LUS and bronchiolitis provided data on the feasibility and characteristics of successful LUS in children that include B lines, small consolidations, pleural abnormalities, and atelectasis[31] and was prognostic of the need for oxygen supplementation in infants found to have posterior and paravertebral interstitial findings. Another study[32] discovered 46% of children discharged with a diagnosis of bronchiolitis had a positive LUS versus none in those with a final diagnosis of asthma,[33] suggesting POCUS could distinguish bronchiolitis from reactive airway disease. Limitations include the availability of skilled sonographers; however, the safety of ultrasound in pediatric patients compared with standard radiography is undeniable.

TREATMENT

Treatment is supportive and includes suctioning, supplemental oxygen, and hydration. Florin and colleagues'[8] review describes a global comparison of treatments citing similar approaches worldwide. Newer evidence of common therapies follows in **Table 2**.

Suctioning

Nasal suctioning provides relief of respiratory distress from the presence of copious secretions. An observational study of 40 infants in an ED setting showed that baseline oxygen saturations increased after suctioning[34] and, in spite of a small population, suggested that overdiagnosis of hypoxemia could lead to unnecessary hospitalizations of children who do not receive suctioning. A retrospective cohort study showed increased LOS for patients who were suctioned at intervals greater than 4 hours and in those who required deep suctioning in the first 24 hours.[35] The association of deep suctioning with longer LOS may reflect a worse disease process in these patients, not necessarily that treatment was ineffective. These results further emphasize the clinical importance for anticipatory guidance of suctioning infants with bronchiolitis after an ED visit for respiratory symptoms. A study of nasal irrigation with saline solution also did find that a single irrigation significantly improved oxygen saturation in infants with bronchiolitis.[36]

Table 2 Bronchiolitis best practices for emergency practitioners	
Evidence-based medicine	EPs must be familiar with recent evidence regarding the therapeutic benefit of bronchiolitis treatments, test utilization, and/or decision to hospitalize.[1] Advocacy to improve diffusion of new information and establish collaborative workgroups to improve overall pediatric care in general EDs requires attention.
Documentation pearls	EPs must document a thorough history on infants with bronchiolitis[1] and know the factors that place an infant at risk for apnea. EPs must consider all risk factors for severe infection with RSV when arranging disposition. Follow up instructions including reasons for Ed return must be clear for patients that are discharged.
Clinical scoring in bronchiolitis	Evidence does not support the sole use of clinical scoring tools when making the decision to admit.[18] The decision to admit must be based on repeated clinical examinations to determine a child's work of breathing and ability to maintain hydration.
Testing[1]	*Viral testing*: Viral testing is not generally indicated but may be considered in children <29 d of age or those requiring admission. *SBI*: Routine testing in otherwise well-appearing children with bronchiolitis is not necessary except in high-risk patients and those <29 d with fever >100.4°F. Urinalysis and urine culture may be considered in febrile RSV-positive infants with only mild respiratory symptoms. *Imaging studies*: Chest radiography is not generally indicated but may be considered in patients who require hospitalization or in whom an alternate cause of respiratory distress is suspected.[29]
Supportive measures: recommended	Supportive care remains the mainstay for treatment of bronchiolitis and includes suctioning, supplemental oxygen, and hydration.[1] Supplemental oxygen may be initiated for patients with saturations <90% while awake. Nasogastric replacement of fluids is an acceptable alternative to intravenous therapy when warranted and may be better tolerated compared with the intravenous route.[41] Continuous pulse-oximetry is not indicated.
Therapies with limited to no benefit	Bronchodilators, hypertonic saline, and corticosteroids are not recommended for standard ED treatment of bronchiolitis. Although helium-oxygen mixtures may be used as a temporizing measure, there are insufficient data to recommend its use. Antibiotics are not indicated unless bacterial coinfection exists.[1]
Newer therapies: insufficient evidence	Oxygen via high-flow humidified nasal cannula may be attempted as a temporizing measure for children in moderate respiratory distress; however, evidence is still limited regarding its efficacy in severe disease.[55]
Disposition	Criteria for safe discharge with reliable families from the ED[56] includes the following: • Ability of a child to maintain saturations higher than 90% on room air while awake (>88% while sleeping) • Respirations <70/min without increased work of breathing • Ability to hydrate • Close urgent PCP follow-up or return to the ED

Abbreviation: PCP, primary care physician.

Supplemental Oxygen, Oximetry, and Capnography

The threshold for which supplemental oxygen therapy is initiated remains globally nonuniform.[9] Arbitrary oxygenation thresholds promote increased hospitalizations and resource utilization if used as the sole proxy for illness severity. Intermittent hypoxemia in otherwise stable infants was not found to cause long-term harm: a Canadian investigation of infants discharged with home pulse-oximetry found no significant difference in unscheduled 72-hour return visits between those who had desaturations lasting 1 minute or more at home versus no desaturations.[37] A British randomized controlled trial (RCT) found a saturation target of 90% to be safe. Continuous pulse oximetry of children under ED observation is not thought to be useful because of the dynamic nature of the disease,[38,39] and spot checks of children with mild to moderate symptoms are reasonable. End-tidal capnometry has not yet been proven to predict children in need of hospitalization to date.[40]

Hydration

Infants and younger children are at increased risk for fluid losses through tachypnea or fever or from poor fluid intake due to congestion. Studies investigating nasogastric versus intravenous fluid administration have found both to be efficacious[41] with fewer attempts for successful nasogastric insertion versus peripheral venous cannulation.

Controversial Treatments Not Currently Recommended in the Clinical Practice Guideline

Nebulized β-agonists
Evidence fails to show consistent benefit in the use of albuterol (or salbutamol) for infants and children with bronchiolitis.[1] Although it is not recommended, its use persists in both outpatient and inpatient settings.[42] A Canadian survey found that physicians commonly gave a trial of either salbutamol or epinephrine to patients with bronchiolitis.[43] The 2014 CPG states that "if a clinical trial of bronchodilators is undertaken, clinicians should note that the variability of the disease process, the host's airway, and the clinical assessments, particularly scoring, would limit the clinician's ability to observe a clinically relevant response to bronchodilators."[1] The risks and benefits of using β-agonists must be weighed because of the adverse effects, including tachycardia, tremors, and hypoxemia.[42] An inpatient multicenter collaborative to decrease overuse of bronchodilators and steroids for bronchiolitis has been found to be effective.[5]

Nebulized epinephrine
The use of nebulized epinephrine for acute bronchiolitis is also not recommended.[1] Although epinephrine may improve clinical symptoms in the short-term, its use as standard ED treatment is controversial, as it would not be prescribed as a home medication. The National Institute for Health and Care Excellence's clinical guidelines do comment that epinephrine may be considered for its short-term benefit for severe respiratory distress.[44] A systematic review and meta-analysis concluded that epinephrine reduces hospitalizations compared with placebo on the day of the ED visit but did not improve inpatient LOS.[45] It is important to stress that the benefits of nebulized epinephrine are small and transient, but one could *consider its use for those patients in severe respiratory distress as a bridge to more definitive treatment*.

Nebulized hypertonic saline
The CPG does not recommend ED use of nebulized hypertonic saline (HS) in infants with acute bronchiolitis.[1] Among infants in a pediatric emergency department with a first episode of acute moderate to severe bronchiolitis, an RCT comparing nebulized 3% HS with nebulized 0.9% Normal saline did not significantly reduce the rate of hospital admission.[46] Another study demonstrated prolonged hospitalization of children younger than 2 years with acute, nonsevere bronchiolitis when given nebulized 3%

HS independent of age, clinical presentation of disease, or inclusion of other treatments in their management.[45]

Systemic corticosteroids

The use of systemic corticosteroids for acute bronchiolitis is not recommended.[1] Inhaled and systemic formulations that are widely used for asthma have not been shown to be effective in infants and children with bronchiolitis. Several RCTs have shown no difference in admission rates, readmission rates, length of hospitalization, or clinical scores for infants.[47]

Combination therapies

Combination therapy including nebulized epinephrine with 3% HS versus nebulized 3% HS alone was studied in infants with moderate bronchiolitis. Hospital LOS and disease severity decreased in patients from the third day of treatment who received nebulized epinephrine with 3% HS.[48] Combination therapies with bronchodilators show mixed results: one study demonstrates improvement with epinephrine for outpatients, whereas a more recent study of dexamethasone with nebulized epinephrine or β-agonists did not show clinical improvement.[49] Although combination epinephrine-dexamethasone may be effective for outpatients,[50] further research is needed.

Heliox

A meta-analysis[51] found that heliox is effective in reducing clinical respiratory scores within an hour after initiation in infants with bronchiolitis; however, it did not reduce intubation rates or length of treatment. Its availability is also not universal.

Antibiotics

Children with clinical bronchiolitis are more likely to receive antibiotics if diagnostic imaging has been performed.[52] Antibiotics should be avoided unless concurrent bacterial pneumonia, urinary tract infection, or otitis media have been identified.

Newer Therapies Not Discussed in the Clinical Practice Guideline

Noninvasive ventilatory strategies: high-flow warm humidified oxygen

Literature is evolving, but so far inconclusive regarding the use of high-flow nasal cannula (HFNC) as a preferable alternative to wall oxygen or continuous positive airway pressure in moderately severe bronchiolitis.[53] The mechanism of action is thought to be via reduction of inspiratory resistance and improvement of pulmonary compliance.[54] Recommendations for initial flow rates are not yet published, but suggestions are to initiate HFNC at 10 L/min with titration to effect. An Australian RCT comparing HFNC with standard cold wall oxygen found no benefit regarding weaning strategies in infants with moderately severe disease but noted a role in rescue therapy from standard treatment to prevent escalation to intensive care treatment in some patients.[55] Complications have been reported, such as pneumothorax. Limitations to its use could include availability of pediatric high-flow equipment at GEDs and knowledge of indications.

Safe discharge from the emergency department

Criteria for safe discharge from the ED include the ability of a child to maintain saturations higher than 90% on room air while awake (>88% while sleeping), respirations less than 70 per minute without increased work of breathing, the ability to hydrate, and close urgent primary care physician (PCP) follow-up or return to the ED.[56] A Swiss study determined that a period of at least 5 hours and up to 25 hours was needed to identify infants at risk of delayed saturation (oxygen saturation <92%) who were more likely to be younger than 3 months, female, with tachypnea and moderate retractions, with a recent ED visit.[57] The same group reported children greater than 3 months of age took longer to manifest desaturations (11 hours). In a study looking at unscheduled return visits, 3 independent factors associated with unscheduled visits were age less than 2 months, male sex, and a previous history of hospital admission.[58] Regardless, the literature stresses the importance of close PCP follow-up and return precautions for children with borderline tachypnea or a risk of poor hydration. Admission is recommended when patient safety cannot be guaranteed.

REFERENCES

1. Ralston SJ, Lieberthal AS, Meissner HC, et al. Clinical practice guideline: the diagnosis, management, and prevention of bronchiolitis. Pediatrics 2014; 134(5):e1502. Available at: http://www.ncbi.nlm.nih.gov/pubmed/25349312.
2. Florin TA, Byczkowski T, Ruddy RM, et al. Variation in the management of infants hospitalized for bronchiolitis persists after the 2006 American Academy of Pediatrics bronchiolitis guidelines. J Pediatr 2014;165(4):92.e1.
3. Carande EJ, Pollard AJ, Drysdale SB. Management of respiratory syncytial virus bronchiolitis: 2015 survey of members of the European Society for Paediatric infectious diseases. Can J Infect Dis Med Microbiol 2016;2016:9139537. Available at: http://search.proquest.com/docview/1846088232.
4. Ralston SL, Garber MD, Rice-Conboy E, et al. A multicenter collaborative to reduce unnecessary care in inpatient bronchiolitis. Pediatrics 2016;137(1): e20150851. Available at: http://www.ncbi.nlm.nih.gov/pubmed/26628731.
5. Gong C, Byczkowski T, McAneney C, et al. Emergency department management of bronchiolitis in the United States. Pediatr Emerg Care 2017. https://doi.org/10.1097/PEC.0000000000001145.
6. Lin M. Acute bronchiolitis management PV card. Academic Life in Emergency Medicine Website; 2016. Available at: http://www.aliem.com/2016/11/pv-card-algorithm-acute-bronchiolitis-management. Accessed Sep 30, 2017.
7. Mansbach JM, McAdam AJ, Clark S, et al. Prospective multicenter study of the viral etiology of bronchiolitis in the emergency department. Acad Emerg Med 2008;15(2):111–8. Available at: http://www.ingentaconnect.com/content/bpl/aem/2008/00000015/00000002/art00001.
8. Florin TA, Plint AC, Zorc JJ. Viral bronchiolitis. Lancet 2017;389(10065):211–24. Available at: http://search.proquest.com/docview/1858172086.
9. Nair H, Nokes DJ, Gessner BD, et al. Global burden of acute lower respiratory infections due to respiratory syncytial virus in young children: a systematic review and meta-analysis. The Lancet 2010;375(9725):1545–55. Available at: http://www.sciencedirect.com/science/article/pii/S0140673610602061.
10. Hasegawa K, Tsugawa Y, Brown DF, et al. Trends in bronchiolitis hospitalizations in the United States, 2000-2009. Pediatrics 2013;132(1):28–36. Available at: http://www.ncbi.nlm.nih.gov/pubmed/23733801.
11. Friedman JN, Rieder MJ, Walton JM. Bronchiolitis: recommendations for diagnosis, monitoring and management of children one to 24 months of age. Paediatr Child Health 2014;19(9):485. http://www.ncbi.nlm.nih.gov/pubmed/25414585.
12. Parker MJ, Allen U, Stephens D, et al. Predictors of major intervention in infants with bronchiolitis. Pediatr Pulmonol 2009;44(4):358–63. Available at: http://www.ncbi.nlm.nih.gov/pubmed/19283838.
13. Prodhan P, Sharoor-Karni S, Lin J, et al. Predictors of respiratory failure among previously healthy children with respiratory syncytial virus infection. Am J Emerg Med 2011;29(2):168–73. Available at: http://www.sciencedirect.com/science/article/pii/S0735675709004215.

14. Schroeder AR, Mansbach JM, Stevenson M, et al. Apnea in children hospitalized with bronchiolitis. Pediatrics 2013;132(5):E1201.

15. Jones L, Hashim A, McKeever T, et al. Parental and household smoking and the increased risk of bronchitis, bronchiolitis and other lower respiratory infections in infancy: systematic review and meta-analysis. Respir Res 2011;12(1):1–11. Available at: http://www.ncbi.nlm.nih.gov/pubmed/21219618.

16. Ravaglia C, Poletti V. Recent advances in the management of acute bronchiolitis. F1000Prime Rep 2014;6:103. Available at: http://www.ncbi.nlm.nih.gov/pubmed/25580257.

17. Luo G, Stone BL, Johnson MD, et al. Predicting appropriate admission of bronchiolitis patients in the emergency department: rationale and methods. JMIR Res Protoc 2016;5(1):e41. Available at: http://www.ncbi.nlm.nih.gov/pubmed/26952700.

18. Destino L, Weisgerber MC, Soung P, et al. Validity of respiratory scores in bronchiolitis. Hosp Pediatr 2012;2(4):202–9. Available at: http://www.ncbi.nlm.nih.gov/pubmed/24313026.

19. Chong S, Teoh OH, Nadkarni N, et al. The modified respiratory index score (RIS) guides resource allocation in acute bronchiolitis. Pediatr Pulmonology 2017; 52(7):954–61.

20. Brand HK, de Groot R, Galama JMD, et al. Infection with multiple viruses is not associated with increased disease severity in children with bronchiolitis. Pediatr Pulmonology 2012;47(4):393–400. Available at: http://www.narcis.nl/publication/RecordID/oai:repository.ubn.ru.nl:2066%2F108342.

21. Meskill SD, Revell PA, Chandramohan L, et al. Prevalence of co-infection between respiratory syncytial virus and influenza in children. Am J Emerg Med 2017;35(3): 495–8. Available at: http://search.proquest.com/docview/1878847623.

22. Stollar F, Alcoba G, Gervaix A, et al. Virologic testing in bronchiolitis: does it change management decisions and predict outcomes? Eur J Pediatr 2014; 173(11):1429–35.

23. Bergroth E, Aakula M, Korppi M, et al. Post-bronchiolitis use of asthma medication: a prospective 1-year follow-up study. Pediatr Infect Dis J 2016;35(4):363–8. Available at: http://www.ncbi.nlm.nih.gov/pubmed/26658529.

24. Librizzi J, McCulloh R, Koehn K, et al. Appropriateness of testing for serious bacterial infection in children hospitalized with bronchiolitis. Hosp Pediatr 2014;4(1): 33–8. Available at: http://www.ncbi.nlm.nih.gov/pubmed/24435599.

25. Piedra FA, Mei M, Avadhanula V, et al. The interdependencies of viral load, the innate immune response, and clinical outcome in children presenting to the emergency department with respiratory syncytial virus-associated bronchiolitis. PLoS One 2017;12(3):e0172953. Available at: http://search.proquest.com/docview/1875113886.

26. Elkhunovich M, Wang V. Assessing the utility of urine testing in febrile infants aged 2 to 12 months with bronchiolitis. Pediatr Emerg Care 2015;31(9):616–20. Available at: http://www.ncbi.nlm.nih.gov/pubmed/25834961.

27. Schuh S, Lalani A, Allen U, et al. Evaluation of the utility of radiography in acute bronchiolitis. J Pediatr 2007;150(4):429–33. Available at: http://www.sciencedirect.com/science/article/pii/S0022347607000078.

28. Johnson LW, Robles J, Hudgins A, et al. Management of bronchiolitis in the emergency department: impact of evidence-based guidelines? Pediatrics 2013;131(Supplement 1):S109. Available at: http://www.ncbi.nlm.nih.gov/pubmed/23457145.

29. Chao JH, Lin RC, Marneni S, et al. Predictors of airspace disease on chest x-ray in emergency department patients with clinical bronchiolitis: a systematic review

and meta-analysis. Acad Emerg Med 2016;23(10):1107–18. Available at: http://onlinelibrary.wiley.com/doi/10.1111/acem.13052/abstract.

30. Pereda MA, Chavez MA, Hooper-Miele CC, et al. Lung ultrasound for the diagnosis of pneumonia in children: a meta-analysis. Pediatrics 2015;135(4):714–22. Available at: http://www.ncbi.nlm.nih.gov/pubmed/25780071.

31. Basile V, Di Mauro A, Scalini E, et al. Lung ultrasound: a useful tool in diagnosis and management of bronchiolitis. BMC Pediatr 2015;15(1):63. Available at: http://www.ncbi.nlm.nih.gov/pubmed/25993984.

32. Varshney T, Mok E, Shapiro AJ, et al. Point-of-care lung ultrasound in young children with respiratory tract infections and wheeze. Emerg Med J 2016;33(9):603–10. Available at: http://www.ncbi.nlm.nih.gov/pubmed/27107052.

33. Dankoff S, Li P, Shapiro AJ, et al. Point of care lung ultrasound of children with acute asthma exacerbations in the pediatric ED. The Am J Emerg Med 2017;35(4):615. Available at: https://search.proquest.com/docview/1885076673.

34. Moschino L, Mario F, Carraro S, et al. Is nasal suctioning warranted before measuring O2 saturation in infants with bronchiolitis? Arch Dis Child 2016;101(1):114–5. Available at: http://www.ncbi.nlm.nih.gov/pubmed/26672100.

35. Mussman GM, Parker MW, Statile A, et al. Suctioning and length of stay in infants hospitalized with bronchiolitis. JAMA Pediatr 2013;167(5):414–21.

36. Schreiber S, Ronfani L, Ghirardo S, et al. Nasal irrigation with saline solution significantly improves oxygen saturation in infants with bronchiolitis. Acta Paediatr 2016;105(3):292–6. Available at: http://onlinelibrary.wiley.com/doi/10.1111/apa.13282/abstract.

37. Principi T, Coates AL, Parkin PC, et al. Effect of oxygen desaturations on subsequent medical visits in infants discharged from the emergency department with bronchiolitis. JAMA Pediatr 2016;170(6):602–8.

38. McCulloh R, Koster M, Ralston S, et al. Use of intermittent vs continuous pulse oximetry for nonhypoxemic infants and young children hospitalized for bronchiolitis: a randomized clinical trial. JAMA Pediatr 2015;169(10):898–904.

39. Schuh S, Freedman S, Coates A, et al. Effect of oximetry on hospitalization in bronchiolitis: a randomized clinical trial. JAMA 2014;312(7):712–8.

40. Jacob R, Bentur L, Brik R, et al. Is capnometry helpful in children with bronchiolitis? Respir Med 2016;113:37–41. Available at: http://www.sciencedirect.com/science/article/pii/S0954611116300257.

41. Oakley E, Bata S, Rengasamy S, et al. Nasogastric hydration in infants with bronchiolitis less than 2 months of age. J Pediatr 2016;178:245.e1.

42. Gadomski AM, Scribani MB. Bronchodilators for bronchiolitis. Cochrane Database Syst Rev 2014;(6). CD001266. Available at: http://www.ncbi.nlm.nih.gov/pubmed/24937099.

43. Plint AC, Grenon R, Klassen TP, et al. Bronchodilator and steroid use for the management of bronchiolitis in Canadian pediatric emergency departments. CJEM 2015;17(1):46–53. Available at: http://www.ncbi.nlm.nih.gov/pubmed/25781383.

44. Caffrey Osvald E, Clarke JR. NICE clinical guideline: bronchiolitis in children. Arch Dis Child Educ Pract Ed 2016;101(1):46. Available at: http://www.ncbi.nlm.nih.gov/pubmed/26628507.

45. Hartling L, Bialy LM, Vandermeer B, et al. Epinephrine for bronchiolitis. The Cochrane database of systematic reviews. 2011(6):CD003123. http://www.ncbi.nlm.nih.gov/pubmed/21678340.

46. Angoulvant F, Bellêttre X, Milcent K, et al. Effect of nebulized hypertonic saline treatment in emergency departments on the hospitalization rate for acute bronchiolitis: a randomized clinical trial. JAMA Pediatr 2017;171(8):e171333.

47. Pinto JM, Schairer JL, Petrova A. Duration of hospitalization in association with type of inhalation therapy used in the management of children with nonsevere, acute bronchiolitis. Pediatr Neonatal 2016;57(2):140. Available at: http://www.ncbi.nlm.nih.gov/pubmed/26464183.

48. Flores-González JC, Dominguez-Coronel MT, Matamala Morillo MA, et al. Does nebulized epinephrine improve the efficacy of hypertonic saline solution in the treatment of hospitalized moderate acute bronchiolitis? A double blind, randomized clinical trial. Minerva pediatrica 2016;68(2):81. Available at: http://www.ncbi.nlm.nih.gov/pubmed/25263242.

49. Bawazeer M, Aljeraisy M, Albanyan E, et al. Effect of combined dexamethasone therapy with nebulized r-epinephrine or salbutamol in infants with bronchiolitis: a randomized, double-blind, controlled trial. Avicenna J Med 2014;4(3):58. Available at: http://www.ncbi.nlm.nih.gov/pubmed/24982826.

50. Plint AC, Johnson DW, Patel H, et al. Epinephrine and dexamethasone in children with bronchiolitis. N Engl J Med 2009;360(20):2079–89. Available at: http://content.nejm.org/cgi/content/abstract/360/20/2079.

51. Liet J, Ducruet T, Gupta V, et al. Heliox inhalation therapy for bronchiolitis in infants. The Cochrane database Syst Rev 2015;(9). CD006915. Available at: http://www.ncbi.nlm.nih.gov/pubmed/26384333.

52. Knapp J, Hall M, Sharma V. Benchmarks for the emergency department care of children with asthma, bronchiolitis, and croup. Pediatr Emerg Care 2010;26(5):364–9. Available at: http://www.ncbi.nlm.nih.gov/pubmed/20404778.

53. Mikalsen IB, Davis P, Øymar K. High flow nasal cannula in children: a literature review. Scand J Trauma Resusc Emerg Med 2016;24(1):93. Available at: http://www.ncbi.nlm.nih.gov/pubmed/27405336.

54. Pham TMT, O'Malley L, Mayfield S, et al. The effect of high flow nasal cannula therapy on the work of breathing in infants with bronchiolitis. Pediatr Pulmonology 2015;50(7):713–20. Available at: http://onlinelibrary.wiley.com/doi/10.1002/ppul.23060/abstract.

55. Kepreotes E, Whitehead B, Attia J, et al. High-flow warm humidified oxygen versus standard low-flow nasal cannula oxygen for moderate bronchiolitis (HFWHO RCT): an open, phase 4, randomised controlled trial. The Lancet 2017;389(10072):930. Available at: https://search.proquest.com/docview/1874438870.

56. Bronchiolitis Guideline Team, Children's Hospital Medical Center: evidence-based care guideline for management of first time episode bronchiolitis in infants less than 1 year of age. 2015.

57. Stollar F, Gervaix A, Barrazone-Argiroffo C. Safely discharging infants with bronchiolitis from an emergency department: a five step guide for pediatricians. PLoS One 2016;11(9):e0163217.

58. Norwood A, Mansbach JM, Clark S, et al. Prospective multicenter study of bronchiolitis: predictors of an unscheduled visit after discharge from the emergency department. Acad Emerg Med 2010;17(4):376–82. Available at: http://www.ingentaconnect.com/content/bpl/aem/2010/00000017/00000004/art00010.

Pediatric Minor Head Injury 2.0

Moving from Injury Exclusion to Risk Stratification

James (Jim) L. Homme, MD

KEYWORDS

- Pediatric minor head trauma • Traumatic brain injury • Clinical decision rule
- PECARN • CATCH • CHALICE • Risk stratification • Shared decision making

KEY POINTS

- Less than 10% of children with minor blunt head trauma who undergo neuroimaging in the emergency department show any form of traumatic brain injury.
- Appropriate application of clinical decision rules for minor TBI decrease neuroimaging rates in children with minor blunt head trauma without missing significant injuries.
- Observation, shared decision making, and further risk stratification of children with minor blunt head trauma not considered very low-risk can aid clinicians in decisions regarding the necessity of neuroimaging.
- Children with minor blunt head trauma and normal neuroimaging or isolated linear skull fractures can likely forego hospitalization owing to very low rates of neurologic deterioration or neurosurgical intervention.

INTRODUCTION

Blunt head trauma (BHT) is a leading cause of trauma-related death and disability in children worldwide. Falls account for the majority of injuries in children less than 13 years of age. Assault, sports-related injuries, and motor vehicle accidents constitute the top 3 causes in children 13 to 18 years old.[1] Every year in the United States there are more than 600,000 emergency department (ED) visits for pediatric head trauma and over the decade of 2001 to 2010 rates of ED visits for BHT have nearly doubled. Fortunately, rates of hospitalization and deaths associated with traumatic brain injury (TBI) have steadily decreased.[2] This apparent paradox highlights the

Disclosures: None.
Pediatric and Adolescent Medicine Residency, Department of Emergency Medicine, Division of Pediatric Emergency Medicine, Mayo Clinic, 200 First Street Southwest, Rochester, MN 55905, USA
E-mail address: homme.james@mayo.edu

Emerg Med Clin N Am 36 (2018) 287–304
https://doi.org/10.1016/j.emc.2017.12.015   **emed.theclinics.com**
0733-8627/18/© 2018 The Author. Published by Elsevier Inc. This is an open access article under the CC BY-NC-ND license (http://creativecommons.org/licenses/by-nc-nd/4.0/).

increasingly concerned populous seeking evaluation, even after minor BHT. Some of this concern likely originates from a heightened awareness of consequence of concussions.[3,4] Certainly, differentiation between concussion and other forms of TBI is a critical aspect of discussions with patients and caregivers seeking care for minor BHT.[5]

For clinicians evaluating BHT, the specter of more severe structural brain injuries looms large even though the vast majority of these patients can be categorized as minor head trauma (Glasgow Coma Scale [GCS] score of 14–15). Enabled by increased availability and speed of current computed tomography (CT) scans and fueled by fear of missing injuries that may result in litigation,[6,7] clinicians opt for imaging for 32% to 53% of children presenting with minor head injury[1] when fewer than 10% show any sort of TBI and only 0.1% require neurosurgical intervention. The use of CT scanning for minor head injury varies significantly between institutions and clinician specialty.[8–10]

CLINICAL DECISION RULES: BRIEF PRIMER FOR CLINICIANS

Clinical decision rules (CDRs) are derived in an attempt to improve on current standard practices in establishing or excluding certain diagnoses. They also create a common "language" that further codifies data used in establishing what is commonly referred to as the "clinical gestalt" regarding the likelihood of a condition. In the current era of CDRs, "clinical gestalt" is often informed by these CDRs, making it difficult to completely separate one from the other.

For CDRs to be useful, they must be accessible to clinicians at the beside, direct appropriate action, and improve on current practice.[11] Additionally, they must be externally valid. Decision rules can take the form of 1-way or 2-way rules. One-way rules typically rule out a condition by identifying low-risk patients who require no further investigation. These rules do not imply that patients who do not meet all criteria of the rule are at high risk of having the condition, a common misunderstanding of how to use the rule. Patients who cannot be "ruled out" by the one-way CDR require additional information for further risk stratification. Two-way rules are designed to direct action toward confirmation or exclusion a condition depending on whether the criteria of the rule are met. Patients meeting all criteria of the rule can forgo testing, whereas those who do meet all the criteria do not require testing.

Despite what the term would imply, CDRs are not meant to be rules that must be followed, but rather viewed as tools that inform clinician decision making. A patient may be "rule negative" with a 1-way rule, but other factors in the presentation warrant further testing. Additionally, all criteria of a 2-way rule may not be met, yet the likelihood of the condition of interest remains low enough, or the benefit of diagnosis does not outweigh the risk of testing, and therefore testing is constrained.

CLINICAL DECISION RULES FOR PEDIATRIC MINOR HEAD TRAUMA: PEDIATRIC EMERGENCY CARE APPLIED RESEARCH NETWORK, CANADIAN ASSESSMENT OF TOMOGRAPHY FOR CHILDHOOD HEAD INJURY, AND CHILDREN'S HEAD INJURY ALGORITHM FOR THE PREDICTION OF IMPORTANT CLINICAL EVENTS

Investigators in the United States (Pediatric Emergency Care Applied Research Network [PECARN]), Canada (Canadian Assessment of Tomography for Childhood Head Injury [CATCH]), and Europe (Children's Head Injury Algorithm for the Prediction of Important Clinical Events [CHALICE]) have independently and prospectively derived CDRs for use in evaluation of children with minor BHT. Comparative details of the derivation studies are summarized in **Table 1**. The decision rules and performance statistics are summarized in **Table 2**.

The primary outcomes, inclusion/exclusion criteria, and outcomes for the studies varied slightly. For PECARN and CATCH, primary outcomes were clinical endpoints, whereas for CHALICE primary outcomes are a composite of clinical and radiologic outcomes. The PECARN primary endpoint was clinically important TBI (ciTBI; see **Table 1**). Notably, there were no deaths reported in the study of 42,412 patients. For CATCH, the primary endpoint was neurosurgical intervention (see **Table 1**) and a secondary outcome was acute injury on CT scan with the exception of nonde-pressed skull and basilar skull fractures. The composite endpoint for CHALICE was clinically significant intracranial injury, neurosurgical intervention, or marked abnor-mality on CT scan (see **Table 1**). Secondary outcomes were presence of skull fracture or need for admission. CT scans were performed in 52.8% of patients in CATCH compared with 35.5% in PECARN and 3.3% in CHALICE. In this study, the admission rate was 6.4% compared with 9.0% in PECARN. Admission rate data were not re-ported in the CATCH study.

CATCH and CHALICE both performed very well in their derivation studies citing high sensitivities, specificities, and negative predictive values (NPVs). PECARN combined derivation and validation into a single study, reporting sensitivity of 100% and an NPV of 100% for those less than 2 years of age and a sensitivity of 96.8% and an NPV of 99.95% for those 2 to 18 years of age from the validation portion of the study.

External validation studies lend some insight into whether there is a compelling reason to use one rule over another. A single-center, prospective validation study of these rules compared with physician gestalt in a large urban children's ED favored PECARN and physician gestalt for sensitivity of detecting ciTBI. PECARN was the only rule that did not miss any patients requiring neurosurgical intervention. Specific-ities vary between approaches with CHALICE having the highest at 85%, followed by PECARN (62%), physician gestalt (50%), and CATCH (44%).[12] Additional prospective and retrospective studies have validated PECARN in Scandinavia and Japan, respec-tively.[13,14] The most recent comparison was performed prospectively in 10 pediatric EDs across Australia and New Zealand including more than 20,000 children.[15] PECARN did not miss any children less than 2 years of age with ciTBI, but did miss a single child greater than 2 years of age who did not require neurosurgery. CATCH missed 13 children with ciTBI with a single child requiring neurosurgery. CHALICE missed 31 children according to its own rule specifications, but when PECARN ciTBI criteria were applied, it only missed 12 children, 2 requiring neurosurgery. PECARN had the highest sensitivity across rules. All 3 had similar NPVs (PECARN: <2 years of age, 100% and 2–18 years of age, 100%; CATCH, 99.4%; CHALICE, 99.8%), although CATCH and CHALICE had higher specificities (56% and 78%, respectively). With a prevalence of ciTBI of 1% in this study, similar to other studies of minor head injury, the positive predictive value for ciTBI of PECARN for those less than 2 years of age was 2.0% and for those 2 to 18 years of age, it was 1.6%; CATCH 2.5% (for neuro-surgical intervention) and for CHALICE it was 7.9% (for clinically significant intracranial injury).

All 3 rules are highly sensitive, weighted toward not missing injuries, although PECARN seems to have a slight edge over CATCH and CHALICE. Specificity favors CATCH and CHALICE, although the general sentiment among clinicians and patients favors the sensitivity of a rule over specificity.[16–18] Using any of these CDRs as a 1-way injury exclusion rules is reasonable, with validation studies slightly favoring PECARN with the lowest miss rate. In practice, these CDRs are most appropriately applied

Table 1
Comparison of derivation studies for PECARN, CATCH, and CHALICE

	PECARN <2 y (N = 10,718)	PECARN 2–18 y (N = 31,695)	CATCH (N = 3866)	CHALICE (N = 22,772)
Inclusion criteria	Age <2 y; presenting within 24 h of head injury	Age 2–18 y; presenting within 24 h of head injury	Age <17 y All of the following: blunt trauma to the head resulting in witnessed LOC, definite amnesia, witnessed disorientation, persistent vomiting (≥2 distinct episodes of vomiting 15 min apart), persistent irritability in the ED (in children <2 y) Initial GCS score in ED ≥13, as determined by treating physician Injury within the past 24 h	Age <16 y; any history or signs of injury to the head
Exclusion criteria	Trivial mechanism of injury, defined by ground-level fall or walking or running into stationary objects and no signs or symptoms of head trauma other than scalp abrasions and lacerations; penetrating trauma Known brain tumors Preexisting neurologic disorder complicating assessment Neuroimaging at an outside hospital before transfer Patient with ventricular shunt Patient with bleeding disorder CSG score <14	Trivial mechanism of injury, defined by ground-level fall or walking or running into stationary objects and no signs or symptoms of head trauma other than scalp abrasions and lacerations Penetrating trauma Known brain tumors Preexisting neurologic disorder complicating assessment Neuroimaging at an outside hospital before transfer Patient with ventricular shunt Patient with bleeding disorder CSG score <14	Obvious penetrating skull injury Obviously depressed fracture Acute focal neurologic deficit Chronic generalized developmental delay Head injury secondary to suspected child abuse Returning for reassessment of previously treated head injury Patients who were pregnant	Refusal to consent

Primary outcome	Clinically important TBI, defined as death from TBI, neurosurgical intervention for TBI (intracranial pressure monitoring, elevation of depressed skull fracture, ventriculostomy, hematoma evacuation, lobectomy, tissue debridement, dura repair, or other), intubation of >24 h for TBI or hospital admission of ≥2 nights for TBI,[a] associated with TBI on CT[b]	Clinically important TBI, defined as death from TBI, neurosurgical intervention for TBI (intracranial pressure monitoring, elevation of depressed skull fracture, ventriculostomy, hematoma evacuation, lobectomy, tissue debridement, dura repair, or other), intubation of >24 h for TBI, or hospital admission of ≥2 nights for TBI,[a] associated with TBI on CT[b]	Need for neurologic intervention, defined as either death within 7 d secondary to the head injury or need for any of the following procedures within 7 d: craniotomy, elevation of skull fracture, monitoring of intracranial pressure, or insertion of endotracheal tube for the management of head injury	Clinically significant intracranial injury, defined as death as a result of head injury, requirement for neurosurgical intervention, or marked abnormality on CT (defined as any new, acute, traumatic intracranial pathology as reported by consultant radiologist, including intracranial hematomas of any size, cerebral contusion, diffuse cerebral edema, and depressed skull fracture)
Secondary outcome	None	None	Brain injury on CT, defined as any acute intracranial finding revealed on CT that was attributable to acute injury, including closed depressed skull fracture (ie, depressed past the inner table) and pneumocephalus, but excluding nondepressed skull fractures and basilar skull fractures	Presence of skull fracture Admission to hospital

Abbreviations: CATCH, Canadian Assessment of Tomography for Childhood Head Injury; CHALICE, Children's Head Injury Algorithm for the Prediction of Important Clinical Events; CT, computed tomography; ED, emergency department; GCS, Glasgow Coma Scale; LOC, loss of consciousness; PECARN, Pediatric Emergency Care Applied Research Network; TBI, traumatic brain injury.

a Hospital admission for TBI defined by admission for persistent neurologic symptoms or signs such as persistent alteration in mental status, recurrent emesis owing to head injury, persistent severe headache, or ongoing seizure management.

b TBI on CT defined by any of the following descriptions: intracranial hemorrhage or contusion, cerebral edema, traumatic infarction, diffuse axonal injury, shearing injury, sigmoid sinus thrombosis, midline shift of intracranial contents or signs of brain herniation, diastasis of the skull, pneumocephalus, or skull fracture depressed by at least the width of the table of the skull.

Table 2
Clinical decision rule variables and validation statistics

Predictor Variables	PECARN <2 y (N = 10,718)	PECARN 2–18 y (N = 31,695)	CATCH (N = 3,866)	CHALICE (N = 22,772)
Mechanism of injury	Severe mechanism of injury (MVC with patient ejection, death of another passenger, or rollover; pedestrian or bicyclist without helmet struck by motorized vehicle; falls >0.9 m; or head struck by high-impact object)	Severe mechanism of injury (MVC with patient ejection, death of another passenger, or rollover; pedestrian/ bicyclist without helmet struck by motorized vehicle; falls >1.5m; or head struck by high-impact object)	Dangerous mechanism of injury (eg, MVC; fall from elevation ≥3 ft (≥91 cm) or ≥5 stairs; or fall from bicycle with no helmet)	High-speed RTA as pedestrian, cyclist, or occupant (defined as accident with speed >40 miles per h or 64 km/h); fall >3 m in height; or high-speed injury from projectile or object
History	LOC for ≥5 s Not acting normally per parent report	Any LOC History of vomiting Severe headache	History of worsening headache	Witnessed loss of consciousness for >5 min ≥3 discrete episodes of vomiting after head injury Amnesia (antegrade or retrograde; >5 min) Suspicion of non-accidental injury (any suspicion by the examining doctor) Seizure in patient with no history of epilepsy

Examination			
GCS score <15 Other signs of altered mental status (agitation, somnolence, repetitive questioning, slow response to verbal communication) Palpable or unclear skull fracture Occipital, parietal, or temporal scalp hematoma	GCS score <15 Other signs of altered mental status (agitation, somnolence, repetitive questioning, slow response to verbal communication) Clinical signs of basilar skull fracture (eg, hemotympanum, "raccoon" eyes, otorrhea o rhinorrhea of CSF, Battle's sign	GCS score <15 at 2 h after injury[a] Irritability on examination[a] Any sign of basal skull fracture (eg, hemotympanum, "raccoon" eyes, otorrhea or rhinorrhea of CSF, Battle's sign) Suspected open or depressed skull fracture[a] Large, boggy scalp hematoma	GCS score <14, or <15 if aged <1 y Abnormal drowsiness (in excess of that expected by examining doctor) Positive focal neurology (motor, sensory, coordination, or reflex abnormality) Signs of basal skull fracture (hemotympanum, "raccoon" eyes, otorrhea or rhinorrhea of CSF, Battle's sign, facial crepitus, or severe facial injury) Suspicion of penetrating or depressed skull injury, or tense fontanelle Presence of bruise, swelling, or laceration >5cm if aged <1 y
Statistics[b]			
Sensitivity (95% CI) 100.0% (90.7–100.0)	99.0% (94.4–100.0)	88.7% (82.2–93.4)	92.3% (89.2–94.7)
Specificity (95%CI) 53.8% (52.3–55.4)	45.8% (44.9–46.8)	56.4% (55.0–57.8)	78.1% (77.5–78.7)
PPV (95% CI) 2.0% (1.4–2.8)	1.6% (1.3–1.9)	5.6% (4.7–6.7)	7.9% (7.2–8.7)
NPV (95% CI) 100.0% (99.8–100.0)	100.0% (99.9–100.0)	99.4% (99.1–99.7)	99.8% (99.7–99.9)

Abbreviations: CATCH, Canadian Assessment of Tomography for Childhood Injury; CHALICE, Children's Head Injury Algorithm for the Prediction of Important Clinical Events; CSF, cerebrospinal fluid; GCS, Glasgow Coma Scale; LOC, loss of consciousness; MVC, motor vehicle crash; NPV, Negative Predictive Value; PECARN, Pediatric Emergency Care Applied Research Network; PPV, Positive Predictive Value; RTA, road traffic accident.

[a] High-risk predictors for CATCH (need for neurological intervention).

[b] Data from Babl prospective validation study.[15]

in a "stepwise" fashion—initially as a 1-way rule out. Children who are not low risk can be risk stratified into higher or lower risk groups based on presence of certain high-risk variables or multiple lower risk variables. It is in this area—risk stratification—where PECARN has distinguished itself from the other 2 rules.

RISK STRATIFICATION OF INTERMEDIATE-RISK PATIENTS

Pediatric patients without any PECARN rule risk factors have a very low risk for ciTBI (<2 years of age, 0.02%; 2–18 years of age, <0.05%) and, therefore, imaging is generally not recommended. Those with certain high-risk factors, such as a GCS of less than 15 or other signs of altered mental status, signs of a palpable skull fracture, or signs of a basilar skull fracture are at higher risk of ciTBI (<2 years of age, 4.4%; 2–18 years of age, 4.3%) and imaging is appropriate for most of these patients. However, 30% of children experiencing minor blunt head injury will fall into the "intermediate-risk" group. Rates of ciTBI for this collective cohort of patients less than 2 years and 2 to 18 years of age are 0.9%. This rate may be sufficiently high for some clinicians or caregivers to warrant CT scanning, whereas others may feel that the potential risks of ionizing radiation,[19] cost of the testing, or possibility for discovery of incidental findings[20] outweigh the small risk of missing an injury. Fortunately, through a series of preplanned secondary analyses of the parent dataset, the PECARN group has offered further insight to the predictive nature of variables. Additionally, investigators also expanded the definition of an isolated variable to exclude other factors that have been associated with TBI, but were not part of the applicable PECARN rule. For each study, the variable in question is excluded from the following list to form the extensive definition: no history of loss of consciousness, acting normally per parent/guardian, pediatric GCS score of 15, no signs of altered consciousness, no palpable skull fracture, no scalp hematoma or other signs of traumatic scalp findings, no signs of basilar skull fracture, no neurologic deficits, no vomiting, no seizure, no headache, and no amnesia. Data from these studies[21–26] are summarized in **Fig. 1**A (<2 years of age) and **Fig. 1**B (2–18 years of age) in the form of a risk matrix that can be used to determine rates of ciTBI based on 1 or 2 PECARN risk factors. The intersection of row and column provide the risk estimate with 95% confidence intervals (CIs) for the variable(s) of concerns. These data "refine" the rule for intermediate-risk patients, allowing clinicians to further risk stratify patients within the intermediate-risk (0.9%) ciTBI group. Data on combination of intermediate-risk and high-risk (final 2 columns) variables are also included in **Fig. 1**. All of these cited studies reached a similar conclusion, namely, that ciTBI is very uncommon in patients with isolated PECARN intermediate-risk variables. Additionally, some patients with nonisolated findings are also at sufficiently low risk of ciTBI that neuroimaging may not be indicated.

VALUE OF OBSERVATION AND SHARED DECISION MAKING

Children with minor BHT present as individuals with unique risk factors as well as caregiver values and preferences. Although CDRs attempt to standardize an approach through population-based data, it also stands to reason that some degree of individualization of care is also reasonable and even optimal. This is most realized in the intermediate-risk patients where more than one rational option exists. For children presenting early in their clinical course, a period of observation can influence imaging rates.[27,28] Observation was more common in patients presenting sooner to the ED after their injury and in patients with an intermediate risk for ciTBI (60% were observed) and resulted in a significant decrease in imaging rate (5% in those observed vs 34% in

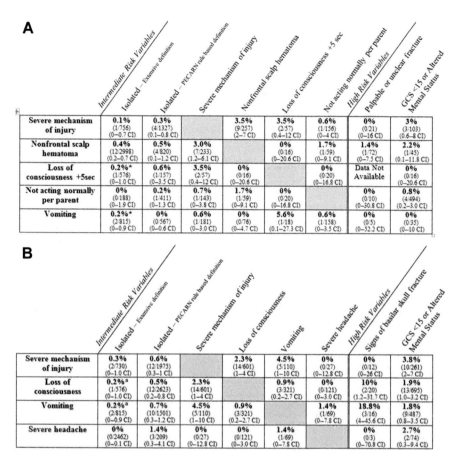

Fig. 1. Risk estimates of ciTBI in children <2 years (*A*) or 2–18 years (*B*) with minor blunt head trauma based on 1 or 2 PECARN variables. [a] Aggregate data for all patients less than 18 years of age. CI, confidence interval; GCS, Glasgow Coma Scale.

those not observed). With each hour of observation, there was an average decrease of 70% in CT scanning. The median ED observation time was 2.5 hours (interquartile range, 1.8–3.3). Although an optimal duration of ED observation after minor BHT remains to be determined, a large retrospective study of children less than 14 years of age with minor head trauma demonstrated that only 5% of children were diagnosed with intracranial hemorrhage (ICH) more than 6 hours after time of injury.[29] Therefore, the necessary ED observation length is likely no more than 6 hours from the time of injury and it is reasonable to consider active observation at home with appropriate caregiver instruction.

Determining observation versus emergent neuroimaging ideally occurs jointly between caregiver and provider through a process of shared decision making. Decision aids are designed to aid in shared decision making when more than one reasonable option exists. Patients are provided with the latest scientific evidence regarding the condition of concern in an accessible format, and clinicians learn about patient values and preferences. Equipped with this knowledge, they work together to determine the course of action. Decision aids have been shown to increase patient knowledge and

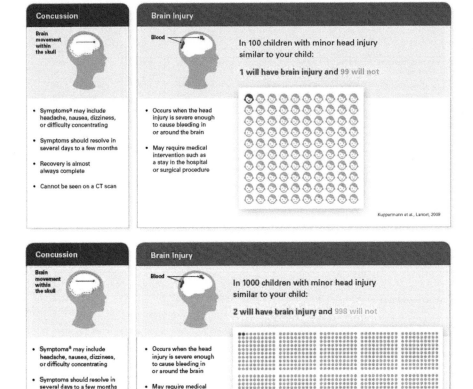

Fig. 2. Head CT Choice clinical decision aids for children with minor blunt head trauma. Decision aids are utilized for knowledge transfer and patient/caregiver preference identification in the process of shared decision making. Examples provided are for ciTBI risk estimates of 1 in 100 and 2 in 1000. [a] This information may not apply to young children who are not yet able to walk or talk. [b] Some symptoms may not apply to young children who are not yet able to walk or talk. CT, computed tomography. (*From* Hess EP, Wyatt KD, Kharbanda AB, et al. Effectiveness of the head CT choice decision aid in parents of children with minor head trauma: study protocol for a multicenter randomized trial. Supplementary Material. Trials 2014;15:253; with permission.)

engagement in decision making, and to improve the accuracy of risk perception.[30] **Fig. 2** provides examples of decision aids (Head CT Choice) developed at the Mayo Clinic (Rochester, MN)[5] and prospectively studied in a multicenter trial (Clinical Trials.gov NCT02063087). In clinical practice, patient/caregiver dyads are provided with a decision aid tailored to the child's specific risk estimates for ciTBI and it is used in the discussion of imaging versus observation. Additional head CT scanning choice

After monitoring your child in the emergency department for a period of time, we will find out if there is any serious bleeding in or around the brain with:

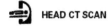 **HEAD CT SCAN**　　or　　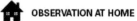 **OBSERVATION AT HOME**

You can have a head CT scan test done to determine if your child has had a brain injury.

If your child's symptoms are the same or better in the next 1–2 d, then there was no serious bleeding in or around the brain.

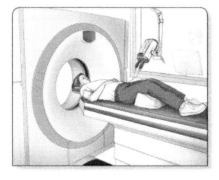

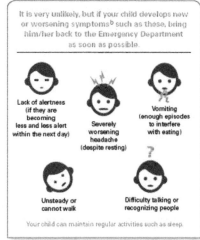

It is very unlikely, but if your child develops new or worsening symptoms[b] such as these, bring him/her back to the Emergency Department as soon as possible.

Lack of alertness (if they are becoming less and less alert within the next day)

Severely worsening headache (despite resting)

Vomiting (enough episodes to interfere with eating)

Unsteady or cannot walk

Difficulty talking or recognizing people

Your child can maintain regular activities such as sleep.

Please circle the issues that are most important to you and your child.

	SPEED OF DIAGNOSIS	RADIATION	SEDATION	COST	POTENTIAL DOWNSIDES	WAIT IN ED
HEAD CT SCAN	Now	Yes	Possible	May increase cost depending on your coverage	May find irrelevant things that lead to more tests	Typically longer
OBSERVATION AT HOME	Delayed	No	No	No added cost	Potential return to ED if symptoms worsen	Typically shorter

After discussing this together, we want to do:

☐ HEAD CT SCAN　　☐ OBSERVATION AT HOME

☐ Let the Emergency Department doctor decide what to do next

You will have the opportunity to revisit this decision with your doctor while you are in the Emergency Department.

Fig. 2. (continued)

decision aids can be accessed for free at http://shareddecisions.mayoclinic.org/decision-aid-information/head-ct-choice-decision-aid/. It is important to note that decision aids were not generated for very low-risk children, because imaging is not indicated. **Fig. 3** shows an example a protocol for minor head trauma that integrates risk stratification and shared decision making in the determination of the need for neuroimaging.

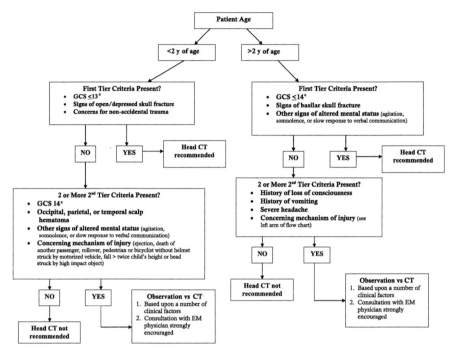

Fig. 3. Example protocol for evaluation of minor blunt head trauma integrating risk stratification and shared decision making in determination of need for neuroimaging. [a] See pediatric Glasgow Coma Scale table. CT, computed tomography; ED, emergency department.

APPLICATION OF THE PEDIATRIC EMERGENCY CARE APPLIED RESEARCH NETWORK RULE TO SELECT PATIENT POPULATIONS
Abusive Head Trauma

Application of the PECARN rule to children where abusive head trauma (AHT) is a strong consideration is not appropriate. The rule was derived based on the assumption that clinical information obtained at the time of the initial ED encounter is accurate. In the case of AHT, the details of the event are likely to be obfuscated, omitted, or simply unknown at the initial time of evaluation. Also, the primary outcome of importance in the PECARN rule, ciTBI, is not necessarily the issue of greatest importance in evaluation of AHT. Although a minor TBI on a CT scan in an accidental setting may not be deemed clinically important, in an AHT evaluation, all findings are clinically relevant, including isolated skull fractures that PECARN did not classify as a TBI on a CT scan.[31] In addition, the decision rule's primary objective is to try and decrease the unnecessary use of CT scanning in low-risk patients. Infants and young children who are victims of abuse are, by definition, at high risk of morbidity and mortality, even in the absence of any neurologic or physical examination findings. In these cases, injury identification outweighs any potential risks of radiation exposure from neuroimaging. In fact, the American Academy of Pediatrics[32] and the American College of Radiology[33] both recommend a head CT scan for all infants and children younger than 2 years with a history or physical examination findings suggestive of or suspicious for abuse. An alternative CDR (Pittsburgh Infant Brain Injury Score) has been derived and validated to guide clinicians evaluating infants with nonspecific signs or symptoms that may be the result of AHT or other intracranial abnormality.[34]

Sports-Related Traumatic Brain Injury

More than 44 million US children ages 5 to 18 participate in organized sports each year.[35] Patients with sports-related TBIs are presenting to EDs in increasing numbers. Analysis of data from a national registry showed an increase of these presentations of 62% between 2001 and 2009.[36] An additional single-center, level I trauma center retrospective review demonstrated a 92% increase over a similar timeframe (2002–2011).[3]

Are sports-related TBIs somehow different than non–sports-related TBI's and should clinicians approach these patients differently? First, it is important for clinicians, patients, and care providers to clearly distinguish concussive TBI from other forms of structural TBI. Concussion diagnoses are made clinically because standard neuroimaging studies can be completely normal in symptomatic patients with concussions. CDRs such as the PECARN TBI rule are not intended to rule in or rule out concussions. For sports participants presenting with BHT, PECARN can be used to evaluate for other forms of TBI. A subset analysis of the PECARN data report on more than 23,000 children ages 5 to 18.[37] In this cohort, sports-related BHT accounted for 14% of TBI with 98% of these patients presenting with GCS scores of more than 14 and more than 90% with GCS scores of 15. Compared with the non–sports-related cohort, these patients undergo neuroimaging at higher rates (53% vs 41%), yet have lower rates of TBI on CT examination (4% vs 7%) and no difference in the rates of ciTBI. Providers cited mechanisms of injury, presence of headache, or history of loss of consciousness as primary drivers for imaging. Parental or referring provider preference was noted as a factor in 20% of cases undergoing imaging. Participation in equestrian, snow, and wheeled sports (ie, skateboard, roller blading, scooters) caries the highest risk of TBI on CT scanning. These authors concluded that children with sports-related TBI should be evaluated with evidence based prediction rules to decrease unnecessary CT scans.

Bleeding Disorders

Patients with either congenital or acquired bleeding disorders are at higher risk of TBI after minor BHT. PECARN investigators analyzed the prediction rules in prospectively enrolled children with bleeding disorders or on anticoagulants.[38] Fifty-six of the 230 children had hemophilia with 60% of them characterized as severe (factor level of <1%). Other forms of bleeding disorders represented in the cohort included von Willebrand disease (19.6%), thrombocytopenia (14.8%), anticoagulation therapy (6.5%), functional platelet disorder (2.6%), and other (0.4%). Eighty-one percent underwent CT scanning with only 2 cases of ICH (1.1%), both of whom did not meet PECARN low-risk criteria and were symptomatic; neither required neurosurgical intervention. Patients with congenital or acquired bleeding disorders may be at increased risk for delayed presentation of bleeding. Enrollment of children in the study was restricted to those with injuries occurring within 24 hours of presentation and, thus, data on delayed presentation are limited. None of the prospectively enrolled patients, however, returned with delayed ICH. The authors concluded that, "although patients with congenital or acquired bleeding disorders are at risk for ICH, the low rate of ICH suggests that they may not routinely require cranial CT imaging after minor BHT in the absence of signs or symptoms of ICH."[38] For children discharged without imaging, clinicians should clearly counsel caregivers on signs or symptoms that should trigger repeat evaluation.

Posttraumatic Seizures

Posttraumatic seizures occur in 0.6% to 4.0% of all children with head trauma with the largest prospective series reporting a rate of 1.3% (95% CI, 1.2%–1.4%).[16,18,39] Rates of TBI on CT scans are increased in the presence of posttraumatic seizures (15.5%;95% CI, 12.3–19.1) and correlate with decreasing GCS (GCS of 15, 6.0% [n = 332]; GCS of 14, 18.9% [n = 37]; GCS of 3–13, 46.4% [n = 97]; PECARN data center), increasing seizure duration, and increased interval time from trauma to seizure onset. Seizure recurrence risk overall is 3.7%, but only 0.3% in children with a GCS of 15. For all children with posttraumatic seizures, strong consideration should be given to neuroimaging owing to their high rates of TBI on CT scanning. Negative CT scans in these can facilitate the discharge of neurologically normal children from the ED because the recurrence risk for seizure is low and none required neurosurgical intervention.[39]

PATIENT DISPOSITION AFTER NORMAL CRANIAL COMPUTED TOMOGRAPHY SCAN, ISOLATED LINEAR SKULL FRACTURES, ISOLATED CEREBRAL CONTUSIONS, OR ISOLATED PNEUMOCEPHALUS

After the decision to image a patient is made, the clinician is faced with what to do with the information obtained. More than 90% of children with minor BHT who undergo imaging will have a normal CT scan.[17] Outcomes for children imaged in the PECARN parent study were studied and reported.[40] For children with a GCS score of 15 and normal CT scans, 83% (n = 10,477) were discharged and 17% (n = 2107) were hospitalized. For children with a GCS score of 14 and normal CT scans, 61% (n = 581) were discharged and 39% (n = 378) were admitted. Repeat imaging occurred in 2% of discharged children with 0.04% (GCS of 15) and 0.20% (GCS of 14) rates of new findings. No discharged children with a normal initial CT scan required neurosurgical intervention. Hospitalized children were 3 times as likely to undergo repeat imaging (6%) with 0.5% (GCS of 15) and 1.0% (GCS of 14) rates of new findings. No admitted children with a normal initial CT scan required neurosurgical intervention. The NPV of a normal CT scan for neurosurgical intervention for children with a GCS score of 15 was 100% (95% CI, 99.97%-100.00%) and for a GCS score of 14 was 100% (95% CI, 99.6%-100.0%). These data show that the natural history for children with a GCS score 14 or 15 and initial CT scan does not include neurologic deterioration or neurosurgical intervention.

Isolated nondepressed skull fractures are commonly encountered in patients imaged for BHT. Retrospective reviews suggest that neurologically normal patients with isolated skull fractures do not require transfer or admission to the hospital.[41–44] PECARN investigators add data supporting these findings,[31] reporting on 350 prospectively enrolled children with isolated linear skull fractures. Twenty-one percent of admitted children underwent repeat imaging with 5 (2.5%) showing new traumatic findings. None of these children required neurosurgical intervention. Of the 149 discharged patients, 13.4% underwent repeat imaging with no new traumatic findings. These data suggest that neurologically normal patients with isolated linear skull fractures not associated with AHT do not require inpatient observation.

Isolated cerebral contusions also pose a disposition conundrum as to whether observed in an intensive care unit setting for neurologic deterioration is warranted. Prospective outcome data from PECARN provides guidance for these children[45] noting that children with a GCS of 14 or 15 and isolated cerebral contusions on CT scan (54 total patients) had no adverse outcomes. Isolated cerebral contusions tended to be small and occur in children with normal mental status. The authors concluded that "in patients with a GCS of 14 or 15 after minor BHT and small isolated cerebral contusions . . . neither [intensive care unit] admission or prolonged hospitalization is generally required." In a related PECARN subanalysis of children with BHT and isolated pneumocephali, with or without a linear skull fracture or basilar skull fractures, CT scans demonstrated pneumocephali in 1% of cases.[46] Of these cases, 37% will have isolated pneumocephali, 78% with associated basilar skull fractures and 15% with associated linear skull fracture. Eighty-three percent of these children were hospitalized with no reported adverse outcomes. The authors conclude that, "The management of these children seems most appropriately aimed at other injuries sustained."

SUMMARY

ED and primary care provider visits for pediatric minor BHT continue to increase. Considerable variability exists in clinician evaluation and management of this generally low- risk population. CDRs should be used to assist providers in identification of very low-risk individuals, eliminating the need for cranial CT scans. The use of periods of observation before imaging can also decrease scanning rates. Outcome data from past retrospective studies as well as prospective data accumulated during the derivation and validation of the PECARN head injury decision rules for children less than 2 years and 2 to 18 years of age can be used to further risk stratify children with minor BHT who are at intermediate or high risk for ciTBI into more discrete categories. Incorporation of decision aids into practice can be useful for increasing caregiver knowledge and accuracy of risk perception and improve provider identification of patient or caregiver preferences. This can help to facilitate shared decision making regarding imaging or observation. For children in whom imaging is performed and is normal or shows only isolated linear skull fractures, the rates of deterioration and neurosurgical intervention are rare and, therefore, hospital admission can likely be avoided.

REFERENCES

1. Quayle KS, Powell EC, Mahajan P, et al. Epidemiology of blunt head trauma in children in U.S. emergency departments. N Engl J Med 2014;371(20):1945–7.
2. Centers for Disease Control and Prevention. TBI data and statistics. Available at: http://www.cdc.gov/traumaticbraininjury/data/index.html. Accessed January 07, 2017.
3. Hanson HR, Pomerantz WJ, Gittelman M. ED utilization trends in sports-related traumatic brain injury. Pediatrics 2013;132(4):e859–64.
4. Fishman M, Taranto E, Perlman M, et al. Attitudes and counseling practices of pediatricians regarding youth sports participation and concussion risks. J Pediatr 2017;184:19–25.
5. Hess EP, Wyatt KD, Kharbanda AB, et al. Effectiveness of the head CT choice decision aid in parents of children with minor head trauma: study protocol for a multicenter randomized trial. Trials 2014;15:253.
6. Wong AC, Kowalenko T, Roahen-Harrison S, et al. A survey of emergency physicians' fear of malpractice and its association with the decision to order computed tomography scans for children with minor head trauma. Pediatr Emerg Care 2011;27(3):182–5.
7. Rohacek M, Albrecht M, Kleim B, et al. Reasons for ordering computed tomography scans of the head in patients with minor brain injury. Injury 2012;43(9):1415–8.

8. Klassen TP, Reed MH, Stiell IG, et al. Variation in utilization of computed tomography scanning for the investigation of minor head trauma in children: a Canadian experience. Acad Emerg Med 2000;7(7):739–44.

9. Larson DB, Johnson LW, Schnell BM, et al. Rising use of CT in child visits to the emergency department in the United States, 1995-2008. Radiology 2011;259(3):793–801.

10. Stanley RM, Hoyle JD, Dayan PS, et al. Emergency department practice variation in computed tomography use for children with minor blunt head trauma. J Pediatr 2014;165(6):1201–6.e2.

11. Green SM. When do clinical decision rules improve patient care? Ann Emerg Med 2013;62(2):132–5.

12. Easter JS, Bakes K, Dhaliwal J, et al. Comparison of PECARN, CATCH, and CHALICE rules for children with minor head injury: a prospective cohort study. Ann Emerg Med 2014;64(2):145–52, 152.e1-5.

13. Lorton F, Poullaouec C, Legallais E, et al. Validation of the PECARN clinical decision rule for children with minor head trauma: a French multicenter prospective study. Scand J Trauma Resusc Emerg Med 2016;24:98.

14. Ide K, Uematsu S, Tetsuhara K, et al. External validation of the PECARN head trauma prediction rules in Japan. Acad Emerg Med 2017;24(3):308–14.

15. Babl FE, Borland ML, Phillips N, et al. Accuracy of PECARN, CATCH, and CHALICE head injury decision rules in children: a prospective cohort study. Lancet 2017;389(10087):2393–402.

16. Dunning J, Daly JP, Lomas JP, et al. Derivation of the children's head injury algorithm for the prediction of important clinical events decision rule for head injury in children. Arch Dis Child 2006;91(11):885–91.

17. Kuppermann N, Holmes JF, Dayan PS, et al. Identification of children at very low risk of clinically-important brain injuries after head trauma: a prospective cohort study. Lancet 2009;374(9696):1160–70.

18. Osmond MH, Klassen TP, Wells GA, et al. CATCH: a clinical decision rule for the use of computed tomography in children with minor head injury. CMAJ 2010;182(4):341–8.

19. Miglioretti DL, Johnson E, Williams A, et al. The use of computed tomography in pediatrics and the associated radiation exposure and estimated cancer risk. JAMA Pediatr 2013;167(8):700–7.

20. Rogers AJ, Maher CO, Schunk JE, et al, Pediatric Emergency Care Applied Research Network. Incidental findings in children with blunt head trauma evaluated with cranial CT scans. Pediatrics 2013;132(2):e356–63.

21. Nigrovic LE, Lee LK, Hoyle J, et al. Prevalence of clinically important traumatic brain injuries in children with minor blunt head trauma and isolated severe injury mechanisms. Arch Pediatr Adolesc Med 2012;166(4):356–61.

22. Dayan PS, Holmes JF, Atabaki S, et al, Traumatic Brain Injury Study Group of the Pediatric Emergency Care Applied Research Network (PECARN). Association of traumatic brain injuries with vomiting in children with blunt head trauma. Ann Emerg Med 2014;63(6):657–65.

23. Dayan PS, Holmes JF, Schutzman S, et al. Risk of traumatic brain injuries in children younger than 24 months with isolated scalp hematomas. Ann Emerg Med 2014;64(2):153–62.

24. Lee LK, Monroe D, Bachman MC, et al. Isolated loss of consciousness in children with minor blunt head trauma. JAMA Pediatr 2014;168(9):837–43.

25. Dayan PS, Holmes JF, Hoyle J Jr, et al. Headache in traumatic brain injuries from blunt head trauma. Pediatrics 2015;135(3):504–12.

26. Nishijima DK, Holmes JF, Dayan PS, et al. Association of a guardian's report of a child acting abnormally with traumatic brain injury after minor blunt head trauma. JAMA Pediatr 2015;169(12):1141–7.
27. Nigrovic LE, Schunk JE, Foerster A, et al. The effect of observation on cranial computed tomography utilization for children after blunt head trauma. Pediatrics 2011;127(6):1067–73.
28. Schonfeld D, Fitz BM, Nigrovic LE. Effect of the duration of emergency department observation on computed tomography use in children with minor blunt head trauma. Ann Emerg Med 2013;62(6):597–603.
29. Hamilton M, Mrazik M, Johnson DW. Incidence of delayed intracranial hemorrhage in children after uncomplicated minor head injuries. Pediatrics 2010;126(1):e33–9.
30. Stacey D, Légaré F, Lewis K, et al. Decision aids for people facing health treatment or screening decisions. Cochrane Database Syst Rev 2017;(4):CD001431.
31. Powell EC, Atabaki SM, Wootton-Gorges S, et al. Isolated linear skull fractures in children with blunt head trauma. Pediatrics 2015;135(4):e851–7.
32. Christian CW. The evaluation of suspected child physical abuse. Pediatrics 2015;135(5):e1337–54.
33. Wootton-Gorges SL, Soares BP, Alazraki AL, et al, Expert Panel on Pediatric Imaging. ACR appropriateness criteria(R) suspected physical abuse-child. J Am Coll Radiol 2017;14(5s):S338–s349.
34. Berger RP, Fromkin J, Herman B, et al. Validation of the Pittsburgh infant brain injury score for abusive head trauma. Pediatrics 2016;138(1) [pii:e20153756].
35. Daneshvar DH, Nowinski CJ, McKee AC, et al. The epidemiology of sport-related concussion. Clin Sports Med 2011;30(1):1–17, vii.
36. Centers for Disease Control and Prevention. Nonfatal traumatic brain injuries related to sports and recreation activities among persons aged ≤19 years– United States, 2001-2009. MMWR Morb Mortal Wkly Rep 2011;60(39):1337–42.
37. Glass T, Ruddy RM, Alpern ER, et al, Pediatric Emergency Care Applied Research Network (PECARN). Traumatic brain injuries and computed tomography use in pediatric sports participants. Am J Emerg Med 2015;33(10):1458–64.
38. Lee LK, Dayan PS, Gerardi MJ, et al, Traumatic Brain Injury Study Group for the Pediatric Emergency Care Applied Research Network (PECARN). Intracranial hemorrhage after blunt head trauma in children with bleeding disorders. J Pediatr 2011;158(6):1003–8.e1-2.
39. Badawy MK, Dayan PS, Tunik MG, et al, Pediatric Emergency Care Applied Research Network (PECARN). Prevalence of brain injuries and recurrence of seizures in children with posttraumatic seizures. Acad Emerg Med 2017;24(5):595–605.
40. Holmes JF, Borgialli DA, Nadel FM, et al, TBI Study Group for the Pediatric Emergency Care Applied Research Network. Do children with blunt head trauma and normal cranial computed tomography scan results require hospitalization for neurologic observation? Ann Emerg Med 2011;58(4):315–22.
41. White IK, Pestereva E, Shaikh KA, et al. Transfer of children with isolated linear skull fractures: is it worth the cost? J Neurosurg Pediatr 2016;17(5):602–6.
42. Greenes DS, Schutzman SA. Infants with isolated skull fracture: what are their clinical characteristics, and do they require hospitalization? Ann Emerg Med 1997;30(3):253–9.
43. Rollins MD, Barnhart DC, Greenberg RA, et al. Neurologically intact children with an isolated skull fracture may be safely discharged after brief observation. J Pediatr Surg 2011;46(7):1342–6.

44. Arrey EN, Kerr ML, Fletcher S, et al. Linear nondisplaced skull fractures in children: who should be observed or admitted? J Neurosurg Pediatr 2015;16(6): 703–8.
45. Varano P, Cabrera KI, Kuppermann N, et al. Acute outcomes of isolated cerebral contusions in children with Glasgow Coma Scale scores of 14 to 15 after blunt head trauma. J Trauma Acute Care Surg 2015;78(5):1039–43.
46. Blanchard A, Cabrera KI, Kuppermann N, et al. Acute outcomes of isolated pneumocephali in children after minor blunt head trauma. Pediatr Emerg Care 2016. [Epub ahead of print].

Pediatric Syncope
High-Risk Conditions and Reasonable Approach

Paul C. Schunk, MD*, Tim Ruttan, MD

KEYWORDS

- Syncope • Pediatric • Brugada syndrome • Long QT • Short QT
- Arrhythmogenic right ventricular cardiomyopathy • Seizures • Breath holding spells

KEY POINTS

- Syncope is a common presenting complaint and although most cases are of a benign cause careful attention must be made not to miss the dangerous and life-threatening causes.

INTRODUCTION

Syncope, classically defined as a transient, self-limited loss of consciousness and postural tone, is a common presenting complaint in the pediatric emergency department (ED). By definition, the recovery from syncope is spontaneous, rapid, prompt, and complete without any neurologic sequelae.[1] Syncope accounts for approximately 126 in 100,000 children coming to medical attention.[1] The approach to syncope and the etiologies differ from the adult population because most pediatric syncope is from non-life-threatening causes, and a minimal evaluation in the ED is appropriate with parental reassurance. Despite this generally benign prognosis, care must be made to find the more uncommon and potentially fatal causes. The primary purpose of the evaluation of the patient with syncope is to determine whether the patient is at increased risk for death and needs either admission to the hospital or an expedited outpatient evaluation.[2]

HISTORY, EXAMINATION, AND TESTING
History

Syncope is a chief complaint where a detailed history is the most important aspect of a safe and efficient evaluation in the pediatric patient.[3] That history might suggest a benign cause, such as a child with a prodrome of lightheadedness after being outside

Disclosure Statement: The author has nothing to disclose.
Department of Pediatric Emergency Medicine, Dell Children's Medical Center, 4900 Mueller Boulevard, Austin, TX 78723, USA
* Corresponding author.
E-mail address: Paul.Schunk@gmail.com

on a hot day, whereas a child with exertional syncope while running is in a higher risk category. Other elements, such as a family history with sudden unexplained death at a young age or congenital deafness, are red flags that may warrant further investigation. Events leading up to the syncopal episode should be carefully noted, and the description of the event itself. The absence of prodromal symptoms, presence of preceding palpitations within seconds of loss of consciousness, lack of a prolonged upright posture, syncope during exercise or in response to auditory or emotional triggers, family history of sudden cardiac death (SCD), abnormal physical examination, and abnormal electrocardiogram (ECG) all should raise concern for a cardiac cause.[4,5] Additionally, standard aspects of the history, such as medication use, can provide clues for QT-prolonging medications, among other potential contributing factors.

The accounts of bystanders are helpful but also potentially misleading. The occurrence of tonic-clonic, seizure-like activity is associated with cardiac and neurologic causes of syncope, and distinguishing between the two etiologies may not be possible. One study found that limb jerking had a sensitivity of 0.686, specificity of 0.877, and a positive likelihood ratio of 5.566 for seizures, making it a moderately helpful but not diagnostic historical feature.[4]

Physical Examination

Certain components of the physical examination are particularly useful in directing the evaluation. Vital signs are a useful clue, although the use of orthostatic vital signs may not be as helpful as often believed. It is estimated that greater than 40% of euvolemic adolescents have positive orthostatic vital signs.[6] In a study of euvolemic adult ED patients it was estimated that 43% met criteria for positive orthostatic vital signs.[7] The presence or absence of positive orthostatic vital signs should not be the sole driver of diagnostic and disposition decisions.

Although challenging in the often noisy and chaotic ED setting, when possible a careful evaluation of the heart for any murmurs, radiation, and change with position of those murmurs should be noted. Specific murmurs are covered in the relevant discussion in this article, but in general any potentially pathologic murmur in the setting of syncope warrants further evaluation by a cardiologist.

A detailed neurologic examination is also paramount to the evaluation of the syncope patient. The presence of focal neurologic symptoms, weakness, ataxia, altered mental status, or slurred speech directs the evaluation toward a more dangerous cause.

Electrocardiogram

Although some studies show only 0.4% of ECGs had a diagnostic yield and there is a high false-positive rate, the low cost and low associated risk makes obtaining an ECG a part of the evaluation of pediatric syncope.[5,8–10] Even the authors of studies critical of the diagnostic yield of ECGs still recommend its use integrated with history and physical examination because of the high sensitivity of all three of these elements combined together.[9] The 2017 American College of Cardiology/American Heart Association guidelines recommended that a detailed medical history, physical examination, family history, and 12-lead ECG should be performed in all pediatric patients presenting with syncope as a Class I recommendation.[5]

SCD is a rare but devastating event. The incidence of SCD during sporting events is infrequent with an incidence of 1 to 2 in 200,000.[11] Despite its rarity, extensive public attention to deaths in otherwise healthy children and the association with exercise has led to a desire to perform some type of risk assessment and screening to decrease the risk of this catastrophic event. In February 2012 the American Medical Society for Sports Medicine held a summit on ECG interpretation in athletes. They developed the Seattle Criteria,[12] and although this was developed as an outpatient preparticipation screening tool rather than one for ED evaluation, an understanding of this tool can highlight potentially concerning ECG findings that warrant further subspecialist evaluation. **Table 1** provides high-risk abnormal ECG findings in athletes.

Table 1
High-risk abnormal ECG findings in athletes

Abnormal ECG Finding	Definition
T-wave inversion	>1 mm in depth in two or more leads V2–V6, II and aVF, or I and aVL (excludes III, aVR, and V1)
ST-segment depression	≥0.5 mm in depth in two or more leads
Pathologic Q waves	>3 mm in depth or >40 ms in duration in two or more leads (except for III and aVR)
Complete left bundle branch block	QRS ≥120 ms, predominantly negative QRS complex in lead V1 (QS or rS), and upright monophasic R wave in leads I and V6
Intraventricular conduction delay	Any QRS duration ≥140 ms
Left axis deviation	−30° to −90°
Left atrial enlargement	Prolonged P wave duration of >120 ms in leads I or II with negative portion of the P wave ≥1 mm in depth and ≥40 ms in duration in lead V1
Right ventricular hypertrophy pattern	R–V1 + S–V5 >10.5 mm AND right axis deviation >120°
Ventricular pre-excitation	PR interval <120 ms with a delta wave (slurred upstroke in the QRS complex) and wide QRS (>120 ms)
Long QT interval[a]	QTc ≥470 ms (male) QTc ≥480 ms (female) QTc ≥500 ms (marked QT prolongation)
Short QT interval[a]	QTc ≤320 ms
Brugada-like ECG pattern	High take-off and downsloping ST-segment elevation followed by a negative T wave in ≥2 leads in V1–V3
Profound sinus bradycardia	<30 bpm or sinus pauses ≥3 s
Atrial tachyarrhythmias	Supraventricular tachycardia, atrial-fibrillation, atrial flutter
Premature ventricular contractions	≥2 per 10-s tracing
Ventricular arrhythmias	Couplets, triplets, and nonsustained ventricular tachycardia

Note: These ECG findings are unrelated to regular training or expected physiologic adaptation to exercise, may suggest the presence of pathologic cardiovascular disease, and require further diagnostic evaluation.

Abbreviation: bpm, beats per minute.

[a] The QT interval corrected for heart rate is ideally measured with heart rates of 60 to 90 bpm. Consider repeating the ECG after mild aerobic activity for borderline or abnormal QTc values with a heart rate less than 50 bpm.

From Drezner JA, Ackerman MJ, Anderson J, et al. Electrocardiographic interpretation in athletes: the 'Seattle criteria'. Br J Sports Med 2013;47(3):123; with permission.

DIFFERENTIAL DIAGNOSIS OF PEDIATRIC SYNCOPE
Other Diagnostic Tests

Reflex laboratory testing is not recommended for evaluation of the syncope patient.[5] Laboratory evaluation should be driven by the history and physical examination and any underlying medical conditions or potential medication complications. Blood glucose, although commonly ordered on many syncope patients, has limited data despite being a part of routine practice of many clinicians. Pregnancy testing of female patients in the reproductive age range is commonly recommended.[5] Other diagnostic testing including echocardiogram, MRI, computed tomography, or electroencephalogram is also not recommended unless compelling clinical evidence is present.[13]

POTENTIALLY LIFE-THREATENING CAUSES OF SYNCOPE

The bulk of the life-threatening causes of syncope are cardiac, and these are explored in more detail below. **Box 1** lists common differential diagnosis in neurocardiogenic syncope. In general, several features should serve as red flags and merit consultation and further evaluation. Any ECG abnormalities, concerning murmur, or a patient with a concerning history (eg, any syncope during exercise, chest pain with syncope, or a concerning family history) all should raise concern for a potential life-threatening cardiac cause and admission or expedited outpatient evaluation should be strongly considered.

CARDIAC: ELECTRICAL PROBLEMS
Brugada Syndrome

Brugada is autosomal-dominant disorder of the cardiac sodium channels that is characterized by syncope, sudden death, and electrocardiographic findings of ST-segment elevation that seems similar to a right bundle branch block in leads V1 to V3.[14,15] Brugada is currently broken down into three subtypes based on the ECG manifestations (**Figs. 1** and **2**).

Type 1: Cove-shaped ST elevation in right precordial leads with J wave or ST elevation of 2 mm (mV) at its peak followed by a negative T wave with little or no isoelectric interval in more than one right precordial leads V1 to V3.
Type 2: The ST segments also have a high take-off but the J amplitude of 2 mV gives rise to a gradually descending ST elevation remaining 1 mV above the baseline

---

Box 1
Common differential diagnosis in neurocardiogenic syncope

Arrhythmias

Channelopathies

Complete heart block

Sick sinus syndrome

Tachyarrhythmias: supraventricular tachycardia, ventricular tachycardia

Wolff-Parkinson-White syndrome

Cardiac: structural

Cardiomyopathy: hypertrophic/dilated

Coronary artery anomalies

Tumor

Left ventricular outflow obstruction

Primary pulmonary arterial hypertension

Eisenmenger syndrome

Mitral valve prolapse

Arrhythmogenic right ventricular dysplasia

Medications

Recreational (illegal)

Antiarrhythmic

Diuretics

Vasodilators

Producing QT prolongation

Neurologic

Seizure

Vertigo

Migraine

Tumor

Psychiatric

Conversion reaction

Panic attack

Hysteria

Hyperventilation

Metabolic

Hypoxia

Hypoglycemia

From Strieper MJ. Distinguishing benign syncope from life-threatening cardiac causes of syncope. Semin Pediatr Neurol 2005;12(1):32–8.

followed by a positive or biphasic T wave that results in a saddle-back configuration.

Type 3: Right precordial ST elevation of less than 1 mm of saddle-back type or coved type.[16]

Syncope or SCD may be the first presentation.[17] Although originally thought to cause mortality in patients in their 30 to 40s[14] reports of children with SCD caused by Brugada have been increasingly noted.[14,15,18–20] Many patients with Brugada syndrome may have a normal ECG and only with drug challenge manifest the classical ECG changes.[21] Syncope and potentially death can result from a variety of factors. One of the most important in the pediatric population is fever.[21] Hyperpyrexia is associated with precipitating cardiac events,[13] and fever control is typically a part of management in patients with known Brugada syndrome.[16,22] It is important to ask about family history of SCD because this may help identify high-risk individuals.[17] Compounding the diagnostic challenge is that patients can have a Brugada pattern on ECG even without symptoms, and patients with Brugada syndrome can also have an ECG that varies over time, which can lead to false-negative screening ECGs even in patients with true Brugada disease.[23] In general, however, any concerning history or ECG findings should be referred to a pediatric cardiologist for complete evaluation and management, potentially including an implantable cardiac defibrillator.[14]

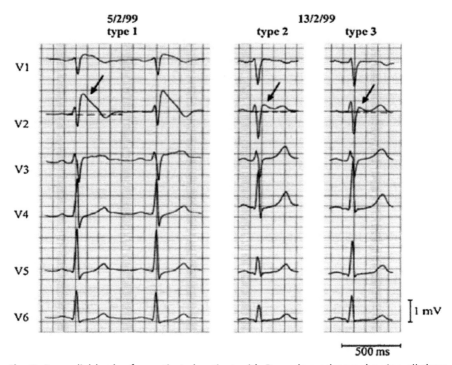

Fig. 1. Precordial leads of a rusticated patient with Brugada syndrome showing all three ECG patterns and dynamic change over an 8-day period. *Arrows* indicate J waves. (*From* Wilde AA, Antzelevitch C, Borggrefe M, et al. Proposed diagnostic criteria for the Brugada syndrome: consensus report. Circulation 2002;106:2515; with permission.)

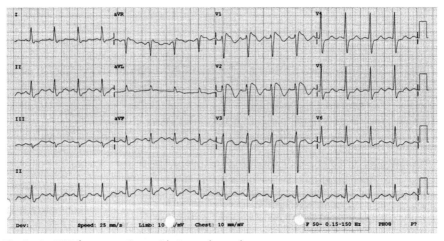

Fig. 2. An ECG from a patient with Brugada syndrome.

Long QT Syndrome

Long QT syndrome (LQTS) is a disease of prolonged ventricular repolarization that can lead to life-threatening events, such as SCD.[24] It is congenital or acquired. The prevalence of congenital LQTS in developed nations is estimated at about 1:5000 to

1:7000, but the condition is frequently overlooked and the true prevalence is likely higher than these estimates.[14] Events typically occur from in utero (rare) until the 40s and uncommonly in older age, with an increased frequency in females.[14]

Current guidelines for congenital LQTS diagnosis in children have values for symptomatic patients with a cardiac arrest or syncope and a QTc greater than 460 ms is required for diagnosis. In asymptomatic individuals a QTc greater than 480 ms is required.[24] Any value greater than 460 ms is potentially abnormal, although even a normal QTC does not completely exclude the diagnosis.[14,24,25] **Fig. 3** is a good example of an ECG with significant LQTS. The syncope of LQTS is sudden and without warning in most cases[14]; a history of palpitations or presyncope is more likely to indicate some other disorder rather than LQTS.[14] Family history can also be helpful because LQTS most frequently has autosomal-dominant transmission and males and females are equally affected genetically, although females seem to have more frequent symptoms than males.[14] Certain historical features, such as deafness, are associated with certain subtypes of LQTS syndrome, and such triggers as swimming or startle events also have associations with different congenital subtypes.[24] Initial treatment is most commonly β-blocker; however, increasingly more patients are having implantable cardiac defibrillators placed.[24]

Acquired LQTS is typically related to medication use, and a variety of factors can precipitate an event. This can either be from a patient with existing congenital LQTS who is given a QT_C-prolonging medication, or, more typically in the ED setting, a patient who is on multiple medications with QTC-prolonging effects. The most commonly recognized implicated medications are psychiatric, although a large number of medications can impact the QT interval.[26] One resource that maintains an updated list of QT_C-prolonging medications is https://crediblemeds.org/healthcare-providers/.

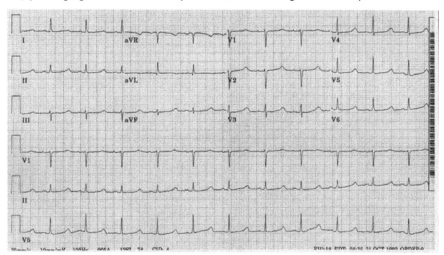

Fig. 3. An ECG in a child with long QT syndrome.

Common Dysrythmias

Wolff-Parkinson-White (WPW) is the presence of accessory conduction pathways in the heart, which is often identified by a delta wave on ECG. WPW syndrome is subsequent tachycardia that can occur because of the presence of those accessory pathways.[27] Electrocardiographic findings suggestive of WPW include a wide QRS complex with slurred upstroke or delta wave indicative of ventricular pre-excitation from the accessory pathway, short PR interval for age, and evidence of repolarization ST-segment/T-wave abnormalities.[28] Approximately 0.2% of the population has the WPW pattern on ECG, and only a small percentage of these go on to develop a tachy-dysrhythmia.[27] It is estimated that less than 0.1% of patients with WPW go on to develop SCD.[27] **Fig. 4** is an ECG from an asymptomatic patient who presented with WPW. **Fig. 5** is an ECG from a patient with a history or WPW who presented in atrial fibrillation; note the delta wave and widened QRS.

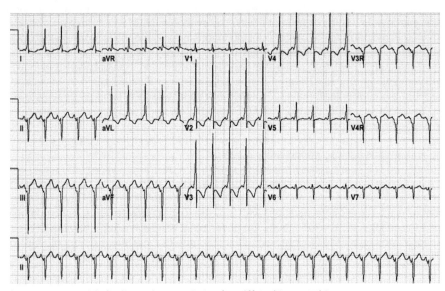

Fig. 4. An ECG with findings characteristic of Wolff-Parkinson-White.

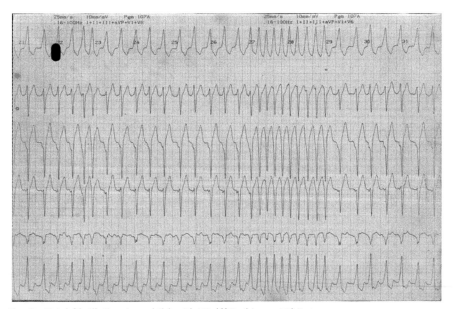

Fig. 5. Atrial fibrillation in a child with Wolff-Parkinson-White.

Short QT Syndrome

Short QT syndrome (SQTS) is rare cardiac electrical abnormality characterized by the presence of ventricular tachyarrhythmias leading to syncope and SCD.[29] There is currently much debate in the literature as to the definition of SQTS and what QTc should be considered abnormal. Current guidelines establish a diagnostic criteria of SQTS with a QTc less than 340.[29,30] **Fig. 6** provides a clinical example. The prevalence and incidence of SQTC is not fully known; most of the studies to date have focused on the screening of adult patients. One explanation of the low reported incidence in pediatrics is that fatal arrhythmias may occur early in life, leading to an underrepresentation of the disease in adults.[31,32] If seen on ECG in a pediatric syncope patient, this should prompt cardiology evaluation.

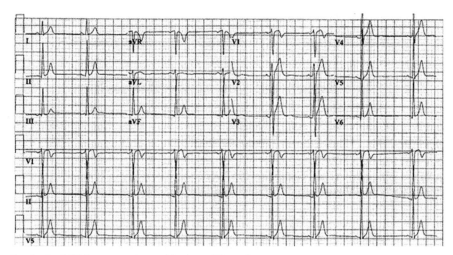

Fig. 6. An ECG from a patient with short QT syndrome.

Arrhythmogenic Right Ventricular Cardiomyopathy

Arrhythmogenic right ventricular cardiomyopathy, previously referred to as arrhythmogenic right ventricular dysplasia, is a progressive pathologic condition that primarily affects the right ventricle.[33] The replacement of the myocardium by fibrofatty tissue predisposes the heart to recurrent ventricular tachydysrhythmias.[18,33–35] It is primarily inherited in an autosomal-dominant condition,[34,35] so family history may help identify higher risk patients for this condition.

The full diagnostic criteria are beyond the scope of this article; however, key ECG findings are repolarization abnormalities of inverted T waves in right precordial leads (V1, V2, and V3) or beyond in individuals older than 14 years of age, epsilon waves in the right precordial leads (V1 to V3), or nonsustained or sustained ventricular tachycardia of left bundle branch morphology with superior axis.[36] **Fig. 7** demonstrates an example of arrhythmogenic right ventricular cardiomyopathy. If arrhythmogenic right ventricular cardiomyopathy is suspected the patient should be placed on activity restriction because of increased risk of SCD during exercise,[34,35] further diagnostic

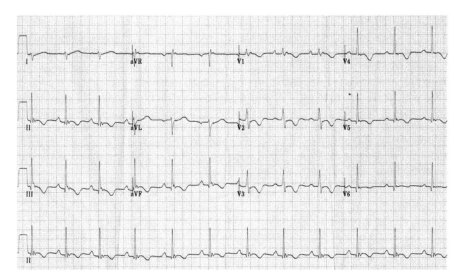

Fig. 7. An ECG from a patient with arrhythmogenic right ventricular cardiomyopathy demonstrating inferolateral T-wave inversion and an Epsilon wave in V1.

testing, and pediatric cardiology versus primary care follow-up depending on severity.

CARDIAC: STRUCTURAL PROBLEMS
Cardiomyopathy/Hypertrophic Obstructive Cardiomyopathy

Hypertrophic obstructive cardiomyopathy is a genetic disorder that causes hypertrophy of the septum causing a structural outflow obstruction.[37] The annual risk of sudden death in patients with hypertrophic cardiomyopathy is estimated to be 0.6% to 1%, and syncope is a major risk factor for subsequent SCD.[2] Any episode of exertional syncope should raise the index of suspicion for hypertrophic obstructive cardiomyopathy, and it is the most common cause of SCD in young competitive athletes.[38]

The classic murmur is described as a mid-systolic to late systolic crescendo decrescendo murmur that increases in intensity with Valsalva and is best heard at the left sternal border.[39,40] In addition to the physical examination, ECG findings suggestive of hypertrophic obstructive cardiomyopathy include so-called "dagger-like" q waves that are deep and narrow in the inferior and lateral leads,[41] t wave inversions,[42] and/or evidence of left ventricular hypertrophy (**Fig. 8**).[43] Patients should not be allowed to continue in sports until cleared by cardiology because of the risk of SCD.

Aortic Stenosis

Aortic stenosis is the most common valvular cardiac abnormality,[1,44] where narrowing of the aortic valve causes decreased blood flow to the aorta and poor coronary perfusion. In the pediatric population, aortic stenosis is usually caused by a bicuspid aortic valve. The cardiac murmur is a harsh, medium-pitched, crescendo-decrescendo systolic murmur and a paradoxically split S2, ejection click, and an S4 gallop.[45]

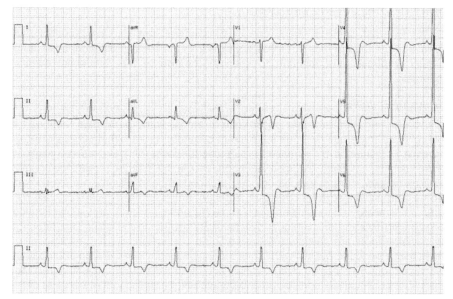

Fig. 8. An ECG from a patient with hypertrophic obstructive cardiomyopathy demonstrating inferolateral T-wave inversion and left ventricular hypertrophy.

CONGENITAL CARDIAC ABNORMALITIES
Myocardial Infarction

Although ischemic cardiac disease in the healthy child is a rare occurrence, it can happen in pediatric patients. History and ECG are paramount in the evaluation. If the history and ECG fits ischemia as it would in an adult patient, do not discount the diagnosis solely because of age. It has been estimated that there is a 2% incidence of ischemic heart disease as a cause of SCD outside of the neonatal and infant population.[46] Special attention should be paid to syncope patients that have chest pain, significant family history of early myocardial infarction, exertional chest pain, or a history of Kawasaki disease. Anomalous origin of the left coronary artery from the pulmonary artery is one congenital lesion that can lead to myocardial ischemia, infarction, and congestive heart failure.

OTHER DANGEROUS CARDIAC ETIOLOGIES
Huffers Ventricular Tachycardia

Inhalant drug abuse has been associated with a condition colloquially called huffers V-tach, which is a cause of syncope. The most commonly abused substances, often by adolescents, are paints, varnishes, glues, gasoline, lighter fluids, and aerosol propellants, which are absorbed within seconds and is quickly distributed to the central nervous system.[47,48] The heart is sensitized to catecholamines and a catecholamine surge (such as being discovered using the drug, causing a startle response) can cause ventricular dysrhythmias. The effect can be transient and the patient may wake up without prolonged resuscitation that could be confused with syncope. It is recommended that if inhalant drug abuse is suspected, avoid sympathomimetics (eg, epinephrine) if possible, to prevent potentially fatal tachyarrhythmia. Tachyarrhythmias may require treatment with β-blockers, such as esmolol.[49]

OTHER LIFE-THREATENING ETIOLOGIES

Similar to adult patients, many causes of syncope can also be potentially life threatening. Although many of these are similar to the adult population, a few merit special emphasis and mention to keep at the top of the differential even in children.

Pulmonary Embolism

Pulmonary embolism is a rare occurrence in the pediatric population, although in recent years there has been an increase in diagnosis rates. Whether this is a true increase in incidence or increase in diagnosis because of improved imaging and recognition is not clear.[50] Close attention should be paid to predisposing risk, such as obesity, central venous catheter, congenital heart disease, nephrotic syndrome, and prolonged total parenteral nutrition, among other typical adult risk factors.[51,52] Vital sign abnormalities, such as tachycardia, hypoxia, and such historical clues as leg swelling or exertional dyspnea can also aid in the diagnosis. Although no decision tools are validated in the pediatric population, current evidence suggests that a pediatric patient with a pulmonary embolism looks like an adult patient with a pulmonary embolism, and historical and clinical features suggesting the diagnosis should be actively considered and pursued and not discounted because of the patient's age.

Pulmonary Hypertension

In the pediatric patient, pulmonary hypertension should be on the differential of the young child with syncope especially with a history of congenital cardiac disease. Pulmonary hypertension is often difficult to diagnose because of its nonspecific presentations of dyspnea, exercise intolerance, and chest pain.[53,54] Any child with a high index of suspicion for pulmonary hypertension should undergo an initial work-up of chest radiographs, electrocardiography, and echocardiography and subsequent specialist evaluation.[55]

Seizures

Although seizures are potentially life threatening, for the purposes of this review the focus is not on life-threatening manifestations, such as status epilepticus, which would likely be obvious to the ED physician. In the context of syncope, recognition of and identification of seizures as a cause of syncope is important, however, because it is a common presenting problem that is in the differential diagnosis of every syncope patient who presents to the ED.

The primary danger is the misdiagnosis of a seizure when the true underlying cause is cardiovascular in origin.[56] Retrospective and prospective studies suggest that one in four patients with epilepsy are misdiagnosed after initial evaluation.[57] Antiepileptic medications may also cause harm to the unhealthy heart because they exert their clinical effect through the manipulation of ion channels.[56] One study of historical features found that cut tongue, head turning, unusual posturing, bedwetting, and blue color by bystanders had the highest likelihood ratios for seizure of 16.46, 13.48, 12.88, 6.45, and 5.81, respectively.[4] Involuntary jerking movements, or myoclonic jerks, are common during syncope of any cause, and can also be confused by seizure activity by bystanders and clinicians alike.[56,57] A detailed history physical examination and ECG are usually be able to elucidate the differences between these two entities; however, caution must be taken when finalizing a diagnosis. **Box 2** illustrates key points on how to distinguish syncope from seizure.

Box 2
Key points on how to distinguish syncope from seizure

	Convulsive Syncope	Epilepsy
Occurs supine	Uncommon	Common
Also has syncope and presyncope	Common	Uncommon
Typical prodrome: diaphoresis, presyncope, warmth	Common	Uncommon
Pallor	Common	Uncommon
Tongue biting	Uncommon	Common
Tongue bite location	Tongue tip	Tongue side
Prodromal cry	Uncommon	Common
Eye deviation	Fixed or upward	Lateral deviation
Incontinence	Uncommon	Common
Muscle movement	Pleiomorphic (see **Box 1**)	Rhythmic and generalized
Convulsion duration	Less than a minute	Often a few minutes
Postictal symptoms	Brief haziness, fatigue, diaphoresis, nausea	Confusion

From Sheldon R. How to differentiate syncope from seizure. Cardiol Clin 2015;33(3):384; with permission.

NON-LIFE-THREATENING ETIOLOGIES
Vasovagal/Neurocardiogenic Syncope/Reflex Syncope

Reflex syncope, also known as vasovagal and neurocardiogenic syncope, is the most common cause of syncope in the pediatric population.[58,59] Syncope associated with recent change of position, poor hydration or nutritional status, or a warm environment is most often reflex syncope.[59] Patients may report a prodrome prior syncopal event, which makes this diagnosis more likely. Patients that present without a prodrome should raise concern for a more serious cause. Patients with reflex syncope may have symptoms of increased vagal tone even after the syncopal event has resolved. These symptoms self-resolve and, without other high-risk factors, require only observation till the patient returns to normal.

Postural Orthostatic Tachycardia Syndrome

Postural orthostatic tachycardia syndrome is defined as the development of orthostatic symptoms associated with an elevated heart rate without orthostatic hypotension.[60] Symptoms of orthostatic intolerance are those caused by brain hypoperfusion and sympathetic overreaction.[60] Patients are most commonly adolescents, and females outnumber males with a 5:1 ratio.[60] Clinical features include palpitations, chest pain, lightheadedness, headache, and nausea.[60] Management typically involves expansion of plasma volume with high salt and high fluid intake. Important in the ED setting is that this is typically a chronic diagnosis and a diagnosis of exclusion, and is challenging to properly diagnose in a single ED snapshot. Patients suspected of this diagnosis may be referred to a cardiologist for further evaluation and management.

Breath-Holding Spells

Breath-holding spells are a common nonepileptic paroxysmal disorder of infancy.[61] They are rare before 6 months of age, peak at 2 years, and commonly abate by 5 years of age.[62] This is an unconscious response on exhalation that is often preceded by emotional stimuli. The child often exhales as if crying and holds a prolonged expiration.[63] Breath-holding spells are categorized by the color change that occurred during the event as cyanotic, pallid, or mixed.[61] Breath-holding spells are differentiated from epilepsy in that epileptic seizures are not usually triggered by anger or injury.[63] Also important is that the child should be developmentally normal with no regression of developmental milestones.

In terms of diagnostics, there is some thought that there may be an association with breath-holding spells and long QT, so an ECG should be considered.[63] If the history is clear, parents can be reassured with no additional diagnostic evaluation beyond a primary care physician follow-up as needed.

Psychiatric

Psychiatric causes of syncope are rare; however, a psychiatric cause should be considered when no other causative etiologies have been found. Psychiatric disease should be considered in not only the patient but with the caregivers. Munchausen syndrome by proxy and nonaccidental trauma should also be considered.

SUMMARY

Although often benign in the pediatric population, syncope can be the first presentation of a serious underlying medical condition. A detailed history and physical examination can identify a potential cause of syncope in many patients.[3] The ECG can help screen for dangerous etiologies. Routine laboratory testing often adds little to the evaluation and is not recommended routinely.[5] Concerning high-risk features, such as early SCD in the family, known or suspected heart disease, congenital cardiac abnormalities, exercise-induced syncope, syncope without prodrome, or an abnormal ECG should prompt a cardiac evaluation for the cause of the syncope. Most syncope patients may be discharged home after a careful and thorough evaluation in the ED.

REFERENCES

1. Kanjwal K, Masudi S, Grubb BP. Syncope in children and adolescents. Adolesc Med State Art Rev 2015;26(3):692–711.
2. Strickberger SA, Benson DW, Biaggioni I, et al. AHA/ACCF Scientific Statement on the evaluation of syncope: from the American Heart Association Councils on Clinical Cardiology, Cardiovascular Nursing, Cardiovascular Disease in the Young, and Stroke, and the Quality of Care and Outcomes Research Interdisciplinary Working Group; and the American College of Cardiology Foundation: in collaboration with the Heart Rhythm Society: endorsed by the American Autonomic Society. Circulation 2006;113(2):316–27.
3. Linzer M, Yang EH, Estes NA 3rd, et al. Diagnosing syncope. Part 1: value of history, physical examination, and electrocardiography. Clinical Efficacy Assessment Project of the American College of Physicians. Ann Intern Med 1997; 126(12):989–96.
4. Sheldon R, Rose S, Ritchie D, et al. Historical criteria that distinguish syncope from seizures. J Am Coll Cardiol 2002;40(1):142–8.
5. Writing Committee Members, Shen WK, Sheldon RS, Benditt DG, et al. 2017 ACC/AHA/HRS guideline for the evaluation and management of patients with syncope: a report of the American College of Cardiology/American Heart Association Task Force on Clinical Practice Guidelines and the Heart Rhythm Society. Heart Rhythm 2017;14(8):e155–217.

6. Stewart JM. Transient orthostatic hypotension is common in adolescents. J Pediatr 2002;140(4):418–24.

7. Koziol-McLain J, Lowenstein SR, Fuller B. Orthostatic vital signs in emergency department patients. Ann Emerg Med 1991;20(6):606–10.

8. Brignole M, Ungar A, Bartoletti A, et al. Standardized-care pathway vs. usual management of syncope patients presenting as emergencies at general hospitals. Europace 2006;8(8):644–50.

9. Steinberg LA, Knilans TK. Costs and utility of tests in the evaluation of the pediatric patients with syncope. Prog Pediatr Cardiol 2001;13(2):139–49.

10. Rodday AM, Triedman JK, Alexander ME, et al. Electrocardiogram screening for disorders that cause sudden cardiac death in asymptomatic children: a meta-analysis. Pediatrics 2012;129(4):e999–1010.

11. Lisman KA. Electrocardiographic evaluation in athletes and use of the Seattle criteria to improve specificity. Methodist Debakey Cardiovasc J 2016;12(2):81–5.

12. Drezner JA, Ackerman MJ, Anderson J, et al. Electrocardiographic interpretation in athletes: the 'Seattle criteria'. Br J Sports Med 2013;47(3):122–4.

13. Redd C, Thomas C, Willis M, et al. Cost of unnecessary testing in the evaluation of pediatric syncope. Pediatr Cardiol 2017;38(6):1115–22.

14. Vincent GM. The long QT and Brugada syndromes: causes of unexpected syncope and sudden cardiac death in children and young adults. Semin Pediatr Neurol 2005;12(1):15–24.

15. Priori SG, Napolitano C, Gasparini M, et al. Natural history of Brugada syndrome: insights for risk stratification and management. Circulation 2002;105(11):1342–7.

16. Vohra J, Rajagopalan S, CSANZ Genetics Council Writing Group. Update on the diagnosis and management of Brugada syndrome. Heart Lung Circ 2015;24(12):1141–8.

17. Wilde AA, Antzelevitch C, Borggrefe M, et al. Proposed diagnostic criteria for the Brugada syndrome: consensus report. Circulation 2002;106(19):2514–9.

18. Campbell RM. The treatment of cardiac causes of sudden death, syncope, and seizure. Semin Pediatr Neurol 2005;12(1):59–66.

19. Suzuki H, Torigoe K, Numata O, et al. Infant case with a malignant form of Brugada syndrome. J Cardiovasc Electrophysiol 2000;11(11):1277–80.

20. Priori SG, Napolitano C, Giordano U, et al. Brugada syndrome and sudden cardiac death in children. Lancet 2000;355(9206):808–9.

21. Khalil Kanjwal M, Hugh Calkins M. Syncope in children and adolescents. Card Electrophysiol Clin 2013;5(4):397–409.

22. Probst V, Denjoy I, Meregalli PG, et al. Clinical aspects and prognosis of Brugada syndrome in children. Circulation 2007;115(15):2042–8.

23. Brugada P. Brugada syndrome: more than 20 years of scientific excitement. J Cardiol 2016;67(3):215–20.

24. Vacanti G, Maragna R, Priori SG, et al. Genetic causes of sudden cardiac death in children: inherited arrhythmogenic diseases. Curr Opin Pediatr 2017;29(5):552–9.

25. Hampel KG, Rocamora Zuñiga R, Quesada CM. Unravelling the mysteries of sudden unexpected death in epilepsy. Neurologia 2017. [Epub ahead of print].

26. Schwartz PJ, Woosley RL. Predicting the unpredictable: drug-induced QT prolongation and torsades de pointes. J Am Coll Cardiol 2016;67(13):1639–50.

27. Kulig J, Koplan BA. Cardiology patient page. Wolff-Parkinson-White syndrome and accessory pathways. Circulation 2010;122(15):e480–3.

28. Chan TC, Sharieff GQ, Brady WJ. Electrocardiographic manifestations: pediatric ECG. J Emerg Med 2008;35(4):421–30.

29. Pereira R, Campuzano O, Sarquella-Brugada G, et al. Short QT syndrome in pediatrics. Clin Res Cardiol 2017;106(6):393–400.
30. Khera S, Jacobson JT. Short QT syndrome in current clinical practice. Cardiol Rev 2016;24(4):190–3.
31. Iribarren C, Round AD, Peng JA, et al. Short QT in a cohort of 1.7 million persons: prevalence, correlates, and prognosis. Ann Noninvasive Electrocardiol 2014; 19(5):490–500.
32. Mazzanti A, Underwood K, Nevelev D, et al. The new kids on the block of arrhythmogenic disorders: short QT syndrome and early repolarization. J Cardiovasc Electrophysiol 2017;28(10):1226–36.
33. Marcus FI, Fontaine GH, Guiraudon G, et al. Right ventricular dysplasia: a report of 24 adult cases. Circulation 1982;65(2):384–98.
34. Azaouagh A, Churzidse S, Konorza T, et al. Arrhythmogenic right ventricular cardiomyopathy/dysplasia: a review and update. Clin Res Cardiol 2011;100(5): 383–94.
35. McNally E, MacLeod H, Dellefave-Castillo L. Arrhythmogenic right ventricular cardiomyopathy. In: Adam MP, Ardinger HH, Pagon RA, et al, editors. GeneReviews [Internet]. Seattle (WA): University of Washington, Seattle; 2017. p. 1993–2017.
36. Marcus FI, McKenna WJ, Sherrill D, et al. Diagnosis of arrhythmogenic right ventricular cardiomyopathy/dysplasia: proposed modification of the task force criteria. Circulation 2010;121(13):1533–41.
37. Shaw KN, Bachur RG. Fleisher & Ludwig's textbook of pediatric emergency medicine. 7th edition. Philadelphia: Wolters Kluwer; 2016. p. xxxii, 1519.
38. Maron BJ, Doerer JJ, Haas TS, et al. Sudden deaths in young competitive athletes: analysis of 1866 deaths in the United States, 1980-2006. Circulation 2009;119(8):1085–92.
39. Naik RJ, Shah NC. Teenage heart murmurs. Pediatr Clin North Am 2014;61(1): 1–16.
40. Hypertrophic obstructive cardiomyopathy (HOCM) topic review. Available at: https://www.healio.com/cardiology/learn-the-heart/cardiology-review/topic-reviews/ hypertrophic-obstructive-cardiomyopathy-hocm. Accessed August 13, 2017.
41. Bent RE, Wheeler MT, Hadley D, et al. Computerized Q wave dimensions in athletes and hypertrophic cardiomyopathy patients. J Electrocardiol 2015;48(3): 362–7.
42. Zorzi A, Calore C, Vio R, et al. Accuracy of the ECG for differential diagnosis between hypertrophic cardiomyopathy and athlete's heart: comparison between the European Society of Cardiology (2010) and International (2017) criteria. Br J Sports Med 2017. [Epub ahead of print].
43. Ellims AH. Hypertrophic cardiomyopathy in the adolescent. Aust Fam Physician 2017;46(8):553–7.
44. Aortic valve stenosis. 2016. Available at: http://www.heart.org/HEARTORG/ Conditions/More/HeartValveProblemsandDisease/Problem-Aortic-Valve-Stenosis_ UCM_450437_Article.jsp - .WZCGQcbMzWY. Accessed August 13, 2017.
45. Baren JM. Pediatric emergency medicine. Philadelphia: Saunders/Elsevier; 2008. p. xxxi, 1320.
46. Gajewski KK, Saul JP. Sudden cardiac death in children and adolescents (excluding sudden infant death syndrome). Ann Pediatr Cardiol 2010;3(2): 107–12.
47. Harris CR. The toxicology handbook for clinicians. Philadelphia: Mosby Elsevier; 2006. p. xvii, 348.

48. Substance Abuse and Mental Health Services Administration, results from the 2013 national survey on drug use and health: summary of national findings, NSDUH series H-48, in HHS publication No. (SMA) 14-4863. Rockville (MD): Substance Abuse and Mental Health Services Administration; 2014.
49. Shannon MW, Borron SW, Burns MJ, et al. Haddad and Winchester's clinical management of poisoning and drug overdose. 4th edition. Philadelphia: Saunders/Elsevier; 2007. p. xxvi, 1559.
50. Fant C, Cohen A. Syncope in pediatric patients: a practical approach to differential diagnosis and management in the emergency department. Pediatr Emerg Med Pract 2017;14(4):1–28.
51. Agha BS, Sturm JJ, Simon HK, et al. Pulmonary embolism in the pediatric emergency department. Pediatrics 2013;132(4):663–7.
52. Stein PD, Kayali F, Olson RE. Incidence of venous thromboembolism in infants and children: data from the National Hospital Discharge Survey. J Pediatr 2004;145(4):563–5.
53. McDivitt JD, Barstow C. Cardiovascular disease update: pulmonary hypertension. FP Essent 2017;454:24–8.
54. Hansmann G. Pulmonary hypertension in infants, children, and young adults. J Am Coll Cardiol 2017;69(20):2551–69.
55. Kula S, Pektaş A. A review of pediatric pulmonary hypertension with new guidelines. Turk J Med Sci 2017;47(2):375–80.
56. Bergfeldt L. Differential diagnosis of cardiogenic syncope and seizure disorders. Heart 2003;89(3):353–8.
57. Duplyakov D, Golovina G, Garkina S, et al. Is it possible to accurately differentiate neurocardiogenic syncope from epilepsy? Cardiol J 2010;17(4):420–7.
58. Anderson JB, Willis M, Lancaster H, et al. The evaluation and management of pediatric syncope. Pediatr Neurol 2016;55:6–13.
59. Sanatani S, Chau V, Fournier A, et al. Canadian Cardiovascular Society and Canadian Pediatric Cardiology Association position statement on the approach to syncope in the pediatric patient. Can J Cardiol 2017;33(2):189–98.
60. Low PA, Sandroni P, Joyner M, et al. Postural tachycardia syndrome (POTS). J Cardiovasc Electrophysiol 2009;20(3):352–8.
61. Rathore G, Larsen P, Fernandez C, et al. Diverse presentation of breath holding spells: two case reports with literature review. Case Rep Neurol Med 2013;2013: 603190.
62. Breukels MA, Plötz FB, van Nieuwenhuizen O, et al. Breath holding spells in a 3-day-old neonate: an unusual early presentation in a family with a history of breath holding spells. Neuropediatrics 2002;33(1):41–2.
63. Breningstall GN. Breath-holding spells. Pediatr Neurol 1996;14(2):91–7.

Pediatric Pain Management

Aarti Gaglani, MD[a], Toni Gross, MD, MPH[a,b],*

KEYWORDS

- Pain • Pediatrics • Emergency • Self-report • Behavioral-observational • Pain scale
- Intranasal • Nonpharmacologic

KEY POINTS

- There are challenges and barriers to pain management in the pediatric emergency department.
- Age-appropriate pain scales and other techniques suitably evaluate pediatric pain.
- Pediatric pain can be treated effectively via pharmacologic and nonpharmacologic methods.

INTRODUCTION

The complaint of pain is a common reason for families to seek care for their children in the emergency department (ED). Alleviating pain is an important component of emergency care, improving the experience for the patient and contributing to improved accuracy of evaluation. Adequate pain control during assessment and procedures can prevent long-term negative consequences, including heightened pain experiences, noncompliance with vaccines, and avoidance of future medical procedures.[1–5] From an operations perspective, rapid time to analgesia has been associated with shorter ED stays for adults.[6]

Pain assessment and management have been identified as a priority by several organizations and accreditation bodies. Standards for pain assessment and treatment were established by The Joint Commission (TJC) in 2001. Current standards require hospitals to have policies for pain assessment and treatment and to ensure staff are educated and compliant with the policies.[7] A 2012 American Academy of Pediatrics (AAP) clinical report provides evidence-based guidance for pain management and anxiolysis in emergency services. It describes pain assessment instruments and includes education tips and treatment protocols.[8] A 2003 National Association of

Disclosure Statement: The author has nothing to disclose.
[a] Division of Emergency Medicine, Phoenix Children's Hospital, 1919 East Thomas Road, Phoenix, AZ 85018, USA; [b] Division of Emergency Medicine, Department of Child Health, Phoenix Children's Hospital, University of Arizona College of Medicine-Phoenix, Phoenix Children's Hospital Emergency Medicine, 1919 East Thomas Road, Phoenix, AZ 85016, USA
* Corresponding author.
E-mail address: tgross@phoenixchildrens.com

Emerg Med Clin N Am 36 (2018) 323–334
https://doi.org/10.1016/j.emc.2017.12.002

Emergency Medicine Service Physicians (NAEMSP) position statement states that the relief of pain should be a priority for every emergency medical services (EMS) system and recommends elements that should be present in prehospital pain management protocols.[9]

PAIN IN THE EMERGENCY DEPARTMENT

Of the 23 million ED visits by patients younger than 15 years in 2013, injury accounted for 30%, and painful conditions such as headache, ear pain, and abdominal pain accounted for an additional 9%.[10] Additionally, children may be subject to several painful procedures during an emergency visit, and considerations for preventing pain during procedures are as important as treating existing pain.

Oligoanalgesia (the undertreatment of pain), is prevalent in both adult and pediatric EDs.[11] Children are prone to oligoanalgesia and frequently experience unnecessary pain with minor illnesses and injuries.[12–14] Pain management begins with appropriate assessment and documentation. Prior to TJC establishment of standards for pain assessment and documentation, ED documentation of pediatric pain scores was reported at 23% to 44% of visits.[15,16] One study in the postmandate era reported pain score documentation in 87% of visits during a 14-month period and a significant association between pain score documentation and the prescription of analgesics.[17] Increased efforts to assess and document pain scores can decrease oligoanesthesia.

The busy environment in the ED can amplify parental and patient anxiety, leading to an increased awareness of pain.[8] Factors inhibiting optimal assessment of pediatric pain include the failure to understand the caregiver's role and decision to seek evaluation, adults' limited understanding of children's pain experience, and sociocultural influence on pain expression.[18] A comparison of pediatric pain assessment by patients, caretakers, and professionals in the ED found that professionals scored pain lower in comparison with guardians and patients, and that guardians were more likely to rate pain similar to the rating given by their child.[19]

Relative unfamiliarity with children of different ages and developmental stages may be a barrier to pain management, as over 80% of children seeking emergency care do so in general EDs treating adults and children.[20] Another factor may be an erroneous belief that infants and neonates do not feel pain, or that children will not remember painful experiences to a significant extent.[21] Additional barriers include difficulty assessing and measuring pain in young patients, unfamiliarity with pain score instruments or scales, distinguishing pain from anxiety, fears of medication adverse events, and concerns of masking serious conditions.[8]

EVALUATION AND ASSESSMENT OF PAIN

Pain assessment tools are commonly defined as one of two types. Observational-behavioral measures aim to reflect a patient's reaction to pain. Self-report measures rely on the patient's ability to quantify and describe his or her pain. Using the appropriate type of tool to assess pain accurately is essential to establishing baseline discomfort and measuring response to treatment.

Self-report scales are currently the standard in the assessment of pain. There are 6 self-report pain scales that have been shown to have well-founded reliability, validity, and feasibility for use in the assessment of acute and chronic pain in children.[22] These include the Faces Pain Scale (FPS), Faces Pain Scale – Revised (FPS-R), Oucher-Photographic, Oucher-Numeric Rating Scale (NRS), Wong-Baker FACES Pain Scale, and Visual Analog Scale (VAS). Multiple studies have found that younger and older children prefer a facial expression pain scale.[23,24] The FPS-R is the recommended scale to use in school-aged children (4–12 years old), as it has better success rates and is preferable for patients compared with the Oucher NRS or VAS.[25] The FPS-R and Color Analog Scale (CAS) have been validated for use in children 4 to 17 years old in the ED setting.[25] NRS is valid for use in children of 8 years and older, who can comprehend numeric order and quantify their degree of pain.[26]

Assessing pain in children younger than 4 years old can be challenging, as most young children have not yet developed the skills to express and quantify the degree of their pain. For this group of patients, clinicians must utilize observational tools to assess pain in addition to physical findings. Observational-behavioral tools for pain assessment should be utilized if the child is preverbal, cognitively impaired, or sedated.[27] Many tools rely on behaviors of the infant or child, whereas some tools consider physiologic signs.

The most commonly used observational tools in infants and toddlers include the FLACC (face, legs, activity, crying, and consolability), revised FLACC, Children's and Infants' Postoperative Pain Scale (CHIPPS), and Children's Hospital of Eastern Ontario Pain Scale (CHEOPS). The FLACC scale can be used when assessing pain in older infants, young children, and developmentally delayed children.[28] A recent study assessing the reliability of this tool specifically in the pediatric ED found the tool to demonstrate high reliability and sensitivity to acute pain assessment in patients who are not undergoing surgery or painful procedures.[29] The Alder Hey Triage Pain Score is an observational tool validated specifically in the ED triage setting.[30]

For the neonatal period, 2 commonly used observational assessment tools are the CRIES (C-crying, R-requires increased oxygen, I-increased vital signs, E-expression, S-sleeplessness) and Neonatal Infant Pain Scale (NIPS). The CRIES tool was found to be valid, reliable, and acceptable by neonatal nurses.[31] The NIPS accounts for facial expression, cry, breathing pattern, arm/leg movement, and arousal state.[32] When compared in the postoperative setting, CRIES, NIPS, and CHIPPS all displayed excellent reliability and validity, but the NIPS was superior to the other 2 scales when considering ease of use and feasibility.[33]

With improved technology, electronic scales are becoming increasingly available for pediatric pain assessment. A digital version of the VAS is a valid, reliable, and responsive tool to measure pain in patients with upper extremity injuries.[34] The agreement between electronic and paper versions of a pictorial pain scale has been shown to be good, but the electronic format was preferred over the paper format by 87.4%.[35] Similar results were demonstrated using a smartphone-based application containing electronic versions of FPS-R and CAS.[36] The use of electronic self-report pain scales may improve patient cooperation and lead to improved pain management. Pain scores obtained via digital scales could potentially be uploaded directly into the electronic health record, allowing for real-time patient reports of pain to measure response to treatment and guide management.

TREATMENT OF PAIN
Nonpharmacologic

The management of acute pain and anxiety should be approached in a stepwise manner, involving both nonpharmacologic and pharmacologic interventions. Nonpharmacologic therapies include physical comfort measures and distraction techniques. The neurodevelopmental stages of neonates, infants, and children affect the way they perceive and cope with pain; therefore, interventions should be tailored to patients based on their age and developmental stage.

For painful traumatic conditions, the utility of basic first aid measures should not be underestimated. Applying splints or using other immobilization techniques to stabilize fractures and dislocations should be done early. Ice or cold packs will decrease swelling and can provide topical analgesia for traumatic injuries. These interventions should be included in prehospital and ED triage pathways.

Parents, play therapists, and child life specialists can also be useful aids in reducing children's pain and anxiety.[37] Evidence supports that the presence of parents may decrease the child's pain and anxiety.[38] However, parental anxiety is associated with pain responses in children.[39,40] Clinicians should prepare parents for what to expect and coach them to use developmentally appropriate strategies to help their child cope with pain.[41]

Distraction techniques are useful to treat pain in preschool- and school-aged children, as well as in adolescents. Younger children are largely not yet able to comprehend verbal reassurance; thus, distraction techniques are likely to be more beneficial.[41] There is strong evidence supporting the use of distraction and hypnosis to reduce pain and distress in children experiencing needle-related pain from toddler age through adolescence.[42] For toddlers, playing peek-a-boo, blowing bubbles, or looking at books are effective methods used for distraction in acute pain.[43] Children demonstrated a higher pain tolerance when provided with interactive and passive video game distraction compared with no distraction.[44] For children aged 6 to 18 years undergoing laceration repairs in the ED, music, video games, cartoon videos, blowing bubbles, and reading books with child life specialists were effective in lowering self-reported anxiety in older children, and lessening parental perception of pain in younger children.[45] Virtual reality as a distraction has been shown to be useful and continues to undergo further study.[46]

Neonates and infants have a positive physiologic response to physical attachment and oral stimulation. Skin-to-skin care (SSC) involves placing the infant skin-to-skin on the parent's chest for 30 minutes prior to and during the painful procedure. SSC is a safe, effective method to reduce distress in term and preterm neonates based on composite pain scores, including behavioral and physiologic indicators.[47] Swaddling simulates the feeling of being held and has also been shown to speed up infant behavioral and physiologic recovery from heel lance.[48]

Sucrose (2 mL of 25% glucose solution (1 mL in each cheek, no more than 2 minutes prior to the painful procedure) has also been recommended for use in neonates (<30 days) for painful procedures performed in the ED, given its low cost, ease of use, accessibility, and low risk of adverse effects.[49,50] Giving sucrose in addition to radiant warmth reduces pain better than sucrose alone.[51]

Non-nutritive sucking and breastfeeding are other forms of nonpharmacologic interventions for infants given their natural sucking response. Breastfeeding infants during painful procedures has been shown to result in lower increases in heart rate and decreased crying time when compared with swaddling, use of a pacifier, maternal holding, and oral sucrose.[52]

Certain nonpharmacologic methods reduce pain during painful procedures, while others improve infant recovery following the procedure. A Cochrane review of 63 studies evaluating nonpharmacologic strategies for painful procedures in neonates and infants reported that interventions resulting in the greatest improvement in pain reactivity were non-nutritive sucking-related interventions (pacifier, mother's nonlactating nipple) and swaddling/facilitated tucking. For improvement in pain-related regulation, the most beneficial techniques were non-nutritive sucking interventions, SSC, swaddling/tucking, and rocking/holding.[53] A combination of interventions should be utilized before, during, and after painful procedures in infants for optimal pain reduction and recovery from pain.[54]

Pharmacologic

When nonpharmacologic therapy alone is inadequate for pain relief, pharmacologic interventions are required. When treating pain, a stepladder approach to analgesics is essential, starting with nonopioid analgesics, and escalating to opioids and adjuvant analgesics with increasing therapeutic intensity. Per the World Health Organization (WHO) guidelines on pharmacologic treatment of pain in children with medical illnesses in 2012, a 2-step approach should be utilized. Acetaminophen and ibuprofen are the drugs of choice in the first step to treat mild pain, followed by opioids to treat moderate to severe pain.[55]

Nonopioid analgesics are beneficial for use in mild pain, as they do not carry the risk of tolerance nor physical dependence that opioids produce.[56] Acetaminophen can be given at any age; however, it carries the risk of liver toxicity in overdose or in patients with pre-existing hepatic insufficiency. When used in conjunction with opioids for postoperative pain, it has been shown to decrease opioid use.[57] Intravenous acetaminophen is US Food and Drug Administration (FDA)-approved for children 2 years and older. Nonsteroidal anti-inflammatory drugs (NSAIDs), such as ibuprofen and naproxen, are also effective in treating mild pain. Ketorolac is the only intravenous NSAID available in the United States, and it may be considered for mild to moderate pain. NSAIDs may cause gastrointestinal and renal side effects, including gastric irritation and acute kidney injury. One study concluded that ibuprofen given to children with acute gastroenteritis and dehydration increased the risk of developing acute kidney injury by more than twofold.[58] NSAIDs should be used with caution in volume-depleted children. Aspirin as an analgesic is avoided in children because of the risk of Reye syndrome.

Moderate pain may require additional analgesics. In these cases, tramadol or opioids may be of benefit. Tramadol is an opioid-related analgesic and causes less respiratory depression than conventional opioids. It should be used with caution in patients with seizure disorders and patients taking psychostimulant or serotonergic medications, as it can lower the seizure threshold and cause serotonin syndrome. The safety and efficacy of tramadol for use in acute pediatric pain are not well-studied.

Opioid analgesics can cause respiratory depression, sedation, and potentially apnea, when used in high doses. They are generally safe for use in children, when used in a ladder approach. Unlike acetaminophen or ibuprofen, opioids do not have a ceiling analgesic effect. Thus, using smaller doses of opioids and titrating to pain relief is the optimal strategy to treat pain and avoid undesirable adverse effects. To determine appropriate dosing of opioids, it is imperative to frequently assess the child's pain response to analgesics.[55] Other adverse effects of opioids include nausea, vomiting, and pruritus due to histamine release, and these effects can be treated with antihistamines and antiemetics.[41]

Oral opioid analgesics include oxycodone, morphine, and hydromorphone. Codeine is no longer recommended for children because of genetic variability in metabolism and the risk of respiratory depression in fast metabolizers. Some oral analgesic preparations include both an opioid and acetaminophen, with fixed opioid-to-acetaminophen dose proportions. This can result in over- or underdosing of acetaminophen, so clinicians should consider prescribing these analgesics separately.[38]

The intranasal route of opioid administration is useful for quick pain relief in children who have moderate-to-severe pain without established intravenous access. Intranasal fentanyl has been found to be an efficacious treatment of acute pain in children as young as 6 month old.[59–61] When compared with intravenous morphine, intranasal fentanyl resulted in comparable pain relief in children with long bone fractures in the ED,[62] and decreased time to administration of opioids.[63] The use of a pain management clinical pathway that included intranasal fentanyl as the primary pain medication was associated with a 25-minute reduction in time to first analgesic in 1 pediatric ED.[64]

Intravenous opioids are used for patients suffering from severe pain and are titrated to effect to avoid adverse events. Morphine and fentanyl are commonly used to treat acute and breakthrough pain in pediatric patients. Hydromorphone is less commonly used, but is useful to treat acute pain in children with chronic pain or opioid tolerance, such as children with sickle cell disease.

ADJUNCTIVE/ADJUVANT THERAPIES

Injectable anesthetics, such as lidocaine with or without epinephrine and bupivacaine, are commonly used for local and regional anesthesia prior to painful procedures. Topical anesthetics, in the form of creams, gels, and jet-injection, have become popular for use alone or as adjunctive therapy for procedures such as venipuncture and laceration repair (**Table 1**).[65] There is also evidence for their use in incision and drainage procedures and performance of lumbar punctures.[66] Cold and vibration stimulation have also been shown to decrease pain and anxiety during venipuncture.[67]

SPECIAL POPULATIONS

The management of pain in certain populations can be particularly challenging. Practitioners should remember that in pervasive developmental disorders, such as autism spectrum disorder, patients may manifest pain with changes in behavior, such as becoming aggressive toward self or others. Sources of pain should be elicited in these patients presenting with behavioral complaints.

Children who are cognitively impaired may be unable to effectively express their pain level because of language delays, increased sensitivity to sound and light, and maladaptive behaviors. For these patients, behavioral pain tools are useful for pain assessment (**Box 1**).[68] These patients may have a heightened level of anxiety because of previous painful experiences.

Children with cognitive impairment frequently have other chronic medical conditions. They experience pain from the same illnesses and injuries as other children, but also often develop related conditions that can cause pain, such as gastroesophageal reflux,

Table 1 Topical anesthetics		
Medication	**Type**	**Comments**
Lidocaine-epinephrine-tetracaine (LET)	Gel	Use on open wounds, causes vasoconstriction, time to effect = 30–60 min, can be compounded by hospital pharmacy, must be refrigerated
Eutectic mixture of lidocaine and prilocaine (EMLA)	Cream	Use on intact skin under occlusive dressing, time to effect = 1 h
Lidocaine 4% (L-M-X)	Cream	Use on intact skin, time to effect = 30 min, approved for use >2 year old, available over the counter
Jet-injected buffered lidocaine (J-tip)	Needle-free jet injection	Time to effect = 1–2 min

Box 1
Pain scales for cognitively impaired children
Noncommunicating Children's Pain Checklist
Echelle Douleur Enfant San Salvador
Pediatric Pain Profile
Revised FLACC
Pain Indicator for Communicatively Impaired Children

constipation, spasticity, osteopenia with pathologic fractures, and poor dentition. Breau and colleagues[69] found that children with severe cognitive impairments suffer from pain at least 1 day per week, and on average 9 to 10 hours per week. They also noted that most of the pain episodes were caused by medical conditions as opposed to medical interventions.[70–73] In managing pain for cognitively impaired children, clinicians should consider the patient's home medications to avoid harmful drug-drug interactions and adverse effects of analgesic therapy that may worsen underlying conditions.

Other patient populations, including children with cancer and blood disorders or children requiring staged surgical procedures, are subjected to multiple potentially painful procedures throughout the course of their life. Each episode builds on the experiential component of future procedures, for both patient and parent. Consideration should be given to institution-wide practice pathways that standardize assessment and treatment across different areas within a health care institution or system, where available.

OPERATIONALIZING QUALITY PAIN MANAGEMENT FOR CHILDREN IN EMERGENCY DEPARTMENTS

All EDs that provide treatment for children should have quality improvement (QI) programs in place for periodic evaluation of pain management practices.[8] QI studies have demonstrated improvements in the proportion of patients receiving analgesia and timeliness to analgesia. Quality and process improvement methods identified key drivers for rapid opioid administration in children with obvious extremity fractures that resulted in a significantly improved timeliness of analgesic delivery.[74] A structured intervention on pain management including provider education, organizational changes, and patient empowerment, resulted in improved rates of analgesic administration, timeliness of analgesic administration, and pain reassessment.[37] An education-based quality improvement initiative significantly improved the frequency of application of topical anesthetics for children undergoing facial or scalp laceration repair.[75] A standardized vaso-occlusive episode (VOE) protocol, using intranasal fentanyl as the first analgesic, provision of a sickle cell disease pain medication calculator, and education of the provider and patient/family, significantly improved care of children with VOE in the ED.[76]

ED overcrowding has been associated with decreased rate and timeliness of analgesic administration in pediatric patients with acute long bone fractures.[77] Studies have demonstrated significant improvements in provision and timely administration of oral analgesics when initiated in triage.[78,79] One study found that triage-administered oxycodone produced greater pain reduction compared with codeine in children with suspected forearm fracture.[80] A list of current practice guidelines from professional organizations is found in **Table 2**.

Table 2
Current practice guideline/principles of pain management

American Academy of Pediatrics	Policy Statement: Relief of Pain and Anxiety in Pediatric Patients in Emergency Medical Systems[8]
Emergency Nurses Association	Position statement: optimizing the treatment of pain in patients with acute presentations[82]
American Academy of Emergency Medicine	Model emergency department pain treatment guidelines[83]
National Association of EMS Physicians	Position statement: prehospital pain management[9]

RECENT ADVANCES AND FUTURE DIRECTIONS IN PAIN MANAGEMENT

Pain assessment and management have become topics of interest and more robustly studied in recent years. A comprehensive analysis of pediatric pain research from 1975 to 2010 demonstrates a considerable surge of pediatric pain literature since 1990, with the most studied topics including pain characterization, pain intervention, and pain assessment.[81] In addition to growing research, national efforts by TJC and the Institute of Medicine have also improved pain recognition and assessment. Further research is necessary to validate the use of certain analgesics and to implement protocols for pediatric pain management in the ED.

SUMMARY

Managing children's pain in the emergency setting is important for multiple reasons, including alleviating patient suffering, improving the success of evaluation and treatment, and preventing future negative health care experiences or avoidance of health care. Assessment of pain in children, especially the very young, can be challenging for practitioners. There are multiple valid assessment tools available to standardize the approach to pain assessment in children. A combination of nonpharmacologic and pharmacologic techniques will optimally treat pain.

REFERENCES

1. Young KD. Pediatric procedural pain. Ann Emerg Med 2005;45:160–71.
2. Tsao JCI, Myers CD, Craske MC, et al. Sensitivity in children's and adolescents' laboratory pain responses. J Pediatr Psychol 2004;29:379–88.
3. Noel M, Chambers CT, McGrath PJ, et al. The influence of children's pain memories on subsequent pain experience. Pain 2012;153:1563–72.
4. Taddio A, Ipp M, Thivakaran S, et al. Survey of the prevalence of immunization non-compliance due to needle fears in children and adults. Vaccine 2012;30: 4807–12.
5. Racine NM, Pillai Riddell RR, Flora DB, et al. Predicting preschool pain-related anticipatory distress: the relative contribution of longitudinal and concurrent factors. Pain 2016;157:1918–32.
6. Sokoloff C, Daoust R, Paquet J, et al. Is adequate pain relief and time to analgesia associated with emergency department length of stay? A retrospective study. BMJ Open 2014;4:e004288.
7. Joint Commission Statement on Pain Management, April 18, 2016. Available at: https://www.jointcommission.org/joint_commission_statement_on_pain_management/. Accessed July 6, 2017.

8. Fein JA, Zempsky WT, Cravero JP, the Committee on Pediatric Emergency Medicine and Section on Anesthesiology and Pain Medicine. Relief of pain and anxiety in pediatric patients in emergency medical systems. Pediatrics 2012; 130:e1391–405.

9. Alonso-Serra HM, Wesley K, for the NAEMSP and Clinical Practices Committee. Prehospital pain management. Prehosp Emerg Care 2003;7:482–8.

10. Rui P, Kang K, Albert M. National Hospital Ambulatory Medical Care Survey: 2013 emergency department summary tables. Available at: http://www.cdc.gov/nchs/data/ahcd/nhamcs_emergency/2013_ed_web_tables.pdf. Accessed August 9, 2017.

11. Cimpello LB, Khine H, Avner JR. Practice patterns of pediatric versus general emergency physicians for pain management of fractures in pediatric patients. Pediatr Emerg Care 2004;20:228–32.

12. Friedland LR, Pancioli AM, Duncan KM. Pediatric emergency department analgesic practice. Pediatr Emerg Care 1997;13:103–6.

13. Brown JC, Klein EJ, Lewis CW. Emergency department analgesia for fracture pain. Ann Emerg Med 2003;42:197–205.

14. Howard RF. Current status of pain management in children. JAMA 2003;290: 2464–9.

15. Drendel AL, Brousseau DC, Gorelick MH. Pain assessment for pediatric patients in the emergency department. Pediatrics 2006;117:1511–8.

16. Eder SC, Sloan EP, Todd K. Documentation of ED patient pain by nurses and physicians. Am J Emerg Med 2003;21:253–7.

17. Kellogg KM, Fairbanks RJ, O'Connor AB, et al. Association of pain score documentation and analgesic use in a pediatric emergency department. Pediatr Emerg Care 2012;28:1287–92.

18. Craig KD, Lilley CM, Gilbert CA. Barriers to optimal pain management in infants, children, and adolescents. Clin J Pain 1996;12:232–42.

19. Maciocia PM, Strachan EM, Akram AR, et al. Pain assessment in the paediatric emergency department: whose view counts? Eur J Emerg Med 2003;10(4): 264–7.

20. Gausche-Hill M, Ely M, Schmuhl P, et al. A National Assessment of Pediatric Readiness of Emergency Departments. JAMA Pediatr 2015;169(6):527–34.

21. Davis PW. Pediatric Sedation and Analgesia. In: Pfenninger JL, Fowler GC, editors. Pfenninger and Fowler's Procedures for Primary Care. 3rd edition. Philadelphia, PA: Mosby Elsevier; 2011. p. 35–58.

22. Stinson JN, Kavanagh T, Yamada J, et al. Systematic review of the psychometric properties, interpretability and feasibility of self-report pain intensity measures for use in clinical trials in children and adolescent. Pain 2006;125:143–57.

23. Miro J, Huguet A. Evaluation of reliability, validity, and preference for a pediatric pain intensity scale: the Catalan version of the Faces Pain Scale–revised. Pain 2004;111(1–2):59–64.

24. Keck JF, Gerkensmeyer JE, Joyce BA, et al. Reliability and validity of the Faces and word descriptor scales to measure procedural pain. J Pediatr Nurs 1996; 11(6):368–74.

25. Tsze DS, von Baeyer CL, Bulloch B, et al. Validation of self-report pain scales in children. Pediatrics 2013;132(4):e971–9.

26. von Baeyer CL, Spagrud LJ, McCormick JC, et al. Three new datasets supporting use of the Numerical Rating Scale (NRS-11) for children's self-reports of pain intensity. Pain 2009;143:223–7.

27. von Baeyer CL, Spagrud LJ. Systematic review of observational (behavioral) measures for children and adolescents aged 3-18 years. Pain 2007;127:140–50.
28. Manworren RC, Hynan LS. Clinical validation of FLACC: preverbal patient pain scale. Pediatr Nurs 2003;29:140–6.
29. Kochman A, Howell J, Sheridan M, et al. Reliability of the faces, legs, activity, cry, and consolability scale in assessing acute pain in the pediatric emergency department. Pediatr Emerg Care 2017;201(33):14–7.
30. Stewart B, Lancaster G, Lawson J, et al. Validation of the Alder Hey Triage Pain Score. Arch Dis Child 2004;89:625–30.
31. Krechel SW, Bildner J. CRIES: a new neonatal postoperative pain measurement score. Initial testing of validity and reliability. Paediatr Anaesth 1995;5(1):53–61.
32. Lawrence J, Alcock D, McGrath P, et al. The development of a tool to assess neonatal pain. Neonatal Netw 1993;12(6):59–66.
33. Suraseranivongse S, Kaosaard R, Intakong P, et al. A comparison of postoperative pain scales in neonates. Br J Anaesth 2006;97:540–4.
34. Sindhu BS, Shechtman O, Tuckey L. Validity, reliability, and responsiveness of a digital version of the visual analog scale. J Hand Ther 2011;24:356–64.
35. Wood C, von Baeyer CL, Falinower S, et al. Electronic and paper versions of a faces pain intensity scale: concordance and preference in hospitalized children. BMC Pediatr 2011;11:87.
36. Sun T, West N, Ansermino JM, et al. A smartphone version of the Faces Pain Scale-revised and the Color Analog Scale for postoperative pain assessment in children. Pediatr Anaesth 2015;25:1264–73.
37. Corwin DJ, Kessler DO, Auerbach M, et al. An intervention to improve pain management in the pediatric emergency department. Pediatr Emer Care 2012;28: 524–8.
38. Ruest S, Anderson A. Management of acute pediatric pain in the emergency department. Curr Opin Pediatr 2016;28:298–304.
39. Frank NC, Blount RL, Smith AJ, et al. Parent and staff behavior, previous child medical experience, and maternal anxiety as they relate to child procedural distress and coping. J Pediatr Psychol 1995;20:277–89.
40. Smith RW, Shah V, Goldman RD, et al. Caregivers' responses to pain in their children in the emergency department. Arch Pediatr Adolesc Med 2007;161:578–82.
41. Krauss BS, Calligaris L, Green SM, et al. Current concepts in management of pain in children in the emergency department. Lancet 2016;387:83–92.
42. Uman LS, Birnie KA, Noel M, et al. Psychological interventions for needle-related procedural pain and distress in children and adolescents. Cochrane Database Syst Rev 2013;10:CD005179.
43. Thrane SE, Wanless S, Cohen SM, et al. The assessment and non-pharmacologic treatment of procedural pain from infancy to school age through a developmental lens: a synthesis of evidence with recommendations. J Pediatr Nurs 2016;31(1): e23–32.
44. Weiss KE, Dahlquist LM, Wohlheiter K. The effects of interactive and passive distraction on cold pressor pain in preschool-aged children. J Pediatr Psychol 2011;36:816–26.
45. Sinha M, Christopher NC, Fenn R, et al. Evaluation of nonpharmacologic methods of pain and anxiety management for laceration repair in the pediatric emergency department. Pediatrics 2006;117(4):1162–8.
46. Gershon J, Zimand E, Pickering M, et al. A pilot and feasibility study of virtual reality as a distraction for children with cancer. J Am Acad Child Adolesc Psychiatry 2004;43:1243–9.

47. Johnston C, Campbell-Yeo M, Disher T, et al. Skin-to-skin care for procedural pain in neonates. Cochrane Database Syst Rev 2017;2:CD008435.
48. Fearon I, Kisilevsky B, Hains SMJ, et al. Swaddling after heel lance: age-specific effects on behavioral recovery in preterm infants. J Dev Behav Pediatr 1997;18: 222–32.
49. Ali S, McGrath T, Drendel AL. An evidence-based approach to minimizing acute procedural pain in the emergency department and beyond. Pediatr Emer Care 2016;32:36–45.
50. Zempsky WT, Cravero JP. The committee on pediatric emergency medicine and section on anesthesiology and pain medicine: relief of pain and anxiety in pediatric patients in emergency medical systems. Pediatrics 2004;114:1248–354.
51. Gray L, Garza E, Zageris D, et al. Sucrose and warmth for analgesia in healthy newborns: an RCT. Pediatrics 2015;135(30):e607–14.
52. Shah PS, Herbozo C, Aliwalas LL, et al. Breastfeeding or breast milk for procedural pain in neonates. Cochrane Database Syst Rev 2012;12:CD004950.
53. Pillai Riddell RR, Racine NM, Gennis HG, et al. Non-pharmacological management of infant and young child procedural pain. Cochrane Database Syst Rev 2015;12:CD006275.
54. Fernandes A, Campbell-Eo M, Johnston C. Procedural pain management for neonates using nonpharmacological strategies. Adv Neonatal Care 2011;11(4):235–41.
55. WHO guidelines on the pharmacological treatment of persisting pain in children with medical illnesses. Geneva (Switzerland): World Health Organization; 2012. Available at: http://www.who.int/medicines/areas/quality_safety/guide_perspainchild/en/. Accessed January 23, 2018.
56. Chiaretti A, Pierri F, Valantini P, et al. Current practice and recent advances in pediatric pain management. Eur Rev Med Pharmacol Sci 2013;17:112–26.
57. Shastri N. Intravenous acetaminophen use in pediatrics. Pediatr Emerg Care 2015;31:444–8.
58. Balestracci A, Ezquer M, Elmo ME, et al. Ibuprofen-associated acute kidney injury in dehydrated children with acute gastroenteritis. Pediatr Nephrol 2015; 30:1873–8.
59. Murphy A, O'Sullivan R, Wakai A, et al. Intranasal fentanyl for the management of acute pain in children. Cochrane Database Syst Rev 2014;10:CD009942.
60. Mudd S. Intranasal fentanyl for pain management in children: a systematic review of the literature. J Pediatr Health Care 2011;25:316–22.
61. Saunders M, Adelgais K, Nelson D. Use of intranasal fentanyl for the relief of pediatric orthopedic trauma pain. Acad Emerg Med 2010;17:1155–61.
62. Borland M, Jacobs I, King B, et al. A randomized controlled trial comparing intranasal fentanyl to intravenous morphine for managing acute pain in children in the emergency department. Ann Emerg Med 2007;49(3):335–40.
63. Schaefer JA, Mlekoday TJ. Time to opioid administration after implementation of an intranasal fentanyl protocol. Am J Emerg Med 2015;33:1805–7.
64. Schacherer NM, Ramirez DE, Frazier SB, et al. Expedited delivery of pain medication for long-bone fractures using an intranasal fentanyl clinical pathway. Pediatr Emerg Care 2015;31:560–3.
65. Lunoe MM, Drendel AL, Levas MN, et al. A randomized controlled trial of jet-injected lidocaine to reduce venipuncture pain for young children. Ann Emerg Med 2015;66:466–74.
66. Ferayorni A, Yniguez R, Bryson M, et al. Needle-free jet injection of lidocaine for local anesthesia during lumbar puncture: a randomized controlled trial. Pediatr Emerg Care 2012;28:687–90.

67. Baxter AL, Cohen LL, McElvery HL, et al. An integration of vibration and cold relieves venipuncture pain in a pediatric emergency department. Ped Emerg Care 2011;27:1151–6.

68. Massaro M, Ronfani L, Ferrara G, et al. A comparison of three scales for measuring pain in children with cognitive impairment. Acta Paediatr 2014; 103(11):e495–500.

69. Breau LM, Camfield CS, McGrath PJ, et al. The incidence of pain in children with severe cognitive impairments. Arch Pediatr Adolesc Med 2003;157:1219–26.

70. McLean SA, Maio RF, Domeier RM. The epidemiology of pain in the prehospital setting. Prehosp Emerg Care 2002;6:402–5.

71. Swor R, McEachin CM, Seguin D, et al. Prehospital pain management in children suffering traumatic injury. Prehosp Emerg Care 2005;9:40–3.

72. Abbuhl FB, Reed DB. Time to analgesia for patients with painful extremity injuries transported to the emergency department by ambulance. Prehosp Emerg Care 2003;7:445–7.

73. Gausche-Hill M, Brown KM, Oliver ZJ, et al. An evidence-based guideline for prehospital analgesia in trauma. Prehosp Emerg Care 2014;18(Suppl 1):25–34.

74. Iyer SB, Schubert CJ, Schoettker PJ, et al. Use of quality-improvement methods to improve timeliness of analgesic delivery. Pediatrics 2011;127(1):e219–25.

75. Sherman JM, Sheppard P, Hoppa E, et al. Let us use LET: a quality improvement initiative. Pediatr Emer Care 2016;32:440–3.

76. Kavanagh PL, Sprinz PG, Wolfgang TL, et al. Improving the management of vaso-occlusive episodes in the pediatric emergency department. Pediatrics 2015;136: e1016.

77. Sills MR, Fairclough DL, Ranade D, et al. Emergency department crowding is associated with decreased quality of analgesia delivery for children with pain related to acute, isolated, long-bone fractures. Acad Emerg Med 2011;18: 1330–8.

78. Boyd RJ, Stuart P. The efficacy of structured assessment and analgesia provision in the paediatric emergency department. Emerg Med J 2005;22:30–2.

79. Campbell P, Dennie M, Dougherty K, et al. Implementation of an ED protocol for pain management at triage at a busy level I trauma center. J Emerg Nurs 2004;30: 431–8.

80. Charney RL, Yan Y, Schootman M, et al. Oxycodone versus codeine for traige pain in children with suspected forearm fracture. Pediatr Emer Care 2008; 24(9):595–600.

81. Caes L, Boerner KE, Chambers CT, et al. A comprehensive categorical and bibliometric analysis of published research articles on pediatric pain from 1975 to 2010. Pain 2016;157:302–13.

82. Emergency Nurses Association. Optimizing the treatment of pain in patients with acute presentations. Available at: http://www.ena.org/docs/default-source/resource-library/practice-resources/position-statements/joint-statements/optimizing treatmentpainacute.pdf?sfvrsn=44291be8_6. Accessed January 10, 2017.

83. American Academy of Emergency Medicine. Model emergency department pain treatment guidelines. Available at: http://www.aaem.org/publications/news-releases/model-emergency-department-pain-treatment-guidelines. Accessed January 10, 2017.

What to Do when Babies Turn Blue

Beyond the Basic Brief Resolved Unexplained Event

Anna McFarlin, MD*

KEYWORDS

- Brief resolved unexplained event (BRUE) • Apparent life-threatening event (ALTE)
- Apnea • Gastroesophageal reflux (GER) • Nonaccidental trauma • Pertussis
- Respiratory syncytial virus (RSV)

KEY POINTS

- Infants who meet low-risk brief resolved unexplained event classification criteria can be briefly observed in the emergency department and discharged after caregiver reassurance and education.
- Infants who demonstrate historical or physical examination elements suggestive of a specific etiology of their event, such as gastroesophageal reflux or trauma, should be evaluated and treated accordingly.
- Patients who demonstrate no specific historical or physical examination clues yet who are high risk should be evaluated for the most common etiologies of apneic events and admitted.

INTRODUCTION

A perceived near death event of an infant is a frightening experience for parents, frequently triggering a visit to the emergency department. Often, on arrival, the baby is well-appearing without any evident cause for the event. This presentation can leave the provider aimless with regard to direction of work-up and the parent dissatisfied with answers regarding the cause of the event. Over the years, many strategies have been developed to assist the provider in the evaluation of these patients.

The term "apparent life-threatening event" (ALTE) was coined in 1986. Before this, these events were categorized as "near-miss sudden infant death syndrome (SIDS)." Once it was discovered that these patients with near-miss events were not actually at increased risk of SIDS, the verbiage was changed to ALTE. Although this change may seem like semantics, the goal was to further define these events and thus aid the

Disclosure Statement: The author has nothing to disclose.
Combined Emergency Medicine-Pediatrics Residency, Children's Hospital of New Orleans, Louisiana State University Health Science Center, 200 Henry Clay Avenue, New Orleans, LA 70118, USA
* 200 Henry Clay Avenue, New Orleans, LA 70118.
E-mail address: amcfar@lsuhsc.edu

Emerg Med Clin N Am 36 (2018) 335–347
https://doi.org/10.1016/j.emc.2017.12.001
emed.theclinics.com

physician to focus the evaluation of these infants. An ALTE was defined as an episode that is frightening to the observer and that is characterized by some combination of apnea (central or obstructive), color change (usually cyanotic or pallid but occasionally erythematous or plethoric), marked change in muscle tone (usually marked limpness), choking, or gagging.

Although ALTE was a vast improvement on near-miss SIDS, it remained imperfect. The ALTE categorization remained subjective and imprecise. Infants who fit the criteria for ALTE are a heterogeneous group that can include both babies who are asymptomatic and those with ongoing symptoms and an abnormal examination. Symptoms concerning to the caregiver, and thus fitting definition of ALTE, can represent simple normal neonatal behaviors such as periodic breathing. Furthermore, by including "life-threatening" in the name, the diagnosis of ALTE can increase parental anxiety when not warranted. Additionally, the increased parental anxiety and perceived risk often compelled physicians to order testing and admission, subjecting the baby to unnecessary testing without addressing actual diagnosable and/or treatable conditions or preventing any future events.[1]

In an effort to further categorize these infants, in 2016 an American Academy of Pediatrics Task Force coined the term "brief resolved unexplained event" (BRUE) to replace the diagnosis ALTE. The goal was to further refine the diagnosis, better assessing the risk of an underlying serious disorder, and providing actual evidence-based recommendations on the management of low-risk infants.

By narrowing the definition of BRUE, a more homogenous patient population is created. This classification allows more specific recommendations for management as well as future study of these patients. It also emphasizes the typical nature of the event by using words such as "brief" and "resolved," hopefully reassuring the parents. However, it also excludes many infants brought to the emergency department for apneic or frightening episodes. Although BRUE has given providers specific guidelines with regard to low-risk infants, it does not attempt to address the evaluation of an infant with such an episode not meeting BRUE classification or meeting a high-risk stratification. Thus, in the absence of evidence-based guidelines, providers may again feel obligated to order aimless workups and admission. This article defines and reviews the most recent BRUE guidelines. Additionally, it attempts to provide some guidance to the provider for patients who fall outside of the low-risk BRUE population. **Fig. 1** outlines a clinical pathway for an infant who presents after such an event.

WHAT IS A BRIEF RESOLVED UNEXPLAINED EVENT?

The clinical practice guidelines that define BRUE focus the event characteristics more specifically. By definition, a BRUE occurs in children younger than 1 year of age. The event must be brief, lasting less than 1 minute. The event should be perceived as life-threatening by the clinician rather than caregiver. The event must also be resolved. Although this definition clearly means that the patient cannot currently be cyanotic or hypotonic, the authors go so far as to say that the patient must be completely asymptomatic on presentation with a completely normal examination, normal vital signs, and a reassuring history. The qualifying event must be unexplained, without any suggestion of causation. For example, infants with fever or nasal congestion on examination may suggest temporary airway obstruction from viral infection. A history of choking or gagging suggests reflux. These common scenarios, even if associated with apnea, would therefore not fall under definition of BRUE, because they have some explanation of cause.

The event should include 1 or more of the following characteristics.

- Cyanosis or pallor. This specifically excludes redness, because it is a common phenomenon in healthy infants when crying, straining, or coughing.

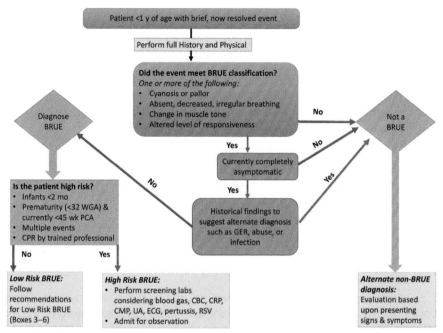

Fig. 1. Clinical pathway for the evaluation of a brief resolved event. BRUE, brief resolved unexplained event; CBC, complete blood count; CMP, complete metabolic panel; CPR, cardiopulmonary resuscitation; CRP, C-reactive protein; ECG, electrocardiogram; GER, gastroesophageal reflux; PCA, postconceptual age; RSV, respiratory syncytial virus; UA, urinalysis; WGA, weeks gestational age.

- Absent, decreased, or irregular breathing.
- A marked change in muscle tone encompassing either hypertonia or hypotonia.
- An altered level of responsiveness.

Although these criteria are similar to the description used to define ALTE, there are significant differences (**Table 1**).

Once an event has been characterized as a BRUE, the provider's attention should be on obtaining a focused history and physical examination followed by risk stratification. The aim of the latest guidelines emphasizes the use of clinical clues to tease out a more precise etiology of the event. The provider should clarify events occurring before, during, and after the event, including infant location, position, and activity. Patients at higher risk would include those infants less than 2 month old, those who are premature (<32 weeks gestational age) and currently less than 45 weeks postconceptual age, those who have had recurrent events, and those who required cardiopulmonary resuscitation by trained medical professional (**Box 1**). See **Box 2** for a differential of apneic events that should be considered when obtaining a history. A further discussion of each of these elements can be found inthe second part of this review Beyond the BRUE.

DISPOSITION AND MANAGEMENT OF THE LOW-RISK INFANT

By narrowing the definition of a BRUE and specifically characterizing a subset of low-risk patients, the BRUE clinical practice guidelines were able to offer specific

Table 1
Characteristics of ALTE and BRUE

	ALTE	BRUE
Color	Any change in color (cyanosis, pallor, erythematous, plethoric)	Cyanosis or pallor
Breathing	Apnea (central or obstructive)	Absent, decreased, or irregular
Tone	Change in tone, choking or gagging	Change in tone (hypertonia or hypotonia) Choking or gagging specifically excluded
Level of responsiveness	Not mentioned	Altered, now at baseline
Assessment of threat	Frightening to the observer	Concerning to provider
Age	No age restriction	<1 y
Duration	Not specified	<1 min

Abbreviations: ALTE, apparent life-threatening event; BRUE, brief resolved unexplained event.

recommendations on this more homogeneous population. They have been split into specific "do not," "need not," "may," and "should" recommendations, which are listed in **Boxes 3–6**, respectively. Further discussion regarding each of these elements can be found in the original clinical practice guidelines.[1] Essentially infants who are diagnosed with a low-risk BRUE require no testing. A brief period of observation with continuous pulse oximetry followed by thorough caregiver education is sufficient. These patients can be safely discharged home with close pediatrician follow-up (within 24 hours). Home apnea monitors are not necessary for discharge because they have never been shown to improve outcomes, are prone to artifact and false alarms, and serve to increase caregiver anxiety and disrupt sleep.

Patients who have episodes that meet the BRUE classification but that are categorized as high risk should likely have further testing and be observed or admitted. These high-risk patients and infants with events that fall outside of the BRUE definition should have relevant testing directed toward their specific symptoms.

BEYOND THE BRIEF RESOLVED UNEXPLAINED EVENT

Although the new BRUE guidelines have given clinicians clear guidance regarding the evaluation, management, and disposition of infants wit low-risk BRUEs, many infants present to the emergency department after an episode that falls outside of the categorization of a low-risk BRUE. Management recommendations as outlined do not

Box 1
High-risk criteria for brief resolved unexplained event

- Infants less than 2 months old
- Infants who are premature (<32 weeks gestational age) and currently less than 45 weeks post conceptual age
- Infants who have had multiple events
- Cardiopulmonary resuscitation by trained medical professional

---

Box 2
Differential diagnosis of apneic events

Child Abuse (particularly intracranial injury)

Cardiopulmonary problems (channelopathies)

Obstructive sleep apnea or central apnea

Gastroesophageal reflux

Serious bacterial illness

Seizures

Respiratory infections (bronchiolitis, pertussis)

Inborn errors of metabolism

Facial or airway dysmorphisms

---

apply in these circumstances. Without clear guidance, the provider may be tempted to order unnecessary testing and admission. The remainder of this article attempts to address the most common causes of apneic episodes or other events that would previously have been categorized as an ALTE, historical and physical elements suggestive of a specific diagnosis, and the appropriate evaluation and management of each of these etiologies.

Gastroesophageal Reflux

Gastroesophageal reflux (GER) is incredibly common, occurring in more than two-thirds of infants. It has been demonstrated to cause apnea and hypoxia related to obstruction, laryngospasm, and aspiration. Before the advent of BRUE, GER was considered the most common etiology of ALTE, attributed in 20% to 54% of patients.[2] Although choking after spitting up is not considered a BRUE, it is consistent with GER and GER management should be initiated, including parental education, guidance, and support.

Box 3
Low-risk brief resolved unexplained event

- Do not admit solely for cardiorespiratory monitoring.
- Do not obtain a blood gas, complete blood count, blood culture, metabolic panel, or cerebrospinal fluid analysis.
- Do not obtain a chest radiograph or neuroimaging (computed tomography scan, ultrasound examination, MRI).
- Do not obtain an echocardiogram.
- Do not obtain an overnight polysomnography (sleep study).
- Do not obtain an electroencephalogram.
- Do not prescribe antiepileptic medications.
- Do not order testing for gastroesophageal reflux (pH probe, upper gastrointestinal series, endoscopy).
- Do not order acid suppression therapy.
- Do not obtain ammonia, urine organic acids, plasma amino acids, or plasma acylcarnitines to detect an inborn error of metabolism.

Box 4
Low-risk brief resolved unexplained event

- Clinicians need not obtain a urinalysis.
- Clinicians need not obtain respiratory viral testing.
- Clinicians need not obtain serum lactic acid, bicarbonate, or glucose to detect an inborn error of metabolism.

The clinical characteristics of an event suggestive of GER include choking, gasping, coughing, vomiting, or gagging. Parents often note recent feeding or milk seen in the infant's nose. If apneic, these infants generally demonstrate an obstructive apnea or very brief central apnea, never ceasing their effort to breathe for long periods. Caregivers often describe that the infant turns red and seems to be struggling to breathe. Other symptoms supportive of a diagnosis of GER include irritability, poor weight gain, and arching of the back. Careful consideration is necessary when attributing an ALTE or BRUE to GER owing to its prevalence in all infants, not just those who have experienced an event.[3]

Although many different types of testing for reflux are available, the results are frequently nondiagnostic and fail to change management of the patient. The North American Society for Pediatric Gastroenterology, Hepatology and Nutrition guidelines do not support invasive testing for a diagnosis of GER disease.[4,5] If done, studies such as a pH probe, upper gastrointestinal series, ultrasound examination, or barium swallow are inadequate to rule out pathologic reflux or to differentiate between physiologic and pathologic reflux. Similarly, a positive study cannot definitively explain BRUE and ALTE symptoms given the high prevalence of GER in the infant population; GER may be coexistent and not causative. ALTE secondary to GER is essentially a clinical diagnosis. Doshi and colleagues[2] demonstrated a high concordance (96%) with a preadmission working diagnosis of GER and discharge diagnosis of GER in patients admitted for ALTE. For these reasons, infants who were previously admitted for ALTE rarely underwent testing for GER, even when suspected.

Management is focused on caregiver education and lifestyle modifications. Patients with a history of ALTE ultimately diagnosed with GER as the causative pathology often return after subsequent events. This pattern underscores the importance of education with a greater emphasis on the natural history of GER, the likelihood of recurrent events, and when to seek medical attention.[1] Parents should be counseled that the incidence of GER peaks at about 4 months of life and typically resolves completely by 12 months.

Recommendations include avoidance of overfeeding. Newborns typically begin feeding 2 to 3 ounces every 2 to 3 hours. Thereafter, most babies are satisfied with 3 to 4 ounces per feeding approximately every 4 hours increasing the amount by 1 ounce per month until they reach a maximum of about 7 to 8 ounces.[6] Caregivers should frequently burp the infant during feeding (every 3–5 min). Secondhand smoke

---

Box 5
Low-risk brief resolved unexplained event

- Clinicians may obtain testing for pertussis.
- Clinicians may obtain an electrocardiogram.

Box 6
Low-risk brief resolved unexplained event

- Clinicians should monitor the infant for 1 to 4 hours in the emergency department with continuous pulse oximetry and serial observations ensuring that vital signs, physical examination, and symptomatology remain stable.
- Clinicians should assess social risk factors to detect child abuse.
- Clinicians should offer resources for CPR training.
  - CPR training has not been shown to increase caregiver anxiety and in fact gives them a sense of empowerment.
  - AAP policy statement on CPR recommends that pediatricians advocate for life support training for all caregivers. As such, this is a perfect opportunity.
- Clinicians should educate caregivers about brief resolved unexplained events.

Abbreviation: CPR, cardiopulmonary resuscitation.
From Tieder J, Bonkowsky J, Etzel R, et al. Brief resolved unexplained events (formerly apparent life-threatening events) and evaluation of lower-risk infants. Pediatrics 2016;137(5):e1–32.

---

should be avoided. Infants who breastfeed have been reported to have fewer incidences of GER.

Infant positioning seems to greatly affect the severity of GER. Caregivers should maintain the infant in an upright position in their arms after feeding (up to 30 min after feeding). In contrast, it has been demonstrated that a semiupright position such as an infant car seat actually exacerbates reflux and thus should be discouraged. Prone positioning has been demonstrated to reduce GER. This is somewhat problematic because infants must not be left prone unsupervised owing to the risk of SIDS. However, prone positioning is acceptable if the infant is observed and awake, particularly in the postprandial period.[7]

Thickening the feeds is commonly recommended to parents of infants with GER. It does not seem to alter esophageal acid exposure or total reflux frequency by pH study.[5] However, the use of a thickened formula may result in fewer visible episodes of reflux and thus may theoretically be helpful in decreasing the incidence of apnea. There are commercially available formulas marketed as antireflux (ie, Enfamil AR). Alternatively, parents may choose to add a thickener, typically rice cereal or oatmeal, to the formula. In response to concerns over arsenic in rice, in 2016 the American Academy of Pediatrics recommended that parents of infants with GER use oatmeal instead of rice cereal.[8] Generally adding 1 tablespoon per 4 to 5 ounces is a reasonable place to start slowly increasing to a maximum of 1 tablespoon per 1 ounce. The provider should remember than adding cereal to formula will considerably increase the caloric density of the formula, resulting in possible excessive energy intake.

A possible cause of frequent vomiting or irritability in infants indistinguishable from that associated with physiologic GER is milk protein sensitivity.[5] Although the emergency provider may defer to the pediatrician to address this possibility, if comfortable and other lifestyle modifications have failed, a 2- to 4-week trial of an extensively hydrolyzed formula may be suggested (ie, Neutramingen or Alimentum). Similarly, in breastfed infants, a 2- to 4-week trial of a maternal exclusion diet that restricts at least milk and egg is recommended.[7] It is important to note that this recommendation is limited to the symptomatic infant, not the "happy spitter."[7]

Last, multiple pharmacologic agents are available to treat GER disease. Although trials have demonstrated a decrease in gastric acid with H2 blockers, no trials have definitively demonstrated reduction in number of apneic events or ALTEs or irritability with acid suppression.[5] No proton pump inhibitor has been approved for use in infants younger than 1 year of age. Additionally, all acid suppressants, whether H2 blockers or proton pump inhibitors, are associated with a number of potential harmful effects in infants, including lower respiratory tract infections, gastroenteritis, candidemia, and necrotizing enterocolitis in preterm infants. Therefore, at this time, there is no role for the initiation of acid suppression in the emergency department for BRUE-, ALTE-, or irritability-associated GER.

In summary, GER is a common cause of choking, gasping, or brief apneic episodes. GER does not require hospitalization for diagnosis or initiation of therapy. The emergency provider should focus on caregiver reassurance and counseling regarding lifestyle modifications.

Nonaccidental Trauma and Child Abuse

Child abuse has been described as a cause of apneic events and ALTE. This diagnosis is often very difficult to make; the history may be misleading and subtle presentations are often missed. Studies have attributed 1% to 11% of all ALTEs to nonaccidental head trauma and, in 1 study, up to 33% of these abused infants with ALTE died.[9–11] One study examining the medical records of 81 infant victims who died of child abuse demonstrated that 75 of them (93%) had a prior history of unusual or unexplained events, most commonly apnea, cyanosis, appearing dazed, or twitching.[12] Another study reports that of all children in their study with abusive head trauma, 31% of them had been seen previously for vague symptoms, misdiagnosed, and discharged.[13] Therefore, a high index of suspicion must be maintained when evaluating children with an ALTE or BRUE.

It is imperative to consider nonaccidental trauma when evaluating an infant who presents after an ALTE or BRUE. Historical elements concerning for child abuse include a developmentally inconsistent history given, a history that is confusing or changing, a delay in care, previous ALTE or BRUE presentations, previous calls to emergency medical services, vomiting, irritability, seizures, bleeding from the nose or mouth, bruising, petechiae, subconjunctival hemorrhage, retinal hemorrhage, a large and full or bulging anterior fontanelle, scalp hematoma or bogginess, head circumference greater than the 95th percentile, a history of rapid head enlargement, oropharynx or frenula damage, and families with a history of a previous ALTE or SIDS.[1,11,14,15]

Brain neuroimaging is indicated in patients with concerning historical or physical findings for child abuse. One might also consider ophthalmologic consultation for evaluation of possible retinal hemorrhages (pathognomonic of intracranial injury) and a skeletal survey with particular attention paid to the ribs.[3,16] Retinal examinations may detect 33% to 60% of head trauma; skeletal surveys may detect 14% of physical abuse.[3] Laboratory findings are not often helpful in identifying infants who have suffered child abuse but, once a head injury concerning for abuse has been identified, further testing is required to identify any other injury. Further laboratory analyses, including a complete blood count, metabolic panel, liver function tests, pancreatic enzymes (amylase and lipase), coagulation studies (prothrombin time, partial thromboplastin time), and a urinalysis, are recommended. Social services and child protection must be notified.

Infants without any concerning findings for nonaccidental trauma and therefore at low risk have a less than 0.3% incidence of abusive head trauma noted on imaging. Although missing abusive head trauma can have significant morbidity and mortality, the yield of imaging all infants is low and is not recommended.[1]

Although head injury is the most commonly described abusive injury presenting as an ALTE, one must also consider other nonaccidental injuries, including intentional intoxication (alcohol or other substances) and intentional suffocation or smothering.

Respiratory Tract Infections

Roughly 8% of ALTEs have been attributed to lower respiratory tract infections. The most commonly cited pathogens are the respiratory syncytial virus (RSV) and pertussis. Authors report an incidence of apnea in 8% to 25% of infants with RSV infection.[1,17] The percentage of infants with apnea and cyanosis was even higher in infants with pertussis than in those with RSV (52.6% vs 10.5%).[18] One study reports an 11-fold increased risk of extreme events in infants with symptoms of a respiratory tract infection (extreme event was defined as apnea for >30 seconds, an SpO_2 of ≤80%, or bradycardia of <60 bpm for ≥10 seconds).[19] Viral infections other than RSV can also lead to prolonged apnea and low oxygenation. Wishaupt and colleagues[17] observed apneas irrespective of the isolated microorganism and hypothesized that they were related to the pathophysiology of the respiratory infection and not to the microorganism itself. Specifically, Ralston and Hill[20] found no significant difference in the rates of apnea with RSV versus influenza or rhinovirus.

The mechanisms remain unclear, but apneas associated with respiratory tract infections have been described as obstructive, central, or mixed. Because infants are obligate nasal breathers, excessive mucus production or plugging may cause obstructive apnea. In contrast, central apnea may be related to autonomic dysfunction, the inflammatory cascade, or immaturity of the brainstem respiratory center.[17,21] Activation of the laryngeal chemoreceptors by inflammatory cytokines can lead to a respiratory pause. This reflex apnea can be prolonged and even fatal.[17,19]

Risk factors for apnea in bronchiolitis are prematurity (postconceptual age of <48 weeks), young postnatal age (<2 months), comorbidity, a history of apnea of prematurity, and a history of previous apnea or cyanosis.[17,19,21] Comorbid conditions include conditions of the respiratory tract, especially anatomic variants, and neurologic disorders that impair muscular strength and/or respiratory regulation by the central nervous system.[20] Although the risk of developing apnea is higher in these risk groups, it must be stressed that healthy infants can also develop apnea with RSV and other respiratory pathogens.[22] The risk of apnea is greatest in the first 3 to 5 days of infection.[23]

The provider should consider respiratory tract infection as a cause of an ALTE in the setting of fever, cough, coryza, wheezing, tachypnea, hypoxia, and auscultatory changes. Most but not all infants with significant lower respiratory tract infections will be symptomatic at the time of ALTE. Apneas may precede other signs of respiratory infections and paroxysmal desaturations have been documented in patients immediately before signs of a viral illness.[17,23] Pertussis can cause paroxysmal cough. Caregivers may describe gagging, gasping, and color change followed by a respiratory pause. Infants with pertussis can be febrile but otherwise asymptomatic initially.[1]

Various diagnostic modalities are available to providers to evaluate for respiratory infection. The decision to test for pertussis should consider potential exposures, vaccination history (including intrapartum immunization of the mother), and awareness of community pertussis activity. The gold standard for the diagnosis of pertussis is culture obtained from nasal swabs or nasopharyngeal aspirates. However, today real-time polymerase chain reaction analysis is available and, depending on laboratory processing, can return results in just a few hours.[18] A definite diagnosis of pertussis changes management; therefore, testing in infants with suspected pertussis is warranted.

A diagnosis of viral respiratory infection is largely clinical. The most recently published clinical practice guideline regarding bronchiolitis emphasizes that clinicians should diagnose bronchiolitis and assess disease severity on the basis of history and physical examination alone; radiographic or laboratory studies should not be obtained routinely.[24] In the patient with clinical signs of bronchiolitis who presents after an apneic event, polymerase chain reaction testing delineating RSV versus a different viral pathogen does not change clinical management or disposition.

Emergency department management of infants status post an apneic event associated with respiratory tract infection is largely supportive. Excessive mucus production or plugging can be temporarily resolved by rinsing the nose with saline or using suction. Patients should be placed on a continuous pulse oximeter. Hypoxia should be addressed with supplemental oxygen. Increased work of breathing may be relieved with high flow. The routine use of albuterol, epinephrine, corticosteroids, hypertonic saline, or empiric antibiotics is not recommended.

All infants with known pertussis, RSV, or bronchiolitis who present with apnea should be admitted for observational monitoring. Respiratory tract infection symptoms with apnea at presentation is an independent risk factor for recurrent ALTE.[25] In fact, clinicians may consider routinely admitting RSV and pertussis infected infants younger than 1 month of age, regardless of clinical findings owing to the high risk of apnea.

Other Serious Bacterial Infections

In rare instances, ALTE can be a presenting complaint of invasive infections such as meningitis, bacteremia, urinary tract infection, and pneumonia. These infants typically seem to be ill or are febrile on presentation, disqualifying their event as a BRUE. In today's post–*Haemophilus influenzae* type B and pneumococcal conjugate vaccine environment, the low-risk, well-appearing infant is exceedingly unlikely to have a serious occult infection. However, urinary tract infections remain a cause of ALTE detected in 2% to 8% of infants.[26,27] This risk is highest in infants less than 2 months of age. Clinical signs worrisome for serious bacterial infections include fever, hypothermia, lethargy, and poor feeding. One study evaluating the risk of serious bacterial illness in infants less than 2 months after an ALTE found that 4 of 182 infants (2.2%) less than 60 days of age had bacteremia or a urinary tract infection. Of these infants, all had multiple events the day of presentation. They were more likely to be premature and hypothermic.[26] These infants would all be considered high risk and therefore not merit low-risk BRUE recommendations. Another study demonstrated no serious bacterial infection in their patient population (0/198). Two infants in this study were diagnosed with enteroviral meningitis. Both of these infants were ill-appearing on examination where one was febrile and the other had seizures and multiple apneic events.[27] A septic evaluation, including a complete blood count, blood culture, urinalysis, and urine culture, is recommended in infants less than 60 days of age with a history of prematurity, an ill appearance, symptoms suggestive of bacterial illness, or multiple events.

Seizures and Breath Holding Spells

Seizures have been shown to occur in 4% to 7% of infants with an ALTE. Clinical features of an ALTE ultimately attributed to seizures would include loss of consciousness, choking, staring, eye deviation, eye fluttering, twitching or convulsions, hypotonia or hypertonia (stiffening), microcephaly or macrocephaly, or other dysmorphic features. Hewertson and colleagues[28] described tachycardia as an additional specific finding in ALTE secondary to seizures rather than bradycardia, which is associated with other causes of ALTE. Seizures in this age group can be the initial presentation of epilepsy or a symptom of a more sinister underlying cause, including trauma, infection, or a metabolic pathology. In a young infant suspected of having a seizure, it is prudent to perform a full evaluation, including a full septic evaluation, neuroimaging, electroencephalography, and neurologic consultation. In patients without concern for seizure, there is no need for neuroimaging, electroencephalography, or empiric antiepileptic medications.

In older infants, breath holding spells may cause apnea. This spell is a reflex typically triggered by a provoking event such as frustration, surprise, anger, or fear. The patient then usually cries followed by a pause, at which time they become pale or blue, and if severe, lose consciousness and become limp. These events are self-limiting and not dangerous. Treatment consists of reassurance and caregiver education. Breath holding spells can begin as early as 6 months of age and are outgrown by midchildhood.

Other Causes of Apparent Life-Threatening Events

Multiple other processes have been implicated in an ALTE. Cardiac conditions that may present as an ALTE include arrhythmias (supraventricular tachycardia), ventricular preexcitation (Wolff-Parkinson-White syndrome), channelopathies (long QT syndrome, Brugada syndrome), and myocarditis or cardiomyopathy (hypertrophic cardiomyopathy, dilated cardiomyopathy). The clinician should consider a cardiac etiology in infants with family history of sudden unexplained deaths in first-degree relatives, diaphoresis, difficulties with feeding, or cyanosis. Clinicians can screen with an electrocardiogram. If the infant has an abnormal electrocardiogram or concerning findings on history and physical examination, one might order an echocardiogram.

Risk factors for obstructive sleep apnea in infants include prematurity, maternal smoking, bronchopulmonary dysplasia, obesity, and craniofacial abnormalities, including laryngomalacia, micrognathia, neuromuscular weakness, Down syndrome, achondroplasia, Chiari malformations, and Prader-Willi syndrome.[1] These patients may have a normal examination or may present with stridor or a history of feeding difficulties. Although the yield is low for low-risk infants with a BRUE and is generally poorly predictive of ALTE recurrence, patients at risk of obstructive sleep apnea may benefit from overnight polysomnography (sleep study).

Last, inborn errors of metabolism have been implicated in up to 5% of ALTEs, most commonly fatty acid oxidation and urea cycle disorders. These conditions are rare but potentially devastating and can present with vague, nonspecific symptoms. Clinicians should evaluate for abnormal growth parameters, a family history of inborn errors of metabolism, developmental disabilities, or SIDS. These infants may demonstrate prolonged or multiple events that can be associated with seizures. They are often still symptomatic on arrival. For infants with symptoms concerning for inborn errors of metabolism, the provider should obtain the patient's newborn screen results, serum lactate (>3 mmol/L clinically significant), metabolic panel specifically with bicarbonate (<20 mmol/L significant), ammonia, and a urinalysis. Other metabolic problems that may be implicated in ALTE include thyroid dysfunction, hypoglycemia, or hypocalcemia (especially with known history of vitamin D deficiency or hypoparathyroidism).

EVALUATION AND DISPOSITION OF THE HIGH-RISK BRIEF RESOLVED UNEXPLAINED EVENT

Most infants who have had a BRUE or ALTE will either be categorized as low risk (and therefore require no work-up or admission) or will have clinical clues that lead the provider to the appropriate evaluation as outlined. However, a small subsection who are high risk by age, prematurity, or recurrence will have an event that cannot be diagnosed easily. In these cases, it is prudent to obtain a blood gas, complete blood count with differential, C-reactive protein, metabolic panel, urinalysis, electrocardiogram, and assessment for pertussis and RSV. Inpatient observation for 24 to 72 hours with a pulse oximeter or cardiorespiratory monitor, ideally a monitor with memory capability, is recommended. The clinician may also consider ammonia, lactate, blood culture, toxicology screen, electroencephalogram, and brain imaging. These basic tests may be helpful in selecting high-risk infants to screen for underlying infection, trauma, pulmonary disease, control of breathing disorders, and inborn errors of metabolism.

SUMMARY

A perceived near death or apneic episode in an infant is a frightening event for both parents, and perhaps provider. The differential diagnosis is broad and includes both benign and life-threatening etiologies. Therefore, these infants often undergo thorough shot-gun work-ups including extensive laboratory tests, images, and admission. Although admitting patients with an ALTE can facilitate further diagnostic testing for an underlying cause, typical hospital charges for an ALTE admission were $15,567.[3] The most recent BRUE guidelines, in part, outline a selection of low-risk infants who can be safely discharged home without extensive testing and admission. Furthermore, these guidelines encourage providers to use a thorough history and physical examination to narrow their diagnostic testing and treat according to likely underlying pathology.

REFERENCES

1. Tieder J, Bonkowsky J, Etzel R, et al. Brief resolved unexplained events (formerly apparent life-threatening events) and evaluation of lower-risk infants. Pediatrics 2016;137(5):e1–32.
2. Doshi A, Bernard-Stover L, Kuelbs C, et al. Apparent life-threatening event admissions and gastroesophageal reflux disease. Pediatr Emerg Care 2012;28: 17–21.
3. Fu L, Moon R. Apparent life-threatening events: an update. Pediatr Rev 2012; 33(8):361–9.
4. Rudolph C, Mazure L, Liptak G, et al. Guidelines for evaluation and treatment of gastroesophageal reflux in infants and children: recommendations of the North American Society for Pediatric Gastroenterology and Nutrition. J Pediatr Gastroenterol Nutr 2001;32(suppl 2):S1–31.
5. Vandenplas Y, Rudolph C, Di Lorenzo C, et al. Pediatric gastroesophageal reflux clinical practice guidelines: joint recommendations of the North American Society for Pediatric Gastroenterology, Hepatology, and Nutrition (NASPGHAN) and the European Society for Pediatric Gastroenterology, Hepatology and Nutrition (ESPGHAN). J Pediatr Gastroenterol Nutr 2009;49(4):498–547.
6. Shelov S, editor. Caring for your baby and young child: birth to age 5. New York: Bantam Books, American Academy of Pediatrics; 2009.
7. Lightdale J, Gremse D. Gastroesophageal reflux: management guidance for the pediatrician. Pediatrics 2013;131(5):e1688–95.
8. Oatmeal: the safer alternative for infants & children who need thicker food. American Academy of Pediatrics; 2016. Available at: healthychildren.org. Accessed February 3, 2018.
9. Altman R, Brand D. Abusive head injury as a cause of apparent life-threatening events in infancy. Arch Pediatr Adolesc Med 2003;157:1011–5.
10. Bonkowsky J, Guenther E, Filloux F, et al. Death, child abuse, and adverse neurologic outcome of infants after an apparent life-threatening event. Pediatrics 2008; 122:125–31.

11. Guenther E, Powers A, Srivastava R, et al. Abusive head trauma in children presenting with an apparent life-threatening event. J Pediatr 2010;157(5):821–5.
12. Meadow R. Unnatural sudden infant death. Arch Dis Child 1999;80:7–14.
13. Jenny C, Hymel K, Ritzen A, et al. Analysis of missed cases of abusive head trauma. JAMA 1999;281:621–6.
14. Parker K, Pitetti R. Mortality and child abuse in children presenting with apparent life-threatening events. Pediatr Emerg Care 2011;27(7):591–5.
15. Vellody K, Freeto J, Gage S, et al. Clues that aid in the diagnosis of nonaccidental trauma presenting as an apparent life-threatening event. Clin Pediatr 2008;47(9): 912–8.
16. Pitetti M, Maffei F, Chang K, et al. Prevalence of retinal hemorrhages and child abuse in children who present with an apparent life-threatening event. Pediatrics 2002;110(3):557–62.
17. Wishaupt J, van den Berg E, van Wijk T, et al. Pediatric apneas are not related to a specific respiratory virus, and parental reports predict hospitalization. Acta Paediatr 2016;105:542–8.
18. Nicolai A, Nenna R, Stefanelli P, et al. Bordetella pertussis in infants hospitalized for acute respiratory symptoms remains a concern. BMC Infect Dis 2013;13: 256–62.
19. Al-Kindy H, Gelinas J, Hatzakis G, et al. Risk factors for extreme events in infants hospitalized for apparent life-threatening events. J Pediatr 2009;154:332–7.
20. Ralston S, Hill V. Incidence of apnea in infants hospitalized with respiratory syncytial virus bronchiolitis: a systematic review. J Pediatr 2009;155(5):728–33.
21. Stock C, Teyssier G, Pichot V. Autonomic dysfunction with early respiratory syncytial virus-related infection. Auton Neurosci 2010;156:90–5.
22. Rayyan M, Naulaers G, Daniels H, et al. Characteristics of respiratory syncytial virus-related apnea in three infants. Acta Paediatr 2004;93:847–9.
23. Arms J, Ortega H, Reid S. Chronological and clinical characteristics of apnea associated with respiratory syncytial virus infection: a retrospective case series. Clin Pediatr 2008;47(9):953–8.
24. Ralston S, Lieberthal A, Meissner H, et al. Clinical practice guideline: the diagnosis, management, and prevention of bronchiolitis. Pediatrics 2014;134(5): e1474–502.
25. Ueda R, Nomura O, Maekawa T, et al. Independent risk factors for recurrence of apparent life-threatening events in infants. Eur J Pediatr 2017;176:443–8.
26. Zuckerbraun N, Zomorrodi A, Pitetti R. Occurrence of serious bacterial infection in infants aged 60 days or younger with an apparent life-threatening event. Pediatr Emerg Care 2009;25(1):19–25.
27. Mittal M, Shofer F, Baren J. Serious bacterial infections in infants who have experienced an apparent life-threatening event. Ann Emerg Med 2009;54(4):523–7.
28. Hewertson J, Poets C, Samuels M, et al. Epileptic seizure-induced hypoxemia in infants with apparent life-threatening events. Pediatrics 1994;94(2):148–56.

Imaging Gently

Amy L. Puchalski, MD*, Christyn Magill, MD

KEYWORDS

• Ionizing radiation • Imaging • Computed tomography (CT) utilization

KEY POINTS

- Ionizing radiation, even at low doses, imparts a small but real risk of malignancy; this impact is greater on pediatric patients. Consider this when deciding to use radiographic studies, such as plain radiography, computed tomography, and fluoroscopy, in pediatric patients.
- Clinical information is vital to the judicious use of radiographic studies.
- Ultrasound and MRI, which do not rely on ionizing radiation, have an increasing role in the evaluation of pediatric patients in the emergency setting.

BACKGROUND

Advances in medical imaging are invaluable in the care of pediatric patients in the emergent setting. The diagnostic accuracy offered by studies using ionizing radiation, such as plain radiography (XR), computed tomography (CT), and fluoroscopy, are not without inherent risks. This article reviews the evidence supporting the risk of ionizing radiation from medical imaging as well as discusses clinical scenarios in which clinicians play an important role in supporting the judicious use of imaging studies.

Biological Effects of Ionizing Radiation

People are exposed to ionizing radiation from a variety of sources. There is natural background exposure, which on average exposes a person living in the United States to 3 mSv per year.[1,2] Additional exposures come from medical imaging, occupational exposure, or industrial accidents. Unfortunately, ionizing radiation causes damage on a cellular level, and evidence supports that it exerts a linear increase in the lifetime cancer risk even at low doses.[2] The energy from ionizing radiation is capable of removing electrons from their atomic orbit, thus, creating ions. Ions either directly damage DNA molecules or cause secondary damage via hydroxyl radicals created from radiated water molecules. Often DNA strands are repaired without consequence; but double-strand breaks or errors in DNA repair can cause permanent alteration in cellular DNA, potentially inducing cancer later in life.[3]

For several reasons, children are more susceptible to the potential increased risk of cancer from ionizing radiation.

Department of Emergency Medicine, Division of Pediatric Emergency Medicine, Carolinas Medical Center, Levine Children's Hospital, 1000 Blythe Boulevard, Charlotte, NC 28203, USA
* Corresponding author.
E-mail address: alpuchalski@gmail.com

Emerg Med Clin N Am 36 (2018) 349–368
https://doi.org/10.1016/j.emc.2017.12.003   emed.theclinics.com
0733-8627/18/© 2017 Elsevier Inc. All rights reserved.

- Actively reproducing tissue is more susceptible to DNA damage.
- A given dose of ionizing radiation is spread over a smaller area in a child, resulting in greater exposure.
- Malignancies have a very long latency; thus, a child has a longer period of life over which to develop a secondary cancer relative to an older adult.

Studies in atomic bomb survivors in Japan after World War II have provided important information in establishing the link between low levels of ionizing radiation exposure and future malignancy.[4,5]

Increasing Utilization of Computed Tomography

There has been a trend toward increased utilization of CT over the last several years, with approximately 62 million performed in 2006, 4 million of which were in children.[3] CT contributes the largest component of medical radiation exposure, accounting for approximately 40% to 67%, though only 5% to 11% of all imaging studies are CT.[2,6]

Evidence of the Role for Computed Tomography Exposure to Future Malignancy

Several studies estimated organ doses as well as estimated lifetime cancer mortality risk per dose of ionizing radiation to determine the potential impact of CT on the future development of malignancy. Brenner and colleagues[7] estimated that for all head CTs done in 1 year on children less than 15 years of age in the United States, 170 deaths from radiation-induced cancer will result. Likewise, 310 deaths may be attributed to all pediatric CTs of the abdomen and pelvis performed each year.[8] Overall, there may be one fatal radiation-induced cancer attributed to every 1000 pediatric CTs. It is important to remember that this only represents less than 0.5% increase to the overall baseline lifetime cancer mortality when balancing the diagnostic value of CT with its risks. Finally, Pearce and colleagues[9] concluded that for each head CT performed in a child less than 10 years old, there could be one extra case of leukemia and one extra brain tumor per 10,000 studies (**Table 1**).

CLINICAL SCENARIOS
Respiratory Illnesses

Respiratory illnesses comprise a significant proportion of the presenting symptoms prompting pediatric patients to seek emergency care. Various clinical guidelines look to reinforce scenarios when exposure to ionizing radiation is not necessary; however, chest XR (CXR) is still performed frequently.[12] **Table 2** summarizes guidelines for CXR utilization, emphasizing that routine CXR is not warranted for bronchiolitis, asthma, or well-appearing, otherwise healthy children with clear signs of pneumonia.

Table 1
Effective radiation doses of imaging studies

Study	Effective Dose (mSv)
Chest XR: Posteroanterior and lateral	0.02–0.1
Pelvis XR	0.6
Cervical spine XR	0.6
Head CT	2–4
Neck CT	3–4
Abdominal/pelvis CT, no contrast	5–8
Chest CT	3–8

Data from[1,3,10,11]

Table 2
Summary of guidelines for chest radiography use in respiratory illness

Clinical Guideline	Pneumonia	Bronchiolitis	Asthma
Source	Pediatric Infectious Diseases Society and the Infectious Diseases Society of America, 2011[13]	American Academy of Pediatrics[14]	National Asthma Education and Prevention Panel[15]
Recommendations	• Children well enough to be treated as outpatients do not routinely require CXR if the provider has clinical suspicion for pneumonia. • Children with hypoxemia or respiratory distress should undergo 2-view CXR. • Admitted patients or those not responding to antibiotic treatment might benefit from CXR to evaluate for complications.	• When bronchiolitis is diagnosed based on history and physical examination, CXR should not be routinely used. • There is no evidence that currently supports its routine use. • CXR should be reserved for those who require ICU admission or in order to evaluate patients with signs of a complication, such as pneumothorax.	• CXR is not needed for routine assessment. • Consider it to evaluate for complications, such as congestive heart failure, pneumothorax, pneumomediastinum, or lobar atelectasis.

Abbreviation: ICU, intensive care unit.

Ultrasound for pneumonia

Ultrasound has a role as an alternative imaging modality in the diagnosis of pneumonia, and its clinical utility is supported in the literature. In 2013, a study compared lung ultrasounds on pediatric patients with clinical suspicion of pneumonia with their CXR.[16] Overall, ultrasound had a sensitivity of 86% and specificity of 89%. The lack of ionizing radiation and ease of use at all experience levels gives this imaging modality great potential for application to the emergency department, outpatient settings, and the developing world.

First time wheezing

Frequently, a CXR is performed on patients presenting with wheezing for the first time solely based on their chief complaint. Several studies show this yields a low percentage of positive results, ranging from 5.7% to 9.0%.[17–19] Generally, those with positive findings have specific clues in their history and physical that would support obtaining a film, including[18,19]

- ↑Heart Rate
- ↑Respiratory Rate
- Localized finding on examination
- Fever
- Saturation less than 95%
- No improvement with inhaled bronchodilators

Selective imaging in first-time wheezing episodes as well as in all asthma exacerbations would certainly yield a decrease in ionizing radiation exposure.

Cervical Spine Trauma

Cervical spine injuries (CSIs) are rare among pediatric victims of blunt trauma, occurring in about 1% of patients, though the significant associated morbidity and mortality often prompts imaging.[20–22] Research to provide guidance on the necessity of

Table 3
Summary of studies assessing need for radiographs in pediatric cervical spine injuries

Study	NEXUS[24]	Canadian C-Spine[25]	Viccellio et al,[21] 2001	PECARN[23,26]
Design	Prospective	Prospective	Prospective	Retrospective case control
Patient population	All ages	>16 y	<18 y	<15 y
Enrollment	>34,000 (3700, 19 y)	8924	3065	540 cases
Significant results	Established clinical prediction rule to avoid XR in CSI • No neurologic abnormalities • Normal level of alertness • Not intoxicated • No midline tenderness to palpation • No distracting injuries 5 of 5 present: sensitivity 99.0%, NPV 99.8% for no CSI Potentially avoid 12.6% of XR in this group	3 Clinical questions to detect clinically important CSI • Is a high-risk factor present mandating XR? These factors include age ≥65 y, paresthesias, or dangerous mechanism. • Is the scenario low risk allowing for assessment of neck range of motion? These scenarios include a low-risk mechanism, absence of midline neck pain, ambulatory at any point, and ability to sit up. • Are patients able to actively rotate their neck 45° to both sides? Sensitivity 100% Specificity 42.5% Applying the rule would result in only 58.2% undergoing XR.	Sought to validate NEXUS criteria in pediatric patients • Sensitivity 100% • NPV 100% Consider applying NEXUS to patients aged >8 y	Identified 8 factors associated with CSI in children • Altered mental status • Focal neurologic findings • Report of neck pain • Torticollis • High-risk MVC • Significant torso injury • Diving as the mechanism • Predisposing factors (trisomy 21, Klippel-Feil, and so forth) Presence of any 1 associated with CSI Sensitivity 98% Age-specific risks 2–7 y • Neck pain • Torticollis • Altered mental status 8–15 y • Diving • Altered mental status
Limitations	Only 44 pediatric patients total with CSI No patients aged <2 y with CSI	Cannot apply to children aged <16 y	Only 4 patients aged <9 y with CSI No patients with CSI aged <2 y Cannot apply to children aged ≤8 y	Only 27 patients aged <2 y; no specific risks identified Needs prospective validations

Abbreviations: MVC, motor vehicle collision; NEXUS, national emergency X-radiography utilization study group; NPV, negative predictive value; PECARN, pediatric emergency care applied research network.

imaging is challenging given the rarity of these injuries, particularly in the younger age groups.[20,23] Anatomic differences in the pediatric cervical spine make application of well-known decision rules primarily validated in adults less reliable. Overall, pediatric patients have greater ligamentous laxity, less well-developed supporting musculature, horizontally oriented facets, and a higher fulcrum of motion, predisposing them to a higher-level injury as well as ligamentous and spinal cord injury.[22]

Clinical decision rules
Table 3 summarizes some of the studies to use in deciding which patients may warrant imaging to assess for CSIs.

Evaluating children less than 3 years of age
Clinically clearing the cervical spine of young, nonverbal children can present a challenge. Two studies offer guidance to situations in which victims less than 3 years of age might be appropriate for clinical clearance and are presented in **Table 4**.

Sensitivity of plain radiographs of the cervical spine
Cervical spine CT is extremely sensitive for bony injury and is the imaging modality of choice in critically injured children. MRI is sensitive for all types of acute CSIs and spinal cord injuries, though accessibility at all centers, time to complete, and frequent need for sedation can be limiting in its acute use.[22] Although CT may be used as the first-line imaging in adult trauma patients, plain XR of the cervical spine still have a role as the initial screening for pediatric patients. A secondary analysis of the Pediatric Emergency Care Applied Research Network (PECARN) cohort previously mentioned found adequate XR had a sensitivity of 90%.[28] When broken down by age, XR in those younger than 8 years had a sensitivity of 83%, increasing to 93% for the 8- to 15-year-old group. Another study of pediatric patients from the National Emergency X-Radiography Utilization Study Group (NEXUS) cohort who had plain XR showed 100% sensitivity for clinically important fractures (**Box 1**).[29]

Table 4 Evaluation of children less than 3 years of age for cervical spine injury		
Study	**Pieretti-Vanmarcke et al,[20] 2009**	**Anderson et al,[27] 2010**
Design	Retrospective review	Prospective cohort
Patient population	Aged <3 y, blunt trauma, 22 trauma registries	Aged <3 y, hospitalized with blunt trauma requiring cervical-spine clearance
Enrollment	>12,000 with blunt trauma 83 with CSI	575 28 with CSI
Significant results	4 independent predictors of CSI • GCS <14 • GCS eye = 1 • Motor vehicle collision • Age >2yr Score 0 or 1-0.07% CSI Score 7 or 8%–21% CSI For every 1 case of CSI, 40 negative CTs were obtained. Consider these variables in addition to other historical and PE factors.	Clearance protocol used • Negative XR • Low-impact mechanism • No focal pain • No neurologic deficit • Sit up and move head without pain All meeting these criteria were clinically cleared. No late injuries were detected.
Limitations	Retrospective Small total number with CSI	Small number with CSI

Abbreviations: GCS, glasgow coma scale; PE, physical exam.

> **Box 1**
> **Cervical-spine imaging summary**
>
> - Use CT or MRI for critically injured patients, an abnormal neurologic examination, or a high-risk mechanism.
> - Consider NEXUS risk factors in children older than 8 years and PECARN for children 2 to 15 years of age.
> - Use XR as the initial imaging in alert patients, a low-risk mechanism, or normal neurologic examination.
> - Consider clinical clearance in appropriate patients with various reassuring clinical and historical factors.

Blunt Abdominal Trauma

Abdominal trauma is second only to blunt head injury as a major cause of morbidity in the pediatric population. Abdominal CT is a frequent imaging modality used in these patients, though often the results do not change management. In one retrospective cohort of more than 1400 children with blunt abdominal trauma (BAT), only 2% overall required surgical intervention, with just 5% of those with positive CT findings undergoing an operative procedure.[30] Two different cohort studies demonstrated that 33% of pediatric patients thought to be at low risk for intra-abdominal injury (IAI) (**Table 5**) after BAT still underwent abdominal CT in their evaluation.[31,32]

Clinical prediction rules

Table 5 summarizes the results of several studies seeking to identify clinical predictors of IAI.

The largest study identifying pediatric patients with BAT at low risk of IAI was performed in 2013 through PECARN.[35] Even when considering those with any IAI, whether intervention was required or not, the rule had a sensitivity of 92.5% with a negative predictive value of 98.9%. Interestingly, 25% of the patients at very low risk per this prediction model underwent abdominal CT, underscoring the potential role of this rule to diminish CT utilization in low-risk patients. In a planned subanalysis of this cohort, the prediction rule was more sensitive in identifying those requiring acute interventions for IAI (97.0% vs 82.8%), whereas clinical suspicion was more specific (78.7% vs 42.5%).[31] This study still requires external validation.

Focused assessment with sonography in trauma examination

Focused assessment with sonography in trauma (FAST) has been used for approximately 30 years, though its adoption into pediatric trauma evaluation has come more slowly than in the adult population.[37] With the benefit of no ionizing radiation exposure, it can be very helpful in rapidly identifying free intra-abdominal fluid, hemothorax, pneumothorax, and pericardial effusions at the bedside (**Figs. 1–6**). However, there are some limitations in the pediatric population, such as underestimating solid organ injury if there is no associated free peritoneal fluid and poor indication of retroperitoneal, bowel, and mesenteric injuries.[37] See **Box 2**.

Test characteristics Studies have reported a wide range of sensitivities and negative predictive values for FAST examinations in pediatrics. The sensitivity to detect intra-abdominal free fluid ranges from 55% to 92% with negative predictive values of 50% to 97% in various studies.[38–42] Although a negative FAST should not be used as the sole indicator of IAI in pediatric patients, a hemodynamically stable child with a positive examination should certainly prompt additional evaluation for IAI.

Table 5
Summary of studies identifying clinical predictors of IAI

Study	Holmes et al,[33] 2002	Karam et al,[34] 2009 BATiC	Streck et al,[32] 2012	Holmes et al,[35] 2013 PECARN
Design	Prospective cohort	Prospective cohort	Retrospective chart review	Prospective, multicenter
Patient population	Children with blunt trauma thought to be at risk for IAI	Children hospitalized with BAT	Aged <16 y seen as a trauma alert	Children in ED with BAT
Enrollment	>100	147	125	>12,000
Significant findings	• Low SBP • Abdominal tenderness • Femur fracture • AST >100 • ALT >125 • >5 RBC/HPF • Hct <30%	• Abnormal FAST • Abdominal pain • Peritoneal signs • Hemodynamic instability • WBC >9.5 • LDH >330 • Lipase >30 • Cr >0.5 BATiC score ≤7 had NPV 97% for IAI Separate validation study[36] Score of 6 has • Sensitivity 100% • Specificity 87% This cutoff would avoid 47% of CTs within the cohort.	4 Clinical variables associated with IAI • Abnormal abdominal examination • AST >200 • Hct <30% • Abnormal CXR Sensitivity 94% NPV 99% Model could potentially eliminate 33% of unnecessary CTs	PE findings to show low risk of IAI requiring intervention • No seat belt sign • GCS 14 or 15 • No abdominal tenderness • No thoracic wall trauma • No complaint of abdominal pain • No diminished breath sounds • No vomiting Sensitivity 97% NPV 99.9% Model would have avoided CT in 25% Not yet externally validated

Abbreviations: ALT, alanine aminotransferase; AST, aspartate aminotransferase; BATiC, blunt abdominal trauma in children; Cr, creatinine; ED, emergency department; FAST, focused assessment with sonography in trauma; Hct, hematocrit; HPF, high-power field; LDH, lactate dehydrogenase; NPV, negative predictive value; RBC, red blood cell; SBP, systolic blood pressure; WBC, white blood cell.

Clinical utility A recently published randomized controlled trial of FAST in the evaluation of blunt pediatric trauma has further evaluated how this test truly impacts the care of pediatric patients with blunt trauma. A group of 925 hemodynamically stable children were evaluated for blunt torso trauma and randomized to standard trauma evaluation with or without the performance of a FAST examination.[43] Overall, the performance of FAST did not result in a decrease in the number of CT scans performed; there was not a difference in the number of missed IAI among the groups.[43] Some studies show combining the results of FAST with either physical examination or laboratory results can improve the sensitivity and specificity for IAI.[40,44]

Appendicitis

Acute appendicitis is the most common pediatric surgical emergency, with a prevalence estimated between 7.0% and 18.5%.[45,46] Ultrasound is the preferred first-line

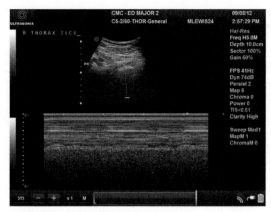

Fig. 1. Normal lung sliding, seashore sign on M-mode of ultrasound.

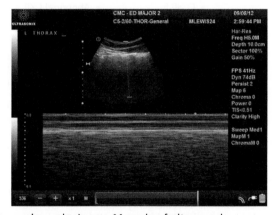

Fig. 2. Pneumothorax, barcode sign on M-mode of ultrasound.

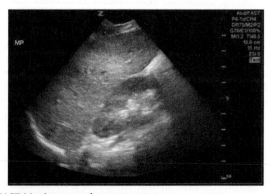

Fig. 3. Negative FAST Morison pouch.

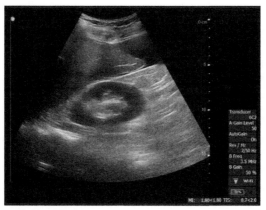

Fig. 4. Positive FAST Morison pouch.

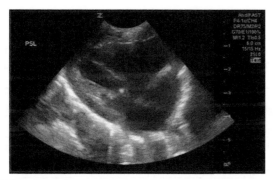

Fig. 5. Negative FAST subcostal.

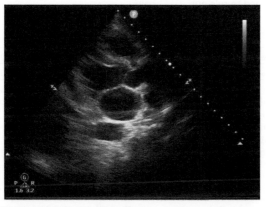

Fig. 6. Positive FAST subcostal. Pericardial effusion visible on left side.

Box 2
Application of focused assessment with sonography in trauma to pediatric blunt abdominal trauma

- FAST can expedite emergent intervention in hemodynamically unstable children without unnecessary exposure to ionizing radiation.

- In hemodynamically stable children with an unconcerning examination, no laboratory abnormalities, and a normal mental status, a negative FAST can provide further reassurance that CT is unlikely to be clinically useful.

- FAST alone has significant limitations to detect solid organ injury, retroperitoneal injury, and IAI without associated free fluid.

- A positive FAST should prompt further evaluation for IAI.

- Repeat FAST along with repeat examination can provide a strategy to reduce unnecessary exposure to CT.

imaging modality in pediatrics, with increasing use of MRI as well (**Figs. 7–9**). Of note, there is essentially no role for abdominal XR in the diagnosis of acute appendicitis.[47] **Table 6** highlights the benefits and limitations of the 3 major imaging modalities in appendicitis.

Intussusception

Ultrasound is the initial imaging modality of choice for diagnosis. An intussusception will look like a target or a doughnut in the transverse view on ultrasound or abdominal

Table 6
Appendicitis imaging modalities

	Ultrasound	CT[47–49]	MRI[50,51]
Use	First-line imaging study for uncomplicated acute appendicitis[46,47]	First-line imaging study for perforated appendicitis	Gaining popularity in use
Strengths	• No radiation • Available to ED physicians at bedside • Best to RULE IN appendicitis, but not as good to rule out	• Highly sensitive and specific • Better for abscess or phlegmon • Atypical abdominal pain • High appendicitis suspicion but indeterminate US	Better than CT to detect perforation
Sensitivity	93.8%–97.1%	—	94%–100%
Specificity	90.6%–96.3%	—	96%–100%
Limitations	• Not available at all facilities[52] • Sonographer experience • Restricted by bowel gas • Obese patients • Not as sensitive as CT	Ionizing radiation exposure (lifetime risk of cancer in 5 y old is 20.4–26.1 per 100,000)[53] Dose attenuation (by up to 50%) protocols and limited-view CT abdomen being explored[54,55]	• Expense • Child cooperation

Abbreviations: ED, emergency department; US, ultrasound.

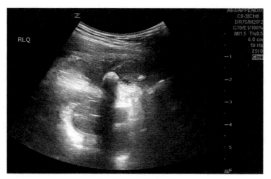

Fig. 7. Appendicitis with appendicolith on ultrasound.

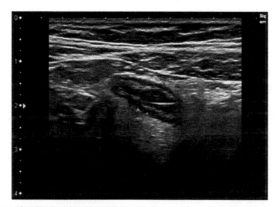

Fig. 8. Acute appendicitis on ultrasound.

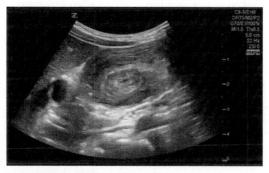

Fig. 9. Intussusception target sign in transverse view.

XR or there will be a pseudokidney sign or a sandwich sign in the long axis view on ultrasound.[56] See **Table 7** for imaging summary.

Ultrasound-guided reduction of intussusception

Ultrasound guidance for reduction by enema has gained popularity compared with fluoroscopy-guided reduction. The rates of successful reduction range between 80% and 100% when symptoms have been present for less than 24 hours versus 9% with symptoms greater than 24 hours.[58,61] Technology and training have reduced the total fluoroscopy and radiation exposure time significantly.[62] Fluoroscopy-guided enema reduction can be safely used when ultrasound is not available.

Nephrolithiasis

The incidence of pediatric nephrolithiasis is steadily increasing, with one study showing an average increase in the annual incidence of 10.6% per year from 1999 through 2008.[63] This study additionally demonstrated an increase in CT utilization for diagnosis from 26% to 45% over the study period.[63] This finding is concerning, as it is estimated for every 1000 naturally occurring cancers in the population, an additional 2 to 3 radiation-induced cancers can be attributed to CT scans done on children to diagnosis a kidney stone.[64] CT remains the most common initial imaging modality obtained, with studies showing 63% to 71% of pediatric patients undergoing CT first for nephrolithiasis.[65,66] Interestingly, hospitals with a care pathway for nephrolithiasis see greater initial ultrasound utilization.[65]

Ultrasound is the recommended initial imaging modality to evaluate pediatric patients with suspected nephrolithiasis.[67,68] If ultrasound is nondiagnostic and suspicion still exists, a CT with its greater sensitivity to detect stones can be considered. The sensitivity of CT for nephrolithiasis is excellent at 95% to 100% with similarly

Table 7
Imaging for intussusception

	Abdominal XR[56]	Ultrasound	Fluoroscopy	CT[56]
Use	If concern for peritonitis or perforation	First-line imaging modality in intussusception without perforation[57,58]	To evaluate reduction in real time	May be found incidentally while scanning for another cause of acute pain
Strengths	Identifies signs of perforation	• No radiation • Identifies predictors for success/failure of enema in real time (see limitations)	Usually available when ultrasound is not	No benefit over ultrasound
Limitations	• Less sensitive and specific than ultrasound[59] • Not recommended for routine workup[60]	• Poor at identifying perforation	• Potential for long duration of procedure • Exposure to ionizing radiation, but much improved from previous	• Exposure to ionizing radiation • Not recommended as a common imaging modality

high specificity of 96% to 98%.[69] Passerotti and colleagues[70] prospectively compared CT and ultrasound in children presenting with symptoms of urolithiasis. Ultrasound in this study had a sensitivity of 76% compared with CT and a specificity of 100%. In summary, ultrasound should be the initial imaging modality used to evaluate for pediatric nephrolithiasis, with the understanding that CT might still be warranted for nondiagnostic studies in patients who continue to show clinical signs of urolithiasis.

Shunt Malfunction

Secondary to head trauma, cerebrospinal fluid (CSF) shunt malfunction is one of the most common neurosurgical emergencies that is encountered in the emergency department.[71] Between 19.9% and 30.0% of children with shunts who present to the emergency department will be diagnosed with shunt malfunction and will need surgical revision.[71,72]

Computed tomography
Until recently, head CT has been the standard-of-care imaging study to evaluate pediatric patients with suspected CSF shunt malfunction. Several studies evaluated the average exposure to ionizing radiation of patients with CSF shunts and found an average of between 1.0 and 2.6 CT scans per patient per year, but only 17% resulted in neurosurgical evaluation within 7 days.[73,74]

Several groups have evaluated a limited head CT protocol with 3 to 4 slices at key anatomic locations.[75] These limited scans showed a 95.7% match compared with full-head CT, and no cases of increased ventricular size were missed (100% positive predictive value). They found a dose reduction of approximately 87%. These results are promising that a limited head CT protocol is feasible.

MRI
Rapid MRI (rMRI) has been shown to be noninferior to head CT for the evaluation of shunt failure.[76,77] The sensitivity is 58.5% and specificity is 93.3% compared with 53.2% and 95.6%, respectively, for head CT.[78] Physicians should consider rMRI instead of head CT to obtain equivalent results without exposing patients to radiation.

Shunt series/plain radiographs
The consensus is that a shunt series has low sensitivity for shunt malfunction, that it is frequently normal even in the presence of an abnormal head CT or MRI, and that it is of low diagnostic benefit.[71,72,79]

Seizure

New-onset afebrile seizure
For the 25,000 to 40,000 children presenting with new-onset afebrile seizures yearly, the decision to obtain emergent imaging is challenging.[80] Imaging studies for these patients are usually unremarkable. Studies report 8% to 22% of patients have abnormal imaging, with 0.8% to 4.0% having findings that require urgent intervention.[80–83] Several studies clarify the risk factors for intracranial abnormalities in children with seizures to help guide appropriate emergent imaging.[81,84–86] The risk factors established in these studies include

- Focal seizure
- High-risk history (congenital heart disease, sickle cell disease)
- Developmental delay

- New focal neurologic deficit
- Status epilepticus
- Age older than 2 years (**Table 8**)

The decision as to whether imaging must be obtained emergently is based on clinical suspicion or concern for an acute process, such as hydrocephalus, mass, or hemorrhage, in which case CT may be the best imaging choice.

Complex febrile seizure

Children presenting with complex febrile seizures raise more clinical suspicion for an acute intracranial process; however, the literature supports that this group overall has a low rate of significant findings on imaging studies as well. Among multiple studies of hospitalized or emergency department patients with complex febrile seizures, less than 1% have findings on CT scan that require urgent intervention.[88,89] Up to 28% to 65% of patients, however, still undergo CT.[88,89] In a prospective hospitalized cohort of children with complex febrile seizures, 9.8% overall had abnormalities on CT scan, with increased rates among those with partial seizures or abnormal electroencephalograms (EEGs).[90] Therefore, emergency providers might consider that most children with complex febrile seizures do not require emergent imaging with ionizing radiation and perhaps can undergo MRI as an alternative if clinical suspicion is high based on risk factors and EEG results.

SUMMARY

Emergency care providers have a significant role to play in supporting judicious use of ionizing radiation in pediatric patients. Clinicians can use various clinical

Table 8
Guidelines for neuroimaging in pediatric patients with seizures

Group	American Academy of Neurology[80]	International League Against Epilepsy[82]	American Academy of Pediatrics[87]
Population	First-time afebrile seizure	First-time afebrile seizure	Febrile seizure

Recommendations	• Clinically significant abnormalities are most often seen with focal seizures or new neurologic findings.
	• MRI is the preferred imaging modality. Consider it for
	  ○ Children aged <1 y
	  ○ Focal seizures
	  ○ Abnormal neurologic examination
	Consider emergent imaging for
	• Persistent postictal neurologic deficits
	• Children who do not return to baseline mental status within several h
		Consider imaging
		• Focal seizures
		• Abnormal neurologic examination
		• History of developmental delay
		• Age <2 y
		MRI is preferred imaging modality if possible
			Routine imaging is not recommended.

Box 3
Summary of imaging considerations for clinical scenarios

Pneumonia: Healthy, well-appearing children with clinical signs of pneumonia can be treated without XR confirmation. Hospitalized and ill-appearing children should undergo CXR.[13]

Bronchiolitis: CXR is not routinely required. Consider it in those requiring ICU care or if there is concern for complications.[14]

Asthma: Routine CXR for uncomplicated exacerbations is not recommended. Consider it in those with possible complications of asthma.[15]

Minor head trauma: Clinical decision rules play a significant role in reducing the use of CT to evaluate children after minor head trauma.[91]

Cervical-spine trauma: Children older than 8 years with a low-risk mechanism can potentially be cleared with NEXUS criteria without further imaging.[21] MRI is the imaging modality of choice in all children with focal neurologic findings. There is not one clear validated screening instrument for young children to rule out CSI.

Blunt chest trauma: CXR is the best initial imaging modality for pediatric blunt chest trauma.[92]

BAT: Many clinical factors play a role in determining the need for CT in pediatric patients with blunt trauma. Use of FAST examination, laboratory information, serial examination, and observation all play a role in judicious use of CT.

Appendicitis: US is the initial imaging modality of choice to diagnose pediatric appendicitis. Serial examinations, laboratory markers, and use of MRI can be used in certain cases as an alternative to CT if US is nondiagnostic.

Intussusception: US is the imaging modality of choice for diagnosis.[58]

Nephrolithiasis: US is the recommended initial imaging modality.[67,68]

Shunt malfunction: Consider rMRI protocols or limited head CT to evaluate ventricular shunt malfunctions.[77,93]

New-onset afebrile seizure: MRI is the preferred imaging modality. Consider emergent CT in the setting of persistent postictal deficits or prolonged postictal period.[80]

Abbreviation: ICU, intensive care unit; US, ultrasound.

---

indicators and clinical prediction rules to guide their decisions to use imaging and when modalities, such as ultrasound and MRI, can be used over CT. Discussion with our colleagues in radiology can likewise assure the best choice with the lowest risk is made for imaging in various scenarios as well as assure that proper protocols are in place to minimize radiation exposure to children when it is needed for diagnostic studies. Collaboration with pediatric and trauma surgery services is vital as well in establishing protocols for imaging in scenarios, such as trauma and appendicitis, as well as when observation instead of imaging is a reasonable option. Finally, establishing clinical pathways that incorporate judicious imaging use in the emergency department can create a significant impact as well **(Box 3)**.

ACKNOWLEDGMENTS

Thank you to Dr Margaret Lewis and Dr Anthony Weekes of the Department of Emergency Medicine, Division of Ultrasound for contributing images for this article. Thank you to Ms Laura Leach, Medical Librarian at Carolinas Medical Center for her assistance with literature searches.

REFERENCES

1. Brody AS, Frush DP, Huda W, et al, American Academy of Pediatrics Section on Radiology. Radiation risk to children from computed tomography. Pediatrics 2007;120(3):677–82.
2. Frush DP, Donnelly LF, Rosen NS. Computed tomography and radiation risks: what pediatric health care providers should know. Pediatrics 2003;112(4):951–7.
3. Brenner DJ, Hall EJ. Computed tomography–an increasing source of radiation exposure. N Engl J Med 2007;357(22):2277–84.
4. Preston DL, Shimizu Y, Pierce DA, et al. Studies of mortality of atomic bomb survivors. Report 13: solid cancer and noncancer disease mortality: 1950-1997. Radiat Res 2003;160(4):381–407.
5. Preston DL, Cullings H, Suyama A, et al. Solid cancer incidence in atomic bomb survivors exposed in utero or as young children. J Natl Cancer Inst 2008;100(6):428–36.
6. Mettler FA, Wiest PW, Locken JA, et al. CT scanning: patterns of use and dose. J Radiol Prot 2000;20(4):353–9.
7. Brenner D, Elliston C, Hall E, et al. Estimated risks of radiation-induced fatal cancer from pediatric CT. AJR Am J Roentgenol 2001;176(2):289–96.
8. Brenner DJ. Estimating cancer risks from pediatric CT: going from the qualitative to the quantitative. Pediatr Radiol 2002;32(4):228–31 [discussion: 242–4].
9. Pearce MS, Salotti JA, Little MP, et al. Radiation exposure from CT scans in childhood and subsequent risk of leukaemia and brain tumours: a retrospective cohort study. Lancet 2012;380(9840):499–505.
10. Smith-Bindman R, Lipson J, Marcus R, et al. Radiation dose associated with common computed tomography examinations and the associated lifetime attributable risk of cancer. Arch Intern Med 2009;169(22):2078–86.
11. Mettler FA, Huda W, Yoshizumi TT, et al. Effective doses in radiology and diagnostic nuclear medicine: a catalog. Radiology 2008;248(1):254–63.
12. Knapp JF, Simon SD, Sharma V. Variation and trends in ED use of radiographs for asthma, bronchiolitis, and croup in children. Pediatrics 2013;132(2):245–52.
13. Bradley JS, Byington CL, Shah SS, et al. The management of community-acquired pneumonia in infants and children older than 3 months of age: clinical practice guidelines by the Pediatric Infectious Diseases Society and the Infectious Diseases Society of America. Clin Infect Dis 2011;53(7):e25–76.
14. Ralston SL, Lieberthal AS, Meissner HC, et al. Clinical practice guideline: the diagnosis, management, and prevention of bronchiolitis. Pediatrics 2014; 134(5):e1474–502.
15. National Asthma Education and Prevention Program. Expert panel report 3 (EPR-3): guidelines for the diagnosis and management of asthma-summary report 2007. J Allergy Clin Immunol 2007;120(5 Suppl):S94–138.
16. Shah VP, Tunik MG, Tsung JW. Prospective evaluation of point-of-care ultrasonography for the diagnosis of pneumonia in children and young adults. JAMA Pediatr 2013;167(2):119–25.
17. Walsh-Kelly CM, Kim MK, Hennes HM. Chest radiography in the initial episode of bronchospasm in children: can clinical variables predict pathologic findings? Ann Emerg Med 1996;28(4):391–5.
18. Walsh-Kelly CM, Hennes HM. Do clinical variables predict pathologic radiographs in the first episode of wheezing? Pediatr Emerg Care 2002;18(1):8–11.
19. Gershel JC, Goldman HS, Stein RE, et al. The usefulness of chest radiographs in first asthma attacks. N Engl J Med 1983;309(6):336–9.

20. Pieretti-Vanmarcke R, Velmahos GC, Nance ML, et al. Clinical clearance of the cervical spine in blunt trauma patients younger than 3 years: a multi-center study of the American Association for the Surgery of Trauma. J Trauma 2009;67(3): 543–9 [discussion: 549–50].

21. Viccellio P, Simon H, Pressman BD, et al. A prospective multicenter study of cervical spine injury in children. Pediatrics 2001;108(2):E20.

22. Leonard JC. Cervical spine injury. Pediatr Clin North Am 2013;60(5):1123–37.

23. Leonard JC, Kuppermann N, Olsen C, et al. Factors associated with cervical spine injury in children after blunt trauma. Ann Emerg Med 2011;58(2):145–55.

24. Hoffman JR, Mower WR, Wolfson AB, et al. Validity of a set of clinical criteria to rule out injury to the cervical spine in patients with blunt trauma. National Emergency X-Radiography Utilization Study Group. N Engl J Med 2000;343(2):94–9.

25. Stiell IG, Wells GA, Vandemheen KL, et al. The Canadian C-spine rule for radiography in alert and stable trauma patients. JAMA 2001;286(15):1841–8.

26. Leonard JC, Jaffe DM, Olsen CS, et al. Age-related differences in factors associated with cervical spine injuries in children. Acad Emerg Med 2015;22(4):441–6.

27. Anderson RC, Kan P, Vanaman M, et al. Utility of a cervical spine clearance protocol after trauma in children between 0 and 3 years of age. J Neurosurg Pediatr 2010;5(3):292–6.

28. Nigrovic LE, Rogers AJ, Adelgais KM, et al. Utility of plain radiographs in detecting traumatic injuries of the cervical spine in children. Pediatr Emerg Care 2012; 28(5):426–32.

29. Cui LW, Probst MA, Hoffman JR, et al. Sensitivity of plain radiography for pediatric cervical spine injury. Emerg Radiol 2016;23(5):443–8.

30. Fenton SJ, Hansen KW, Meyers RL, et al. CT scan and the pediatric trauma patient–are we overdoing it? J Pediatr Surg 2004;39(12):1877–81.

31. Mahajan P, Kuppermann N, Tunik M, et al. Comparison of clinician suspicion versus a clinical prediction rule in identifying children at risk for intra-abdominal injuries after blunt torso trauma. Acad Emerg Med 2015;22(9):1034–41.

32. Streck CJ, Jewett BM, Wahlquist AH, et al. Evaluation for intra-abdominal injury in children after blunt torso trauma: can we reduce unnecessary abdominal computed tomography by utilizing a clinical prediction model? J Trauma Acute Care Surg 2012;73(2):371–6 [discussion: 376].

33. Holmes JF, Sokolove PE, Brant WE, et al. Identification of children with intra-abdominal injuries after blunt trauma. Ann Emerg Med 2002;39(5):500–9.

34. Karam O, Sanchez O, Chardot C, et al. Blunt abdominal trauma in children: a score to predict the absence of organ injury. J Pediatr 2009;154(6):912–7.

35. Holmes JF, Lillis K, Monroe D, et al. Identifying children at very low risk of clinically important blunt abdominal injuries. Ann Emerg Med 2013;62(2):107–16.e2.

36. de Jong WJ, Stoepker L, Nellensteijn DR, et al. External validation of the blunt abdominal trauma in children (BATiC) score: ruling out significant abdominal injury in children. J Trauma Acute Care Surg 2014;76(5):1282–7.

37. Richards JR, McGahan JP. Focused assessment with sonography in trauma (FAST) in 2017: what radiologists can learn. Radiology 2017;283(1):30–48.

38. Coley BD, Mutabagani KH, Martin LC, et al. Focused abdominal sonography for trauma (FAST) in children with blunt abdominal trauma. J Trauma 2000;48(5):902–6.

39. Holmes JF, Brant WE, Bond WF, et al. Emergency department ultrasonography in the evaluation of hypotensive and normotensive children with blunt abdominal trauma. J Pediatr Surg 2001;36(7):968–73.

40. Suthers SE, Albrecht R, Foley D, et al. Surgeon-directed ultrasound for trauma is a predictor of intra-abdominal injury in children. Am Surg 2004;70(2):164–7 [discussion: 167–8].

41. Holmes JF, Gladman A, Chang CH. Performance of abdominal ultrasonography in pediatric blunt trauma patients: a meta-analysis. J Pediatr Surg 2007;42(9): 1588–94.

42. Fox JC, Boysen M, Gharahbaghian L, et al. Test characteristics of focused assessment of sonography for trauma for clinically significant abdominal free fluid in pediatric blunt abdominal trauma. Acad Emerg Med 2011;18(5):477–82.

43. Holmes JF, Kelley KM, Wootton-Gorges SL, et al. Effect of abdominal ultrasound on clinical care, outcomes, and resource use among children with blunt torso trauma: a randomized clinical trial. JAMA 2017;317(22):2290–6.

44. Sola JE, Cheung MC, Yang R, et al. Pediatric FAST and elevated liver transaminases: an effective screening tool in blunt abdominal trauma. J Surg Res 2009; 157(1):103–7.

45. Blumfield E, Nayak G, Srinivasan R, et al. Ultrasound for differentiation between perforated and nonperforated appendicitis in pediatric patients. AJR Am J Roentgenol 2013;200(5):957–62.

46. Binkovitz LA, Unsdorfer KM, Thapa P, et al. Pediatric appendiceal ultrasound: accuracy, determinacy and clinical outcomes. Pediatr Radiol 2015;45(13):1934–44.

47. Coca Robinot D, Liebana de Rojas C, Aguirre Pascual E. Abdominal emergencies in pediatrics. Radiologia 2016;58(Suppl 2):80–91.

48. Bachur RG, Dayan PS, Bajaj L, et al. The effect of abdominal pain duration on the accuracy of diagnostic imaging for pediatric appendicitis. Ann Emerg Med 2012; 60(5):582–90.e3.

49. Bachur RG, Hennelly K, Callahan MJ, et al. Advanced radiologic imaging for pediatric appendicitis, 2005-2009: trends and outcomes. J Pediatr 2012;160(6): 1034–8.

50. Dillman JR, Gadepalli S, Sroufe NS, et al. Equivocal pediatric appendicitis: unenhanced MR imaging protocol for nonsedated children-a clinical effectiveness study. Radiology 2016;279(1):216–25.

51. Duke E, Kalb B, Arif-Tiwari H, et al. A systematic review and meta-analysis of diagnostic performance of MRI for evaluation of acute appendicitis. AJR Am J Roentgenol 2016;206(3):508–17.

52. Glass CC, Saito JM, Sidhwa F, et al. Diagnostic imaging practices for children with suspected appendicitis evaluated at definitive care hospitals and their associated referral centers. J Pediatr Surg 2016;51(6):912–6.

53. Doria AS. Optimizing the role of imaging in appendicitis. Pediatr Radiol 2009; 39(Suppl 2):S144–8.

54. Adibe OO, Amin SR, Hansen EN, et al. An evidence-based clinical protocol for diagnosis of acute appendicitis decreased the use of computed tomography in children. J Pediatr Surg 2011;46(1):192–6.

55. Davis J, Roh AT, Petterson MB, et al. Computed tomography localization of the appendix in the pediatric population relative to the lumbar spine. Pediatr Radiol 2017;14:14.

56. Waseem M, Rosenberg HK. Intussusception. Pediatr Emerg Care 2008;24(11): 793–800.

57. Ko HS, Schenk JP, Troger J, et al. Current radiological management of intussusception in children. Eur Radiol 2007;17(9):2411–21.

58. Gfroerer S, Fiegel H, Rolle U. Ultrasound-guided reduction of intussusception: a safe and effective method performed by pediatric surgeons. Pediatr Surg Int 2016;32(7):679–82.

59. Henderson AA, Anupindi SA, Servaes S, et al. Comparison of 2-view abdominal radiographs with ultrasound in children with suspected intussusception. Pediatr Emerg Care 2013;29(2):145–50.

60. Tareen F, Mc Laughlin D, Cianci F, et al. Abdominal radiography is not necessary in children with intussusception. Pediatr Surg Int 2016;32(1):89–92.

61. Vujovic D, Lukac M, Sretenovic A, et al. Indications for repeated enema reduction of intussusception in children. Srp Arh Celok Lek 2014;142(5–6):320–4.

62. Cullmann JL, Heverhagen JT, Puig S. Radiation dose in pneumatic reduction of ileo-colic intussusceptions–results from a single-institution study. Pediatr Radiol 2015;45(5):675–7.

63. Routh JC, Graham DA, Nelson CP. Trends in imaging and surgical management of pediatric urolithiasis at American pediatric hospitals. J Urol 2010;184(4 Suppl): 1816–22.

64. Kuhns LR, Oliver WJ, Christodoulou E, et al. The predicted increased cancer risk associated with a single computed tomography examination for calculus detection in pediatric patients compared with the natural cancer incidence. Pediatr Emerg Care 2011;27(4):345–50.

65. Ziemba JB, Canning DA, Lavelle J, et al. Patient and institutional characteristics associated with initial computerized tomography in children presenting to the emergency department with kidney stones. J Urol 2015;193(5 Suppl):1848–53.

66. Tasian GE, Pulido JE, Keren R, et al. Use of and regional variation in initial CT imaging for kidney stones. Pediatrics 2014;134(5):909–15.

67. Fulgham PF, Assimos DG, Pearle MS, et al. Clinical effectiveness protocols for imaging in the management of ureteral calculous disease: AUA technology assessment. J Urol 2013;189(4):1203–13.

68. Riccabona M, Avni FE, Blickman JG, et al. Imaging recommendations in paediatric uroradiology: minutes of the ESPR workgroup session on urinary tract infection, fetal hydronephrosis, urinary tract ultrasonography and voiding cystourethrography, Barcelona, Spain, June 2007. Pediatr Radiol 2008;38(2): 138–45.

69. Lipkin M, Ackerman A. Imaging for urolithiasis: standards, trends, and radiation exposure. Curr Opin Urol 2016;26(1):56–62.

70. Passerotti C, Chow JS, Silva A, et al. Ultrasound versus computerized tomography for evaluating urolithiasis. J Urol 2009;182(4 Suppl):1829–34.

71. Mater A, Shroff M, Al-Farsi S, et al. Test characteristics of neuroimaging in the emergency department evaluation of children for cerebrospinal fluid shunt malfunction. CJEM 2008;10(2):131–5.

72. Lehnert BE, Rahbar H, Relyea-Chew A, et al. Detection of ventricular shunt malfunction in the ED: relative utility of radiography, CT, and nuclear imaging. Emerg Radiol 2011;18(4):299–305.

73. Antonucci MC, Zuckerbraun NS, Tyler-Kabara EC, et al. The burden of ionizing radiation studies in children with ventricular shunts. J Pediatr 2017;182:210–6.e1.

74. Cohen JS, Jamal N, Dawes C, et al. Cranial computed tomography utilization for suspected ventriculoperitoneal shunt malfunction in a pediatric emergency department. J Emerg Med 2014;46(4):449–55.

75. Park DB, Hill JG, Thacker PG, et al. The role of limited head computed tomography in the evaluation of pediatric ventriculoperitoneal shunt malfunction. Pediatr Emerg Care 2016;32(9):585–9.

76. Boyle TP, Nigrovic LE. Radiographic evaluation of pediatric cerebrospinal fluid shunt malfunction in the emergency setting. Pediatr Emerg Care 2015;31(6): 435–40 [quiz: 441–3].

77. Boyle TP, Paldino MJ, Kimia AA, et al. Comparison of rapid cranial MRI to CT for ventricular shunt malfunction. Pediatrics 2014;134(1):e47–54.

78. Yue EL, Meckler GD, Fleischman RJ, et al. Test characteristics of quick brain MRI for shunt evaluation in children: an alternative modality to avoid radiation. J Neurosurg Pediatr 2015;15(4):420–6.

79. Desai KR, Babb JS, Amodio JB. The utility of the plain radiograph "shunt series" in the evaluation of suspected ventriculoperitoneal shunt failure in pediatric patients. Pediatr Radiol 2007;37(5):452–6.

80. Hirtz D, Ashwal S, Berg A, et al. Practice parameter: evaluating a first nonfebrile seizure in children: report of the quality standards subcommittee of the American Academy of Neurology, the Child Neurology Society, and the American Epilepsy Society. Neurology 2000;55(5):616–23.

81. Dayan PS, Lillis K, Bennett J, et al. Prevalence of and risk factors for intracranial abnormalities in unprovoked seizures. Pediatrics 2015;136(2):e351–60.

82. Gaillard WD, Chiron C, Cross JH, et al. Guidelines for imaging infants and children with recent-onset epilepsy. Epilepsia 2009;50(9):2147–53.

83. Aprahamian N, Harper MB, Prabhu SP, et al. Pediatric first time non-febrile seizure with focal manifestations: is emergent imaging indicated? Seizure 2014; 23(9):740–5.

84. Al-Rumayyan AR, Abolfotouh MA. Prevalence and prediction of abnormal CT scan in pediatric patients presenting with a first seizure. Neurosciences (Riyadh) 2012;17(4):352–6.

85. Lyons TW, Johnson KB, Michelson KA, et al. Yield of emergent neuroimaging in children with new-onset seizure and status epilepticus. Seizure 2016;35:4–10.

86. Hsieh DT, Chang T, Tsuchida TN, et al. New-onset afebrile seizures in infants: role of neuroimaging. Neurology 2010;74(2):150–6.

87. Subcommittee on Febrile Seizures, American Academy of Pediatrics. Neurodiagnostic evaluation of the child with a simple febrile seizure. Pediatrics 2011;127(2): 389–94.

88. Teng D, Dayan P, Tyler S, et al. Risk of intracranial pathologic conditions requiring emergency intervention after a first complex febrile seizure episode among children. Pediatrics 2006;117(2):304–8.

89. Kimia AA, Ben-Joseph E, Prabhu S, et al. Yield of emergent neuroimaging among children presenting with a first complex febrile seizure. Pediatr Emerg Care 2012; 28(4):316–21.

90. Rasool A, Choh SA, Wani NA, et al. Role of electroencephalogram and neuroimaging in first onset afebrile and complex febrile seizures in children from Kashmir. J Pediatr Neurosci 2012;7(1):9–15.

91. Kuppermann N, Holmes JF, Dayan PS, et al. Identification of children at very low risk of clinically-important brain injuries after head trauma: a prospective cohort study. Lancet 2009;374(9696):1160–70.

92. Holmes JF, Sokolove PE, Brant WE, et al. A clinical decision rule for identifying children with thoracic injuries after blunt torso trauma. Ann Emerg Med 2002; 39(5):492–9.

93. Kim I, Torrey SB, Milla SS, et al. Benefits of brain magnetic resonance imaging over computed tomography in children requiring emergency evaluation of ventriculoperitoneal shunt malfunction: reducing lifetime attributable risk of cancer. Pediatr Emerg Care 2015;31(4):239–42.

Inborn Errors of Metabolism in the Emergency Department (Undiagnosed and Management of the Known)

Emily C. MacNeill, MD[a],*, Chantel P. Walker, MD[b]

KEYWORDS

- Inborn errors of metabolism • Emergency department • Metabolic crisis

KEY POINTS

- When concerned about an inborn error of metabolism, practitioners have to draw appropriate laboratory work before instituting therapies, such as glucose.
- After drawing the diagnostic studies, it is vital to shut down catabolism with the administration of a continuous infusion of glucose.
- Most children with an inborn error of metabolism require subspecialty care at a dedicated children's hospital and may require emergent transfer.

INTRODUCTION

Inborn errors of metabolism (IEM) present a unique challenge to the emergency medicine physician. IEM represents a large number of individual illnesses each with their own specific risks and treatments, they are individually rare, and mastery of the pathophysiology is complex and outside the normal approach of emergency medicine. The importance of understanding some basic approaches and therapies, however, cannot be overstated. Although individually rare, cumulatively they are fairly common, occurring 1 in 784 to 2555 infants.[1,2] Patients with IEM can present in extremis and failure of the emergency medicine provider to consider the diagnosis and initiate therapy can lead to death or permanent disability. With modern medical advancements, many of these children can otherwise thrive, so it is incumbent on clinicians to have a basic understanding of these diseases.

Disclosure Statement: Neither author has any financial relationship to disclose.
[a] Emergency Medicine, Carolinas HealthCare System, 1000 Blythe Boulevard, 3rd Floor MEB, Charlotte, NC 28203, USA; [b] Pediatric Emergence Medicine, Carolinas HealthCare System, 1000 Blythe Boulevard, 3rd Floor MEB, Charlotte, NC 28203, USA
* Corresponding author. 1000 Blythe Boulevard, 3rd Floor MEB, Charlotte, NC 28203.
E-mail address: emily.macneill@carolinas.org

Emerg Med Clin N Am 36 (2018) 369–385
https://doi.org/10.1016/j.emc.2017.12.014
0733-8627/18/© 2018 Elsevier Inc. All rights reserved.

This article groups presentations and illnesses together in such a way that makes it easier for providers to consider the possible diagnoses and initiate appropriate therapies. The initial portion focuses on the undifferentiated patient: when to consider IEM as a potential diagnosis, what laboratory studies are needed, and what general therapies to consider. The second half concentrates on the patient with a known disorder and the various therapies and the rationale behind them. After reading this article, emergency medicine providers should feel more comfortable diagnosing and managing children with IEM.

THE UNDIAGNOSED PATIENT
When to Consider Inborn Errors of Metabolism

IEM should be considered with any sick neonate, children in extremis without clear cause, and children with unexpected laboratory abnormalities. It is easy to assume that, with advancements in neonatal screening, all children with IEM have a diagnosis and treatment plan before presentation with life-threatening illness. This is not the case.[3] Additionally, one must keep in mind that although most metabolic crises present in the neonatal period, there are diseases that present later in life after accumulation of toxic compounds, and there are patients with partial defects leading to subtler presentations later in childhood.

Clinical Manifestations

Neurologic
Regardless of IEM type, most patients present with primarily neurologic symptoms: irritability/lethargy, vomiting, hypotonia, and sometimes seizures. These symptoms can be secondary to elevated ammonia levels from urea cycle disorders, profound metabolic acidosis from the organic acidemias, or hypoglycemia from fatty acid oxidation disorders or carbohydrate metabolism disorders. It is unusual for an IEM to present with a single neurologic symptom because all brain functions are affected by metabolic derangements (eg, hypotonia from an aminoacidopathy is accompanied by irritability and lethargy).[4–6] Exceptions to this rule include some of the seizure disorders, such as pyridoxine-dependent seizures.[5] Infants with IEM can seem clinically like infants with sepsis where altered mental status may be secondary to hypoperfusion, hypoglycemia, and or acidosis. To further confound the issue, sepsis and IEM can occur in the same patient. They key to differentiating these pathologies is in not anchoring to a single diagnosis, watching response to therapies closely, and obtaining thorough laboratory investigations.

Hyperammonemia as a cause of altered mental status deserves special mention. The accumulation of ammonia affects neurotransmitter systems causing acute and chronic neurologic damage. Acutely, the brain undergoes directly triggered cell death and indirectly stimulated cerebral edema, which can present clinically as vomiting, lethargy, seizures, or coma.[7] Both hypothermia and hyperthermia can result making this diagnosis worthy of consideration alongside sepsis in an irritable neonate with temperature instability.

In addition to the wide array of ammonia-accumulating metabolic disorders that cause acute neurologic decompensation, there are "milder" forms of these illnesses that present with episodic psychiatric symptoms, learning disabilities, and stroke-like episodes.[7,8]

Respiratory
Patients with IEM in metabolic crisis present with tachypnea for one of two reasons. First, metabolic acidoses cause tachypnea. Infants have an immature renal buffering

system reducing their ability to excrete acid; thus, respiratory compensation is an essential mechanism for managing acidosis.[9,10] The lack of physiologic reserve, however, makes this compensatory mechanism less effective especially as the infant becomes more ill. Second, hyperammonemia may cause a central hyperventilation and tachypnea, although the resultant laboratory findings are more consistent with a primary respiratory alkalosis.[9]

Gastrointestinal

Vomiting is another common symptom of metabolic crisis and can be secondary to neurologic stress or intolerance of nutrition as can happen in protein and carbohydrate metabolism derangements. Hepatic disease is found in many of the IEM especially those that involve glycogen metabolism and tyrosinemia.[11] Keep in mind that primary liver disease causes metabolic derangements that can mimic IEM including galactose in the urine, hyperammonemia, and abnormal plasma and urine organic acids.[12]

Cardiac

Primary cardiac dysfunction is a less common presentation for metabolic crisis, but there are a few facts to keep in mind. Fatty acid oxidation defects can cause a primary arrhythmia or conduction abnormality and most cardiac dysrhythmias have been reported at some point with IEM.[13,14] More likely, however, practitioners see a global cardiac dysfunction secondary to acidosis and metabolic stress. This is important to keep in mind during fluid resuscitation that may cause problems if done overaggressively.

Treating the Undifferentiated Patient

In the emergency department (ED), there are basic tenets of treatment that decrease morbidity and mortality. The consideration that IEM is a possibility is the first step. Thorough history taking is important; prenatal complications, such as HELLP, consanguinity, and other children who died during infancy, can all indicate IEM. After that, it is important to

- Run diagnostic testing
- Shut down catabolism
- Administer supportive care
- Remove toxic metabolites
- Consider sepsis

Diagnostic Testing

To make an accurate diagnosis of an IEM, blood samples must be drawn before initiating therapy; especially glucose, because administration quickly obfuscates laboratory findings. Although this may seem like a low priority in a sick or dying child, consider that accurate diagnosis is imperative for preventing further metabolic catastrophes and, in the perimortem setting, diagnosis can help parents make appropriate family planning decisions. The most common blood tests drawn are shown in **Box 1**. Remember that some of the blood (3–5 mL) needs to be placed in a heparinized tube and placed on ice immediately.

Far more important than memorizing descriptions of laboratory abnormalities is a global understanding of what anomalies are seen and why they occur, and a general comprehension of what needs to be addressed immediately (**Fig. 1** for a general overview). After a child is stabilized, formal consultation with a metabolism expert will yield more nuanced recommendations.

Box 1
Common blood tests ordered when considering an IEM diagnosis. This requires 10 mL blood (3–5 mL in heparinized tubes) and 10 mL urine

Venous blood gas

Blood sugar

Comprehensive metabolic panel

Clotting studies

Ammonia level (heparinized tube on ice)

Urinalysis

Plasma amino acids (heparinized tube on dry ice)

Urine organic acids, orotic acids, and amino acids (on ice)

Plasma-free and acylcarnitines (heparinized tube)

Urine-reducing substances (on ice)

Blood glucose

For the purposes of this review, IEM is divided into two distinct groups: those that present with hypoglycemic episodes and those that do not (**Fig. 2**) (note that this does not affect the treatment of the undifferentiated patient where glucose administration is warranted regardless of level). When an infant presents with profound hypoglycemia, one should consider problems with processing glucose or fatty acids.[3,13] Defects in the ability to correctly metabolize amino acids rarely lead to severe hypoglycemia.

Blood gas with lactate level

The blood gas can be the first indication that there is an underlying IEM. Infants who present ill from any cause likely have a mild metabolic acidosis but severe acidosis or an anion gap should alert the physician that there might be an underlying IEM. Elevated lactates can contribute to a gap acidosis and its contribution is calculated with a simple correction (sodium - chloride - bicarbonate - lactate should equal

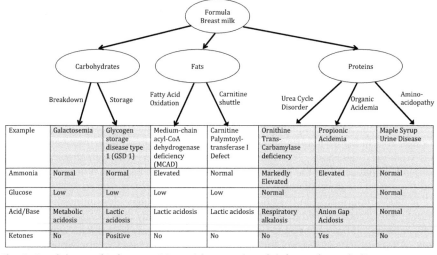

Example	Galactosemia	Glycogen storage disease type 1 (GSD 1)	Medium-chain acyl-CoA dehydrogenase deficiency (MCAD)	Carnitine Palymtoyl-transferase I Defect	Ornithine Trans-Carbamylase deficiency	Propionic Acidemia	Maple Syrup Urine Disease
Ammonia	Normal	Normal	Elevated	Normal	Markedly Elevated	Elevated	Normal
Glucose	Low	Low	Low	Low	Normal		Normal
Acid/Base	Metabolic acidosis	Lactic acidosis	Lactic acidosis	Lactic acidosis	Respiratory alkalosis	Anion Gap Acidosis	Normal
Ketones	No	Positive	No	No	No	Yes	No

Fig. 1. Breakdown of infant nutrition with examples of defects of metabolism.

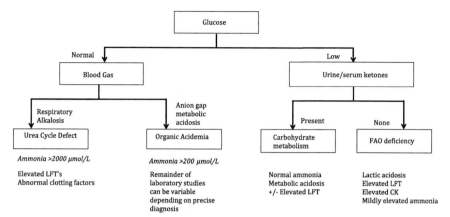

Fig. 2. Flowchart for diagnosis of metabolic diseases from laboratory findings. CK, creatine kinase; FAO, fatty acid oxidation; LFT, liver function tests.

8–16 mEq/L).[8] Gap acidoses from lactate are seen in pyruvate disorders, glycogen storage disease (GSD) type 1, and disorders of gluconeogenesis. If a gap remains after accounting for lactate, one should consider organic acidemias.

Clinicians should be on the lookout for respiratory alkalosis. This is highly unusual in an infant not on a ventilator and suggests an exogenous drive for hyperpnea, which is caused by toxic levels ammonia ions that directly stimulate the respiratory center.[9]

Urinalysis

In addition to screening for infection, providers should look carefully at ketones and reducing substances. Infants maintain a low level of ketosis but this is usually not measurable in the urine and the presence of ketones, although not specific, does point to a significant metabolic derangement. Also concerning is the inappropriate absence of ketones in the setting of hypoglycemia. When the blood sugar drops, fatty acids should undergo breakdown to form acetoacetate and β-hydroxybutyrate that the infant brain can use for fuel. The inability to form ketones despite marked hypoglycemia is highly suggestive of a fatty acid oxidation defect.[8]

The other simple urine evaluation is for the presence of reducing substances, a test that looks for the presence of other sugars in the urine that can reduce a cupric ion.[15] In a young infant, they should raise the suspicion for galactosemia fructosuria, or organic acidurias.[8]

Ammonia

Measuring an ammonia level is imperative in young infants who present with nonspecific neurologic decline and should be done simultaneously with a septic evaluation. An elevated ammonia level is not only indicative of IEM, it also requires immediate reduction to prevent irreversible brain damage. Levels that should alert a practitioner to a potential IEM are greater than 200 μmol/L; lower elevations are seen in healthy neonates in times of stress.[16] Children with urea cycle disorders can present with levels greater than 2000 μmol/L.[6] Differentiating between a urea cycle disorder and an organic acidemia in a patient with an elevated ammonia level is done based on the presence or absence of an anion gap metabolic acidosis. It is not the ammonia level that dictates clinical outcome but the duration of elevation.[7] Thus, stabilization, administration of scavenger molecules, and rapid transfer to a facility that can perform dialysis is life and brain saving.[16]

Treatment

The treatment of IEM in the undifferentiated patient is simplified into three main categories: (1) providing energy while shutting down catabolism, (2) correcting electrolyte and/or acid base imbalances, and (3) removing toxic metabolites. **Table 1** provides common drug dosages.

Shut down catabolism

Children with IEM require glucose administration for two functions: as an energy source for cellular function, and to shut off catabolic processes. As such, a simple bolus of glucose is insufficient and a normal glucose level in the blood should not reassure the provider that exogenous glucose is unnecessary. In fact, infants may need such a high quantity of glucose that insulin might be required to prevent hyperglycemia while avoiding cellular starvation. Additionally, it is imperative to remember that infants are highly prone to hypoglycemia because of high glucose use (almost twice that of an adult), an underdeveloped response to lower blood sugars (including glycogenolysis and gluconeogenesis), and smaller glycogen stores.[17]

Table 1
Common drugs used in the treatment of IEM

Drug	Dose	Effect	Use
10% Dextrose	2–4 mL/kg	Correct hypoglycemia and shut down catabolism	All
Insulin	0.05–0.1 U/kg/h	Anabolic hormone; correct hyperglycemia from exogenous glucose replacement	All
Intralipid	3 g/kg/d IV	Match calorie requirement during time of physiologic stress	All
Sodium bicarbonate	1–2 mEq/kg	Correction of metabolic acidosis	Organic acidemias
Carnitine	50–400 mg/kg IV bolus	Replaces carnitine loss, helps fatty acid oxidation	Organic acidemia; FAO
Ammunol (sodium benzoate/sodium phenylacetate)	250 mg/kg IV over 1–2 h; then 250 mg/kg IV over 24 h	Allows urinary excretion of ammonia	Hyperammonemia >200
Arginine	200–600 mg/kg IV	Scavenges ammonia	UCD
Biotin	10 mg IV/PO	Metabolize amino acids	Organic acidemia
Thiamin	25–100 mg IV	Amino acid metabolism	MSUD
Vitamin K	1–2 mg IM infant; 5–10 mg IM child	Reverse coagulopathy found in some carbohydrate disorders	Carbohydrate disorders

Abbreviations: FAO, fatty acid oxidation; IM, intramuscular; MSUD, maple syrup urine disease; UCD, urea cycle disorder.

Hypoglycemia, even mild, should be avoided in all infants who present to the ED because it can cause irreversible neurologic damage.[18] If the patient presents with hypoglycemia, the provider should take immediate action to correct it in the form of a 10% dextrose solution.[19,20] After correction, glucose should be administered continuously with D10 electrolyte solution at a maintenance rate.[21] For some pathologies, such as fatty acid oxidation deficiencies, a 15% dextrose–containing solution may be necessary.

There are other tools one can use to promote anabolism. Insulin is an anabolic hormone and its administration is helpful in preventing lipolysis, although glucose levels must be closely monitored and glucose administration may need to be increased.[21] Intralipid can also be administered because energy deficits need to be avoided at all costs and, in stress states, caloric requirements are 20% higher than at baseline.[22]

Correct acidosis
Correcting acidosis in young infants must be considered carefully. Severe acidosis can lead to cardiac dysfunction and cardiovascular collapse. In the setting of an organic acidemia, the burden of acid in the blood is not going to correct with hydration and cardiac effects are of significant concern. However, rapid and/or frequent boluses of bicarbonate in a severely dehydrated child may cause massive fluid shifts, cerebral edema, and even hemorrhage.[22] If a patient seems to have compromised hemodynamics in the setting of a profound acidosis that does not improve with fluid resuscitation, sodium bicarbonate is warranted.[23] Acidosis refractory to resuscitative efforts may require dialysis.

Remove toxic metabolites
There are two main subgroups of IEM that require emergent attention to the removal of toxic metabolites: branched chain organic acidurias and urea cycle disorders. Hyperammonemia should be treated with a combination of intravenous (IV) sodium benzoate and IV sodium phenylacetate (Ammonul) and arginine hydrochloride. This drug forms complexes that circumvent the urea cycle and allow for ammonia elimination in the urine. If the ammonia level is greater than 500 mmol/L hemodialysis should be initiated. Again, it is the duration of hyperammonemia, not the level, which causes devastating neurologic damage.[16]

Carnitine
Carnitine is an important cofactor for many biochemical pathways and is part of the mainstay of therapy for numerous IEM. In defects of fatty acid oxidation, carnitine halts lipolysis and helps convert important toxic compounds into usable forms for the Kreb cycle. Generally, this medication is safe to administer and is of benefit in various IEM's. Some of the fatty acid oxidation defects are secondary to issues with absorption or function of carnitine, which is integral in the transport of fatty acids into the mitochondria and their breakdown into acetyl coenzyme A (CoA; an important energy source during times of catabolic stress).[24] In organic acidemias, native carnitine binds to excess organic acids and is excreted in the urine leading to a secondary carnitine deficiency. To optimize the remainder of a patient's metabolism, carnitine should be administered.[4]

Infections
Sepsis should always be considered in the ill infant. Sepsis can mimic metabolic disease, it can provide the tipping point that leads to an emergent presentation in a child with an inborn error of metabolism, and children with IEM are more susceptible to infection (especially those with liver disease).[12]

Remember that *Escherichia coli* are a concern in patients with galactosemia and antibiotics should be emergently initiated to cover this potential infection.[11]

APPROACH TO SUSPECTED OR KNOWN DIAGNOSES
Disorders of Fat Metabolism

Fatty acid oxidation disorders
These disorders are caused by defects in the β-oxidation of fatty acids (medium chain, long chain, or very long chain acyl CoA dehydrogenase) or abnormalities in carnitine metabolism (eg, carnitine palmitoyltransferase deficiency). The hallmark of these disorders is hypoketotic/nonketotic hypoglycemia with fasting and most have similar presentations and treatment plans.

Presentation Metabolic crisis (hypoglycemia and acidosis) occurs in early infancy or early childhood. Most symptoms are prompted by prolonged fasting or decreased oral intake where there is normally reliance on fatty acids for energy. Patients present primarily with cardiac and neurologic signs and symptoms. Neonates can present with arrhythmias and conduction abnormalities and older infants commonly present with cardiomyopathy with recurrent nonketotic hypoglycemia. Fatty acid oxidation disorders also affect the central nervous system through lack of ketones (essential brain energy source during fasting) and accumulation of free fatty acids that cross the blood-brain barrier and cause neurologic damage.[13] Clinical features include hypothermia, hypotonia, seizures, coma, lethargy, hepatomegaly, rhabdomyolysis, myopathy, dysmorphic facies, and developmental delay (**Table 2**).[25]

Management

- Rapid recognition and correction of hypoglycemia (which also improves hyperammonemia). Delays cans lead to sudden death or worsening cardiac arrhythmias.[25]
- Carnitine: altered mental status may take a few hours to resolve even if glucose is stable because toxic metabolites need time to be metabolized.

Disorders of Carbohydrate Metabolism

Glycogen storage diseases
There are 11 inherited disorders of glycogen metabolism that result in accumulation of glycogen in various tissues depending on the affected enzyme. They are thought of in

Table 2	
Laboratory findings in fatty acid oxidation disorders	
CBC	Normal
BMP	Hypoglycemia, anion gap metabolic acidosis
Ammonia	Elevated
Blood gas	Metabolic acidosis
Lactic acid	Elevated
UA	NO ketones, myoglobinuria
AST/ALT	Elevated
CK	Elevated

Abbreviations: ALT, alanine aminotransferase; AST, aspartate aminotransferase; BMP, basic metabolic panel; CK, creatine kinase; UA, urinalysis.

two groups: those that affect hepatic metabolism of glycogen causing hypoglycemic events with build-up of glycogen, and those that effect glycogen breakdown in muscles leading to muscle breakdown but euglycemia. This article focuses on the illnesses where the liver is affected (GSD type 1 or von Gierke disease and GSD type III or Cori disease) because these lead to presentations of acute metabolic crisis.

Etiology GSD type 1 (von Gierke disease) is the most common GSD where either glucose-6-phosphatase or glucose-6-phosphate transporter is deficient resulting in derangements of glycogenolysis and gluconeogenesis. GSD type III causes glycogen accumulation in the liver and cardiac and skeletal muscle.

Presentation Despite three subtypes GSD type I–affected individuals present with profound hypoglycemia after a short period of fasting. Other abnormalities include hepatomegaly, nephromegaly, hyperlipidemia, and growth retardation.[26,27] Impaired myeloid function leading to neutropenia and macrophage dysfunction occurs in some cases. Patients with GSD type III develop hypertrophic cardiomyopathy; however, heart failure is rare (**Table 3**).[28]

Management

- Recognition and rapid correction of hypoglycemia
- Sodium bicarbonate for extreme acidosis or extremis
- Long term, patients require cornstarch or continuous feedings to prevent hypoglycemic episode
- Monitor for liver disease

Galactosemia
Etiology Galactose-1-phosphate uridyltransferase is deficient, rendering affected individuals unable to metabolize lactose into its components: glucose and galactose. Galactose and its intermediates accumulate, leading to osmotic effects in cells and eventual liver and brain dysfunction.

Presentation Patients are normal at birth; however, with lactose ingestion, galactose accumulates, causing vomiting, lethargy, and jaundice to develop around Day 5 to 10 of life. Poor weight gain, hepatomegaly, and marked encephalopathy ensue if untreated.[26] Some infants develop cataracts. An infant with severe liver dysfunction

Table 3
Laboratory findings in glycogen storage diseases

	GSD Type 1	GSD Type III
CBC	Neutropenia	Normal
BMP	Hypoglycemia, NGMA	Hypoglycemia, NGMA
Ammonia	Normal	Normal
Blood gas	Metabolic acidosis	Metabolic acidosis
Lactic acid	Elevated	Normal
UA	Ketones, myoglobinuria	Ketones
AST/ALT	Normal	Markedly elevated
Uric acid	Markedly elevated	Normal

Abbreviations: ALT, alanine aminotransferase; AST, aspartate aminotransferase; CBC, complete blood count; NGMA, nongap metabolic acidosis.

and coagulopathy with elevated bilirubin should be strongly considered to have galactosemia. Most countries have newborn testing but the United Kingdom and the Netherlands do not (**Table 4**).[26]

Management

- Immediate discontinuation of all lactose-containing formulas or breastfeeding
- Rapid recognition and treatment of hypoglycemia
- Evaluate for *E coli* sepsis (blood, urine, and cerebrospinal fluid cultures) and start antibiotics
- Monitor liver function

Hereditary fructose intolerance

Etiology Aldolase B is deficient resulting in accumulation of fructose-1 phosphate. The liver is unable to perform gluconeogenesis and glycogenolysis resulting in severe hypoglycemia after ingestion of fructose, sucrose, or sorbitol. These substances are found mainly in apples, grapes, watermelon, asparagus, peas, zucchini, and honey.[29]

Presentation Infants and toddlers present once solid foods are introduced into the diet with vomiting, poor oral intake, abnormal movements, seizures, and pallor.[30] Continued fructose intake leads to severe liver dysfunction with hepatomegaly and coagulopathy. Some patients do not present until school age because the hypoglycemia associated with fructose ingestion may be masked due to ingestion of other glucose-containing food items (**Table 5**).[26]

Management

- Address hypoglycemia
- Avoidance of fructose (also named levulose or invert sugar) and sorbitol, which both are found in medications as additives
- Treat coagulopathy with intramuscular vitamin K administration
- Clotting factor replacement only if life-threatening hemorrhage is suspected

Fructose bisphosphatase deficiency

Etiology Fructose-1,6 bisphosphatase is absent/deficient. This enzyme is important in gluconeogenesis. Glycolysis is not affected, so pyruvate, lactate, and acetyl CoA build up in cells.

Table 4 Laboratory findings in galactosemia	
CBC	Normal
BMP	Hypoglycemia, NGMA
Ammonia	Normal
Blood gas	Metabolic acidosis
Lactic acid	Elevated
UA	+reducing substances, ketones
Bilirubin	Elevated
AST/ALT	Elevated in rhabdomyolysis
Blood culture	*Escherichia coli*

Abbreviations: ALT, alanine aminotransferase; AST, aspartate aminotransferase; CBC, complete blood count; NGMA, nongap metabolic acidosis.

Table 5
Laboratory findings in hereditary fructose intolerance

CBC	Normal
BMP	Hypoglycemia, NGMA
Ammonia	Normal
Blood gas	Metabolic acidosis
Lactic acid	Markedly elevated
UA	Elevated protein
Bilirubin	Elevated
AST/ALT	Elevated
Albumin	Low
PT/PTT/INR	Abnormal

Abbreviations: ALT, alanine aminotransferase; AST, aspartate aminotransferase; CBC, complete blood count; INR, international normalized ratio; NGMA, nongap metabolic acidosis; PT, prothrombin time; PTT, partial thromboplastin time.

Presentation Neonates present with life-threatening hypoglycemia with metabolic acidosis precipitated by fasting. Apnea, hyperventilation, hypotonia, lethargy, tachycardia, and tachypnea occur. If the disease progresses without treatment hepatomegaly occurs with hypoglycemic episodes **(Table 6)**.[31]

Management

- Address hypoglycemia and severe metabolic acidosis with IV glucose, fluids, and sodium bicarbonate
- Treat coagulopathy with intramuscular vitamin K administration

Pyruvate disorders
Etiology Deficient pyruvate dehydrogenase or pyruvate carboxylase cause excess pyruvate in multiple tissues. Both disorders lead to abnormal increase in lactate resulting in severe metabolic acidosis.[8]

Table 6
Laboratory findings in fructose-1,6 bisphosphatase deficiency

CBC	Normal
BMP	Hypoglycemia, anion gap metabolic acidosis
Ammonia	Normal
Blood gas	Metabolic acidosis
Lactic acid	Markedly elevated
UA	Ketones
Bilirubin	Elevated
Uric acid	Elevated
Albumin	Low
PT/PTT/INR	Abnormal

Abbreviations: ALT, alanine aminotransferase; AST, aspartate aminotransferase; CBC, complete blood count; INR, international normalized ratio; PT, prothrombin time; PTT, partial thromboplastin time.

Presentation Pyruvate dehydrogenase has X-linked inheritance so neonatal males are mostly affected. Both disorders have hypotonia, seizures, lethargy, apnea, and encephalopathy in the newborn period (**Table 7**).

Management

- Correct metabolic acidosis with IV glucose, IV fluids, and sodium bicarbonate
- Thiamin, a pyruvate dehydrogenase cofactor, should be administered at a dose of 10 mg/kg/d
- Biotin, a cofactor for pyruvate carboxylase, should also be administered at a dose of 5 to 20 mg/d[22]

Disorders of Protein Metabolism

For the undifferentiated infant, there is usually a period of normal growth until toxic metabolites begin to accumulate, in hours to days. These infants commonly present with a severe metabolic encephalopathy that mimics sepsis. Other signs and symptoms include poor feeding, vomiting, irritability, abnormal movements (pedaling, boxing, myoclonic jerks), abnormal tone, and abnormal posturing (opisthonus).[11]

Aminoacidopathy
Etiology Aminoacidopathies are a heterogeneous group of illness in which defects in amino acid breakdown lead to accumulation of intact amino acids. Three of the most common aminoacidopathies include phenylketonuria (PKU), where a deficiency in phenylalanine hydroxylase leads to an accumulation of phenylalanine; maple syrup urine disease (MSUD), where branched chain α-ketoacid dehydrogenase is deficient resulting in accumulation of leucines and valine; and homocystinuria and tyrosinemia, where fumarylacetoacetase deficiency causes toxic buildup of tyrosine.

Presentation The clinical presentations of these illnesses vary from slow progressive neurotoxicity in the case of PKU, to rapid neurologic decline in the first weeks of life in MSUD, to primarily liver failure signs in tyrosinemia. Children with PKU, if adequately managed, have the opportunity to live full and productive lives, but if undetected or poorly managed, develop irreversible neurologic sequelae, such as microcephaly, developmental delay, intellectual disability, and/or seizures. PKU screening is performed in all states in the United States, because of the opportunity to intervene and drastically improve quality of life. Children with MSUD present more acutely with signs of neurologic stress once protein feeds begin. These include poor feeding, encephalopathy, and abnormal movements and can progress to coma and death.[22]

Table 7 Laboratory findings in pyruvate disorders	
CBC	Normal
BMP	Anion gap metabolic acidosis, no hypoglycemia
Ammonia	Normal
Blood gas	Metabolic acidosis
Lactic acid	Markedly elevated
UA	Normal
ALT/AST	Elevated ALT

Abbreviations: ALT, alanine aminotransferase; AST, aspartate aminotransferase; CBC, complete blood count.

Homocystinuria does not present with acute metabolic crisis or global neurologic alterations, although it can have acute thrombotic events.[3] Children with tyrosinemia can present with neurologic symptoms and episodes of liver failure. Other derangements include clotting disorders, ascites, bacterial peritonitis, gastrointestinal bleeds, and renal tubular acidosis (**Table 8**).[32]

Management The management for the aminoacidopathies depends on the cause. PKU rarely requires emergency management, although seizures and altered mental status can require supportive care. For MSUD

- Halt protein intake
- Shut down catabolism with insulin, glucose, and lipid emulsion infusion
- Avoid hyponatremia; use isotonic fluids only during the resuscitation phase[3]
- Consider mannitol or hypertonic saline for signs of cerebral edema
- Some phenotypes respond to thiamine supplementation[22]
- If severe neurologic presentation, patient must be treated with emergent toxin removal procedures (hemodialysis and/or exchange transfusion)

For tyrosinemia

- Stop all protein intake
- Start oral nitisinone 2-(2-nitro-4-(trifluoromethyl)benzoyl)cyclohexane-1,3-dione (NTBC) at a dose of 0.5 mg/kg/dose every 12 hours in suspected cases because this halts ongoing liver damage and may prevent need for liver transplantation[12,33]
- Supportive care for liver failure

Organic acidurias (acidemias)

Etiology Organic acidurias are characterized by the inability to breakdown deaminated amino acids. This causes profound metabolic acidosis with an anion gap in the cases of isovaleric aciduria, biotinidase deficiency, methylmalonic acidemia (MMA), and propionic acidemia (PA), and primary neurologic crisis in the case glutaric acidemia (GA). Although these disorders are screened for in newborn screening, there

Table 8 Laboratory findings in common aminoacidopathies			
	PKU	**MSUD**	**Tyrosinemia 1**
CBC	Normal	Normal	Normal
BMP	Normal	AGMA	NGMA
Ammonia	Normal	Elevated	Normal
Blood gas	Normal	MA	MA
Lactic acid	Normal	Elevated	Elevated
UA	Mousy odor	Ketones, maple syrup odor	Reducing substances sulfur odor "sweaty feet"
Ketones	Positive	Positive	Positive
AST/ALT Bilirubin	Normal	Normal	Elevated
Symptoms	Global neurologic decline	Episodic acute neurologic signs	Liver failure, renal tubular acidosis ± encephalopathy

Abbreviations: AGMA, anion gap metabolic acidosis; ALT, alanine aminotransferase; AST, aspartate aminotransferase; BMP, basic metabolic panel; CBC, complete blood count; MA, metabolic acidosis; NGMA, nongap metabolic acidosis; UA, urinalysis.

are children who have false-negative tests and those that present in crisis before availability of newborn screening results.

Presentation The catabolic state is dangerous for children with organic acidemias. Isovaleric aciduria, MMA, and PA present in crisis with neurologic deterioration associated with anion gap metabolic acidosis. Neurologic symptoms in these three classical organic acidurias can range from hypotonia and abnormal movements (boxing or paddling motions) to lethargy, seizures, and coma. Stroke can occur with MMA and PA.[3,34] Children with GA can present differently because crises are primarily neurologic and do not carry the profound laboratory abnormalities that can clue providers into a diagnosis. For these patients, catabolic crises occur during times of physiologic stress (gastroenteritis, febrile illnesses, vaccinations, surgeries) and can lead to profound, irreversible neurologic damage. Patients present with dystonia, movement disorders, hypotonia, and evidence of basal ganglia damage on imaging. Some patients come to medical attention because of subdural hemorrhage, caused by widening of the subarachnoid space. Children with GA are vulnerable to crises until age 6 (**Table 9**).[35–38]

Management

- Stop catabolism; IV glucose replacement and insulin
- Carnitine supplementation
- Alkalanization of urine with sodium bicarbonate
- Seizure treatment with phenobarbital or phenytoin (do not use valproate)
- Treat dystonia with benzodiazepines[39]
- Treat hyperammonemia with sodium benzoate/sodium phenylacetate and arrange for emergent dialysis for levels greater than 500 mmol/L
- Consider vitamin B_{12} and biotin administration because these are indicated in MMA
- Dialysis for refractory metabolic acidosis

Urea cycle disorders
Derangements in any of the six enzymes responsible for the degradation of nitrogenous waste leads to elevated ammonia. Affected individuals present within hours to days after birth with vomiting, altered mental status, and encephalopathy that can

Table 9
Laboratory findings in organic acidurias

	Glutaric Aciduria	Methylmalonic Acidemia	Propionic Acidemia
CBC	Normal		Pancytopenia
BMP	AGMA	AGMA	AGMA
Ammonia	Normal	Elevated	Elevated
Lactic acid	Elevated	Mildly elevated	Mildly elevated
Uric acid	Normal	Elevated	Elevated
Unique presenting features	Subdural hemorrhage (can be confused for nonaccidental trauma)	Stroke	Pancreatitis

Abbreviations: AGMA, anion gap metabolic acidosis; BMP, basic metabolic panel; CBC, complete blood count.

Table 10
Laboratory findings in ornithine transcarbamylase deficiency

CBC	Thrombocytopenia
BMP	Normal
Ammonia	Markedly elevated
Blood gas	Respiratory alkalosis
Lactic acid	Normal
UA	Normal
AST/ALT	Elevated
PT/PTT/INR	Abnormal

Abbreviations: ALT, alanine aminotransferase; AST, aspartate aminotransferase; CBC, complete blood count; INR, international normalized ratio; PT, prothrombin time; PTT, partial thromboplastin time.

lead to coma. In the neonatal onset of disease, ammonia levels are usually at least 150 μmol/L and range from 500 to 2000 μmol/L. Prolonged fasting or excessive protein intake may precipitate a hyperammonemic crisis. In some forms, individuals present later in life with recurrent bouts of gastric (vomiting, abdominal pain) and neurologic (seizure, encephalopathy, behavior issues, psychiatric issues) symptoms.

The two main urea cycle disorders ED clinicians should be aware of are ornithine transcarbamylase deficiency (OTC) and citrullinemia. Citrullinemia differs from OTC in that most affected infants present with liver failure within the first 1 to 3 months of life. ED management is the same for both.

Ornithine transcarbamylase deficiency

Presentation The classic infantile form of OTC presents early with poor feeding, vomiting, tachypnea, lethargy, hypotonia, and apnea (**Table 10**).

Management

- Reduce catabolism with glucose and insulin[22]
- Treat hyperammonemia: sodium benzoate/sodium phenylacetate and arrange for emergent dialysis for levels greater than 500 mmol/L[38]

REFERENCES

1. Campeau PM, Scriver CR, Mitchell JJ. A 25-year longitudinal analysis of treatment efficacy in inborn errors of metabolism. Mol Genet Metab 2008;95:11–6.
2. Deodato F, Boenzi S, Rizzo C, et al. Inborn errors of metabolism: an update on epidemiology and on neonatal-onset hyperammonemia. Acta Paediatr 2004; 93(445):18–21.
3. Rice GM, Steiner RD. Inborn errors of metabolism (metabolic disorders). Pediatr Rev 2016;37(1):3–17.
4. Baumgartner MR, Hörster F, Dionisi-Vici C. Proposed guidelines for the diagnosis and management of mathylmalonic and propionic acidemia. Orphanet J Rare Dis 2014;9:130.
5. Saudubray JM, Nassogne MC, de Lonlay P, et al. Clinical approach to inherited metabolic disorders in neonates: an overview. Semin Neonatol 2002;7:3–15.
6. Ellaway CJ, Wilcken B, Christodoulou J. Clinical approach to inborn errors of metabolism presenting in the newborn period. J Paediatr Child Health 2002;38: 511–7.

7. Gropman AL, Summar M, Leonard V. Neurologic implications of urea cycle disorders. J Inherit Metab Dis 2007;30:865–9.

8. Enns GM, Packman S. Diagnosing inborn errors of metabolism in the newborn: laboratory investigations. Neoreviews 2001;2(8):e191–200.

9. Enns GM. Neurologic damage and neurocognitive dysfunction in urea cycle disorders. Semin Pediatr Neurol 2008;15:132–9.

10. Shaw AM. Bicarbonate and chloride equilibrium and acid-base balance in the neonate. Neonatal Netw 2008;27(4):261–6.

11. Burton BK. Inborn errors of metabolism: a guide to diagnosis. Pediatrics 1988; 102(6):1–9.

12. Clayton PT. Inborn errors presenting with liver dysfunction. Semin Neonatol 2002; 7:49–63.

13. Roe CR. Inherited disorders of mitochondrial fatty acid oxidation: a new responsibility for the neonatologist. Semin Neonatol 2002;7:37–47.

14. Chou JY, Jun HS, Mansfield BC. Type I glycogen storage diseases: disorders of the glucose-6-phosphatase/glucose-6-phosphate transporter complexes. J Inherit Metab Dis 2015;38(3):511–9.

15. Naumova NN, Schappert J, Kaplan LA. Reducing substances in urine: a paradigm for changes in a standard test. Ann Clin Lab Sci 2006;36(4):447–8.

16. Leonard JV, Morris AAM. Urea cycle disorders. Semin Neonatol 2002;7:27–35.

17. Hoe FM. Hypoglycemia in infants and children. Adv Pediatr 2008;55:367–84.

18. Burns CM, Rutherford MA, Boardman JP, et al. Patterns of cerebral injury and neurodevelopmental outcomes after symptomatic neonatal hypoglycemia. Pediatrics 2008;122:65–74.

19. Ghosh A, Banerjee I, Morris A. Recognition, assessment and management of hypoglycemia in childhood. Arch Dis Child 2016;101:575–80.

20. Sweet CB, Grayson S, Polak M. Management strategies for neonatal hypoglycemia. J Pediatr Pharmacol Ther 2013;18(3):199–208.

21. de Baulny HO. Management and emergency treatments of neonates with a suspicion of inborn errors of metabolism. Semin Neonatol 2002;7:17–26.

22. El-Hattab AW. Inborn errors of metabolism. Clin Perinatol 2015;42:413–39.

23. Kwon KT, Tsai VW. Metabolic emergencies. Emerg Med Clin North Am 2007;25: 1041–60.

24. Vishwanath VA. Fatty acid beta-oxidation disorders: a brief review. Ann Neurosci 2016;23(1):51–5.

25. Saudubray JM, Martin D, De Lonlay P, et al. Recognition and management of fatty acid oxidation defects: a series of 107 patients. J Inherit Metab Dis 1999;22(4): 488–502.

26. Levy P. Inborn errors of metabolism part 2: specific disorders. Pediatr Rev 2009; 30(4):e22–8.

27. Dagli A, Sentner CP, Weinstein DA. Glycogen storage disease type III. In: Pagon RA, Adam MP, Ardinger HH, et al, editors. GeneReviews® [Internet]. Seattle (WA): University of Washington, Seattle; 2016. p. 1993–2017. Available at: https://www.ncbi.nlm.nih.gov/books/NBK26372/.

28. Kishnani PS, Austin SL, Arn P, et al. Glycogen storage disease type III diagnosis and management guidelines. Genet Med 2010;12(7):446–63.

29. Zeratski K. Fructose intolerance: which foods to avoid. 2016. Available at: https://www.mayoclinic.org/fructose-intolerance/expert-answers/FAQ-20058097. Accessed June 27, 2017.

30. Mayatepek E, Hoffmann B, Meissner T. Inborn errors of carbohydrate metabolism. Best Pract Res Clin Gastroenterol 2010;4(5):607–18.

31. Buhrdel P, Bohme HJ, Didt L. Biochemical and clinical observations in four patients with fructose-1,6-diphosphatase deficiency. Eur J Pediatr 1990;149:574–6.
32. Sniderman King L, Trahms C, Scott CR. Tyrosinemia type I. In: Pagon RA, Adam MP, Ardinger HH, et al, editors. GeneReviews® [Internet]. Seattle (WA): University of Washington, Seattle; 2017. p. 1993–2017. Available at: https://www.ncbi.nlm.nih.gov/books/NBK1515/.
33. de Laet C, Dionisi-Vici C, Leonard JV, et al. Recommendations for the treatment of tyrosinaemia type 1. Orphanet J Rare Dis 2013;8:8.
34. Dionisi-Vici C, Deodato F, Röschinger W, et al. 'Classical' organic acidurias, propionic aciduria, methylmalonic aciduria and isovaleric aciduria: long term outcome and effects of expanded newborn screening using tandem mass spectrometry. J Inherit Metab Dis 2006;29:383–9.
35. Kolker S, Sauer SW, Hoffman GF, et al. Pathogenesis of CNS involvement in disorders of amino and organic acid metabolism. J Inherit Metab Dis 2008;31: 194–204.
36. Bjugstad KB, Goodman SI, Freed CR. Age at symptom onset predicts severity of motor impairment and clinical outcome of glutaric acidemia. J Pediatr 2000; 137(5):681–6.
37. Strauss KA, Puffenberger EG, Robinson DL, et al. Type I glutaric aciduria, part 1: natural history of 77 patients. Am J Med Genet C Semin Med Genet 2003; 121C(1):38–52.
38. Nassogne MC, Héron B, Touatt G, et al. Urea cycle defects: management and outcome. J Inherit Metab Dis 2005;28:407–14.
39. Vester MEM, Bilo RAC, Karst WA, et al. Subdural hematomas: glutaric aciduria or abusive head trauma? A systematic review. Forensic Sci Med Pathol 2015;11: 405–15.

Section 2: Critical

Pediatric Emergency Noninvasive Ventilation

Chad D. Viscusi, MD[a,b,]*, Garrett S. Pacheco, MD[a,b]

KEYWORDS

- Noninvasive ventilation • Acute respiratory failure • Infants • Children

KEY POINTS

- Noninvasive ventilation (NIV) is a powerful tool often initiated early in the management of pediatric acute respiratory failure (ARF).
- NIV includes the following 2 positive pressure modalities: continuous positive airway pressure and bilevel positive airway pressure, which treat hypoxemic and hypercapnic respiratory failure, respectively.
- Humidified high-flow nasal cannula, although not classically considered a mode of NIV, provides another mean of treating hypoxemic ARF in infants and children.
- Commonly encountered pediatric respiratory diseases, such as bronchiolitis and asthma, may benefit from the early utilization of NIV.

INTRODUCTION (BACKGROUND AND DEFINITIONS)

Respiratory illness is one of the most common reasons parents seek emergency medical care for their children. Although many of these children will have a benign and self-limited process, some will present with respiratory distress or frank respiratory failure. The ability to promptly recognize respiratory failure and appropriately, quickly, and safely initiate ventilatory support are vital skills for any professional providing care to sick or injured children. This article reviews the use of noninvasive ventilation (NIV) in the emergency care of infants and children with acute respiratory failure (ARF). The authors discuss the physiology, highlight the evidence, and provide a practical approach to the use of this powerful technique.

Historically, pediatric ARF has been managed with endotracheal intubation (ETI) and invasive mechanical ventilation (IMV). However, ETI and IMV are associated with a variety of significant complications in children[1,2] (**Box 1**).

Disclosure Statement: The authors have no significant financial or other conflicts of interest to disclose.
[a] Department of Emergency Medicine, University of Arizona College of Medicine, 1501 N. Campbell Avenue, Tucson, AZ 85724, USA; [b] Department of Pediatrics, University of Arizona College of Medicine, 1501 N. Campbell Avenue, Tucson, AZ 85724, USA
* Corresponding author. Department of Emergency Medicine, University of Arizona College of Medicine, 1501 N. Campbell Avenue, Tucson, AZ 85724, USA.
E-mail address: cviscusi@aemrc.arizona.edu

Box 1
Risks and complications associated with conventional invasive acute respiratory failure management

ETI

Oropharyngeal injury

Laryngeal injury

Tracheal injury

Hypoxia, bradycardia

Subglottic stenosis

IMV

Ventilator-associated pneumonia

VILI: barotrauma

VILI: volutrauma

Need for heavy sedation, paralysis

Inability to speak, eat

Abbreviation: VILI, ventilator-induced lung injury.

NIV is the application of mechanical respiratory support without the use of an invasive endotracheal tube. The use of NIV in children has increased significantly in recent years in hopes of improving respiratory physiology while avoiding the risks of ETI and IMV and is now used widely in the management of acute and chronic respiratory failure in patients of all ages.[3–5] Much of the historical evidence supporting the safety and efficacy of NIV in children comes from the study of neonatal apnea and respiratory distress syndrome and the management of obstructive sleep apnea and chronic respiratory failure of neuromuscular disorders.[6,7] Evidence suggests that early NIV decreases the work of breathing, improves oxygenation and ventilation while avoiding complications associated with ETI (see **Box 1**). Additional advantages of NIV include preservation of spontaneous respiration and airway protective reflexes (swallowing, coughing), maintenance of the ability to speak, and the provision of enteral feeding in select circumstances. NIV has become, at many institutions, the first-line intervention in the emergency management of ARF in children.[3,5]

GENERAL PHYSIOLOGY

The primary objective of NIV used in the emergency management of pediatric acute respiratory distress and ARF is to improve oxygenation and ventilation while decreasing the work of breathing and the associated metabolic demands. There are 2 basic types of noninvasive positive pressure ventilation currently in use: continuous positive airway pressure (CPAP) and bilevel positive airway pressure (BiPAP); although not historically considered a form of NIV, high-flow nasal cannula (HFNC) oxygen therapy has emerged as another powerful tool in the emergency armamentarium for noninvasive management of pediatric ARF.

Continuous Positive Airway Pressure

CPAP provides a constant positive distending airway pressure throughout the entire respiratory cycle of spontaneously breathing patients. CPAP is most appropriate for type 1 (hypoxic) respiratory failure and is well suited to infants and small children with significant tachypnea. CPAP recruits collapsed alveoli, increasing lung volume and functional residual capacity; assists with inspiratory work by unloading respiratory musculature and improving flow; and prevents both obstructive apnea by stenting the upper airways and central apnea via respiratory stimulation. Through these mechanisms, CPAP improves oxygenation and decreases the work of breathing.[8,9]

Bilevel Positive Airway Pressure

BiPAP delivers a preset inspiratory positive airway pressure (IPAP) greater than a baseline expiratory positive airway pressure (EPAP), synonymous with positive end expiratory pressure (PEEP), to spontaneously breathing patients when triggered by their inspiratory effort or preset backup mandatory respiratory rate (RR). This active ventilation strategy can generate a tidal volume based on the magnitude of difference between IPAP and EPAP. BiPAP is preferred for type 2 (hypercapnic) as well as type 1 (hypoxic) respiratory failure and represents a higher level of support than CPAP.

High-Flow Nasal Cannula

HFNC oxygen therapy has emerged as a very effective and well-tolerated respiratory support technique, most beneficial to those with respiratory distress or type 1 respiratory failure. Heated, humidified HFNC therapy fully supplies patients' resting minute ventilation and oxygenates the nasopharyngeal dead space. HFNC provides oxygen at optimal warmth and humidity. It has been reported to improve liquefaction of secretions and mucociliary clearance; to inhibit inflammatory reactions and nasopulmonary bronchoconstriction triggered by cold, dry air; to provide PEEP; and to decrease RR and the work of breathing.[10,11] The amount of PEEP generated by HFNC is variable. The continuous high flow can provide a positive pharyngeal pressure, and some studies report obtaining PEEP in newborns as high as 2 to 5 cm H_2O and older children up to 4.0 ± 2.00 cm H_2O.[12,13] However, effective end-expiratory alveolar pressure is variable and difficult to predict compared with the traditional NIV modes of CPAP and BiPAP and can be compromised by a leak from the mouth opening and from around the nasal prongs.

INDICATIONS/RELATIVE AND ABSOLUTE CONTRAINDICATIONS

Practitioners of pediatric emergency care will encounter many patients with respiratory distress and some with respiratory failure. Being able to rapidly recognize the signs of both is a critically important skill (**Table 1**). NIV is typically initiated for children

Table 1	
Recognizing pediatric respiratory distress and failure	
Respiratory Distress	**Respiratory Failure**
Tachypnea	Severe dyspnea/distress/apnea
Retractions (intercostal, subcostal, suprasternal)	Hypoxia: Fio_2 >50% for SpO_2 >92%
Grunting (attempt to create PEEP)	Hypercarbia: Pco_2 >50 mm Hg
Nasal flaring	Respiratory acidosis with pH <7.35
Head bobbing	Accessory muscle exhaustion
Accessory muscle use	Decreased level of consciousness

Data from Vitaliti G, Wenzel A, Bellia F, et al. Noninvasive ventilation in pediatric emergency care: a literature review and description of our experience. Expert Rev Respir Med 2013;7(5):545–52; and Richards AM. Pediatric respiratory emergencies. Emerg Med Clin North Am 2016;34(1):77–96.

with impending or ARF as bridge therapy until the acute illness improves or as a treatment modality to prevent ETI, IMV, and the associated risks.[8] It is recommended that in the absence of contraindications, NIV should be considered as the first-line management for pediatric ARF unless in fulminant acute respiratory distress syndrome (ARDS) or in immediate need of ETI.[8,14] Contraindications to the initiation of NIV are related to the absence of spontaneous respiration, compromise of airway protection, or the inability to achieve a good interface fit or ventilator synchrony (**Table 2**).

MECHANICS/SETTINGS/INTERFACES/VENTS/SYNCHRONY
Interfaces

The selection of a well-fitting, appropriately sized, comfortable interface is critical to achieving successful NIV while minimizing air leaks and maximizing patient comfort and synchrony with the ventilator. Despite the fact that interface tolerance is a major factor in NIV success, there are little comparative data on interfaces for infants and children.[15] Typical interfaces are listed in **Box 2**. The smallest interface with the least air leak should be chosen to minimize dead space.[9] For infants, a nasal cannula, nasal prong, or nasal mask is the best first interface choice,[16] whereas older children and young adults achieve better ventilation and less mask leak with full oronasal face masks. The use of total face masks and helmets is less common; but some data, including one randomized controlled trial (RCT), suggest feasibility, better tolerance, lower risk of skin injury, and less air leak when CPAP is administered by a helmet interface in infants and younger children.[17–19]

Ventilators

CPAP and BiPAP can be delivered by critical care and portable ventilators; however, a critical care ventilator is preferable in the emergency setting. Should conversion to IMV be necessary, the intensive care unit (ICU) ventilator can be used for preoxygenation before ETI. It is best to familiarize yourself with the equipment available at your institution and ensure that a ventilator with specific functionality for NIV, such as leak compensation, is used.[5]

Initial settings

Initial setting recommendations are largely based on clinical experience and expert consensus as there are no consistent data on optimal NIV settings (**Fig. 1**). Additionally, the initial settings chosen should be disease and device specific. In general, support should start low to allow patient acclimation and then increase according to the

Table 2
Relative and absolute contraindications

Absolute Contraindications	Relative Contraindications
Cardiopulmonary arrest	Hemodynamic instability, vasopressors
Coma, severely decreased LOC	Recent airway or upper GI surgery
Inability to protect airway	Active upper GI bleeding
Inability to fit interface or mask	Inability to cooperate, tolerate
Facial deformity, trauma, burns	Excessive secretions
Undrained pneumothorax	Cyanotic congenital heart disease

Abbreviations: GI, gastrointestinal; LOC, level of consciousness.
Data from Nava S, Hill N. Non-invasive ventilation in acute respiratory failure. Lancet 2009;374(9685):250–9; and Bello G, De Pascale G, Antonelli M. Noninvasive ventilation: practical advice. Curr Opin Crit Care 2013;19(1):1–8.

Box 2 **Interface types**
Nasal cannula or prongs
Nasal mask
Oronasal face mask
Total face mask
Helmet

physiologic needs and patient tolerance. Fraction of inspired oxygen (Fio_2) delivery should be sufficient to achieve a peripheral capillary oxygen saturation (SpO_2) greater than 92%. Settings for CPAP start between 3 and 5 cm H_2O and increase as needed and tolerated to 4 to 8 cm H_2O. When initiating BiPAP, start with IPAP 6 to 8 cm H_2O/ EPAP 3 to 5 cm H_2O and increase as needed and tolerated to 10 to 15 cm H_2O/6 to 10 cm H_2O.[8] Monitor carefully for an air leak and patient-ventilator synchrony. There are limited data on optimal flow rates for HFNC oxygen therapy. One study reported that a 2-L/kg/min flow provides the equivalence of 3- to 5-cm H_2O CPAP.[20] The authors recommend 2 L/kg/min for the first 10 kg of body weight and an additional 0.5 L/kg/min for each kilogram greater than 10 kg.[21] The manufacturer of the HFNC device typically labels equipment or packaging with the recommended maximum flow rate. First set the flow to decrease the patients' work of breathing, and then set the temperature to 36°C to 37°C. Finally, set Fio_2 at 0.40 and titrate to achieve an SpO_2 greater than 92%.

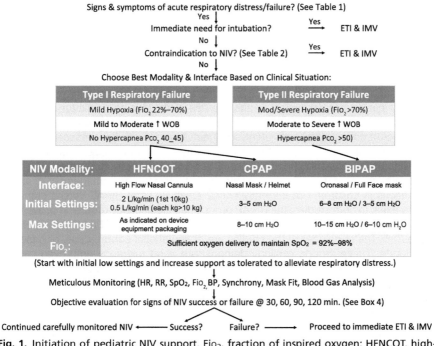

Fig. 1. Initiation of pediatric NIV support. Fio_2, fraction of inspired oxygen; HFNCOT, high-flow nasal cannula oxygen therapy; HR, heart rate; SpO_2, peripheral capillary oxygen saturation.

Synchrony and sedation

The most common causes of ventilator asynchrony in children are intolerance of the interface, auto-triggering, and insufficient inspiratory effort to trigger ventilation.[22] Therefore, setting appropriate sensitivity of the inspiratory and expiratory triggers is vital to NIV synchrony in children.[8] Sedation should rarely be used and only with great caution in children with ARF. Patient agitation, interface intolerance, or ventilator asynchrony may, in actuality, be a manifestation of the air hunger associated with significant hypoxia and the increased work of breathing.[5] Every effort should be made to clearly address these issues before any consideration is given to sedative administration. Optimal sedative choice must preserve central respiratory drive and airway protective reflexes, while exerting minimal impact on muscular strength and tone.[5,23]

PEDIATRIC EMERGENCY DEPARTMENT NONINVASIVE POSITIVE PRESSURE VENTILATION: THE DATA AND SPECIFIC CLINICAL SCENARIOS

NIV has become increasingly prevalent in the pediatric emergency department (PED) and pediatric ICU (PICU) as supportive therapy for ARF. In 2008, the first pediatric RCT of NIV plus standard therapy versus standard therapy alone as support for undifferentiated ARF in children was published. The results showed a significantly improved heart rate (HR) and RR, improved Po_2/Fio_2 ratio, and a lower rate of ETI (28% vs 60%) in the NIV cohort.[24] The trend toward improvement in vital signs (HR, RR, SpO_2), the work of breathing, and respiratory acidosis (pH, Pco_2) with NIV has been demonstrated in other studies as well.[22,25] NIV also seems to protect children from ETI, with published success rates ranging from 64% to 84%,[14,23,24,26–28] with the lower percentages in infant patients with hypoxic respiratory failure.[2,29,30]

Asthma

Asthma is a chronic respiratory condition consisting of bronchial smooth muscle spasm, airway inflammation, and increased mucous production[31] that can lead to smaller airway obstruction, respiratory distress, and ARF. ETI is risky in status asthmaticus, as these patients do not tolerate apnea well. Further, IMV can be challenging because of air trapping, dynamic hyperinflation (auto-PEEP) with the subsequent danger of cardiovascular collapse, and the risk of developing ventilator-associated pneumonia (VAS). In asthma, NIV seems to unload respiratory muscles, offset intrinsic PEEP, recruit collapsed alveoli, stent small airways, decrease resistance to airflow, minimize air-trapping, and possibly even directly bronchodilate/decrease bronchial hyperresponsiveness and improve delivery of aerosolized bronchodilators.[32,33]

Data are emerging that NIV may be safe and effective for the management of status asthmaticus in children, but currently only 2 small RCTs of BiPAP versus standard therapy exist. In both studies, the BiPAP groups had significantly greater improvement in clinical status (improved RR and clinical asthma score) without any major adverse events.[34,35] The remainder of the studies are observational cohort, case, or case series reports. These reports similarly demonstrate good tolerance, improved clinical and laboratory respiratory parameters, and safety with no major complications during the use of NIV in the care of children with status asthmaticus.[36–38] However, recent systematic reviews caution that the current data are not yet conclusive, especially regarding the ability of NIV to prevent ETI/IMV; further high-quality research is needed (although simple randomization may no longer be ethical because of the lack of clinical equipoise).[39,40]

The use of HFNC in the management of pediatric status asthmaticus has been associated with significantly reduced work of breathing, RR, and respiratory time fraction.[20] HFNC's ability to effectively improve the expiratory time may decrease dynamic hyperinflation in patients with obstructive lung disease, such as asthma. In addition to improvement in physiologic parameters, HFNC has also been shown to reduce ETI in patients with status asthmaticus.[11,41] Some HFNC devices also allow for the administration of in-line nebulized short-acting beta agonists.[42]

Bronchiolitis

A major cause of seasonal illness and hospitalization for children less than 2 years of age, bronchiolitis is typically caused by a viral acute lower respiratory tract infection manifesting a clinical syndrome of rhinorrhea, congestion, cough, crackles, wheezes, and dyspnea. Airway inflammation, increased mucous production, and mucous plugging obstruct bronchial airways, resulting in hypoxia and respiratory distress that can progress to respiratory failure in a small number of infants and children.

Although recent Cochrane and systematic reviews have concluded that because of the lack of high-quality RCTs there is currently insufficient evidence to determine the effectiveness of either CPAP or HFNC therapy for bronchiolitis,[43–45] there has been a definite clinical movement toward routine use of NIV (CPAP and HFNC), with HFNC frequently chosen as the first-line therapy for infants with severe bronchiolitis.[46] This widespread clinical practice adoption of NIV is based on data from several observational studies and 2 small RCTs that support the safe use of NIV in bronchiolitis. In 2008, the first RCT noted a significant decrease in Pco_2 while on CPAP but observed no significant differences in secondary outcomes of HR, RR, need for IMV, or length of stay, although the study was likely underpowered to detect these effects.[16] A 2008 retrospective review of infants with severe bronchiolitis noted a significantly reduced ETI rate during the period when NIV was available and that the use of NIV was associated with less VAP and a shorter duration of oxygen requirement.[47] In 2012, another retrospective review revealed a significant increase in the use of NIV (2.8%/y) and a decrease in ETI (1.9%/y) over the study period (83.2% NIV success). The presence of a comorbidity (prematurity, chronic lung disease, neuromuscular disease, immune deficiency, congenital heart disease) was associated with a higher likelihood of NIV failure.[4] The second RCT, published in 2013, compared 6 cm H_2O nasal CPAP (nCPAP) with conventional oxygen therapy. CPAP rapidly reduced the clinical respiratory distress score, the need for oxygen, and the inspiratory muscle work (assessed by measuring esophageal pressures) associated with acute severe RSV bronchiolitis.[48] In 2014, 2 additional retrospective cohort reviews were published. One demonstrated that nCPAP for severe RSV was independently associated with a shorter duration of ventilation, even after adjusting for disease severity and comorbidity.[49] Another larger review found that those receiving CPAP had a shorter length of ventilation, shorter length of stay, and significantly lower cost of care.[50] These studies suggest that initiating early NIV in severe bronchiolitis is safe and well tolerated and provide evidence of decreased work of breathing and improved ventilation physiology. A large, well-designed RCT is needed to confirm the impact of NIV on these clinically important outcomes.

HFNC oxygen therapy has become a reasonable alternative to NIV for the treatment of acute bronchiolitis, where it has been shown to reduce rates of ETI.[11,51–54] However, a 2014 Cochrane review concluded that although the median SpO_2 at 8 and 12 hours was higher in the HFNC group, there was no significant difference in total oxygen therapy duration or total length of stay. The absence of adverse events or need for IMV in either group suggests that HFNC may be safe and feasible, although it has not yet been demonstrated to be equivalent or superior to NIV.[44] In fact, a recent study suggested that nCPAP was more efficient than HFNC for initial respiratory support in young infants hospitalized for moderate to severe bronchiolitis.[55] In the authors' experience, a carefully monitored trial of HFNC is reasonable to initiate early for infants or children with increased work of breathing, difficulty clearing nasal secretions, and mild hypoxia due to acute bronchiolitis. In fact, many institutions have a bronchiolitis treatment protocol that suggests initiation of HFNC based on a clinical respiratory distress score.[52,56]

Pneumonia and Acute Respiratory Distress Syndrome

The data supporting the effective use of NIV for significant pediatric airspace disease, such as pneumonia or ARDS, are less consistent and suggest that NIV be used with caution. A report from the 2015 Pediatric Acute Lung Injury Consensus Conference proposed that NIV (BiPAP via oronasal or full face mask preferred) might be considered as an early treatment option in children at risk for ARDS or with early ARDS, if carefully monitored by highly trained staff in an appropriate setting. They emphasize that ETI and IMV should be undertaken for those children with moderate to severe disease and those who do not show clinical improvement as measured by RR, HR, oxygen requirement, Pco_2, and the work of breathing.[57] This cautious recommendation is based on the high NIV failure rates reported in children with moderate to severe ARDS (67.8% in a 2015 study).[5] Others have also reported NIV failure rates in the setting of ARDS between 50% and 78%.[58,59] Therefore, the authors think that early ETI and IMV is a better choice for patients with moderate to severe ARDS. There are currently no high-quality data regarding the utility of HFNC use in ARDS; therefore, the authors cannot make recommendations regarding its use in this circumstance.

Although NIV is being used to support children with acute pneumonia, this deserves careful consideration and close monitoring as well. Although a small prospective RCT of NIV versus standard therapy in patients with viral and bacterial pneumonia in 2008 did show decreased ETI in the NIV group, nearly 28% of the NIV group with pneumonia still required ETI and IMV.[24] Pneumonia also emerged as an independent risk factor for NIV failure by an 2012 observational prospective study of NIV use in children with ARF.[60] A recent study in the *Lancet* randomized children younger than 5 years with severe pneumonia to 5 cm H_2O bubble CPAP, standard nasal cannula 2 L/min, or HFNC (2 L/kg/min). Those who received CPAP had less NIV treatment failure (6% vs 24%) and a significantly lower rate of death (4% vs 15%) than those who received low-flow oxygen therapy. Mortality rates were similar in the CPAP and HFNC groups.[61] Several other noncontrolled trials and retrospective reviews report an improvement in clinical and laboratory parameters without major adverse events in children with pneumonia.[14,29,59,62] The impact on ETI was variable. NIV may be a useful tool in the management of mild to moderate pneumonia with careful monitoring, but more data are needed. There are several ongoing studies examining the use of HFNC that, it is hoped, will guide our practice; but currently there are insufficient data for the efficacy of HFNC in children with pneumonia.

Monitoring (The Golden Two Hours)

Concurrent with the initiation of NIV must be the initiation of meticulous patient monitoring. In fact, children managed with NIV may actually require more careful observation during the first 2 hours of therapy than do their IMV counterparts. Children should have nothing by mouth and be placed on continuous cardiorespiratory monitoring and SpO_2. The lung examination (adventitious sounds, prolonged expiratory time), HR, RR, work of breathing, patient tolerance/synchrony, interface leak, and periodic blood gas analysis must all be monitored and documented. Venous or capillary blood gas obtained 30 minutes after ventilation start and each hour thereafter will allow close

Pco_2 and pH monitoring. Delaying ETI for the child who truly needs IMV can have serious consequences, and those children with a good response to NIV typically manifest improvement within the first 2 hours.

Predictors of Success/Failure

Some children started on NIV will ultimately fail and require ETI and IMV. The likelihood of success or failure depends on multiple factors, including the patients' underlying medical conditions; the cause, severity, and type of the respiratory failure; the timing of NIV implementation; and the level of experience of the health care team.[5,63] Those who successfully avoided ETI were more likely to have a good early response to NIV (decreased RR, Pco_2, Fio_2, and work of breathing) during the first 2 hours of NIV than were their counterparts who ultimately required IMV. Similarly, patients with bronchiolitis who benefited from HFNC demonstrated a decrease in RR and HR within 90 minutes of the start of HFNC therapy.[52] Therefore, meticulous monitoring of respiratory status and blood gas values during the first hours of NIV in children is of critical importance.

Several studies have attempted to identify specific independent predictors of NIV failure (**Box 3**). NIV failure is associated with apnea and pneumonia[60]; ARDS[14]; higher Pediatric Risk of Mortality or Pediatric Logistic Organ Dysfunction scores[14,16,26,27]; failure to result in decreased RR, Pco_2, or work of breathing during the first hours of NIV[14,27]; and significant hypoxemia or lack of improvement in the Pao_2/Fio_2 ratio. Predictors of HFNC failure in bronchiolitis include increased Pco_2, failure to reduce RR or normalize HR, and failure to decrease Fio_2 less than 0.5 in the first 1 to 2 hours.[56,64]

Complications

Overall, NIV is a safe strategy for the management of ARF in infants and children.[8] However, as with any ventilation therapy, there are a few adverse effects and serious complications of which to be cognizant. **Box 4** outlines the reported complications and, where applicable, methods to minimize the risk of the complication.

Box 3
Predictors of failure

- High severity of illness (eg, PRISM, PELOD score)
- Younger age
- More severe respiratory distress or apnea
- Lack of improvement in RR or work of breathing
- Higher initial oxygen requirement or inability to reduce Fio_2
- Poor tolerance of interface
- High mean airway pressure
- pH less than 7.25 after 1 to 2 hours of NIV
- Multisystem organ dysfunction
- Moderate to severe ARDS or pneumonia
- ARF related to underlying process: immunosuppression, malignancy, sepsis
- Acute severe neurologic compromise/coma, inability to protect airway

Abbreviations: PRISM, Pediatric Risk of Mortality; PELOD, Pediatric Logistic Organ Dysfunction.
  Data from Refs.[5,14,25,27,28,59,62,64]

Box 4
Complications of noninvasive ventilation

- Inadequate oxygenation or ventilation → gradually increase Fio_2, flow, pressure support
- Interface-related pressure damage → use hydrocolloid patch application
- Nasal cannula or prong mucous obstruction → decreased by humidification, suctioning
- Nasal dryness, congestion → minimize with humidification, heating
- Gastric insufflation/abdominal distension/vomiting/aspiration
- VILI: barotrauma/volutrauma → rare with NIV, less likely than IMV
- Air leak: pneumothorax/pneumomediastinum → very uncommon

Abbreviation: VILI, ventilator-induced lung injury.
  Data from Abadesso C, Nunes P, Silvestre C, et al. Non-invasive ventilation in acute respiratory failure in children. Pediatr Rep 2012;4(2):e16; and Gay PC. Complications of noninvasive ventilation in acute care. Respir Care 2009;54(2):246–57. (discussion: 257–8).

Complications reported by the use of HFNC oxygen therapy are rare and similar to those reported with CPAP and BiPAP, including gastric insufflation, eye irritation, inability to continuously monitor capnography, air leak (eg, pneumothorax, pneumomediastinum), and failure to recognize treatment failure that delays ETI. Compared with NIV, HFNC has improved patient comfort and fewer skin injuries.

SUMMARY

NIV has seen widespread use in the PED and PICU management of acute respiratory distress and seems to be claiming the position of the first-line therapy for pediatric ARF at many institutions.[3,5] Although there is a paucity of RCT high-quality evidence, the safety, tolerance, and efficacy of NIV in this application is supported by multiple observational studies. Early institution of NIV in carefully selected children may alleviate or preclude worsening of ARF, with reported rates of NIV success in preventing ETI and IMV between 75% and 90%. The authors recommend a meticulously monitored NIV trial for the management of acute respiratory distress or ARF in any infant or child with no contraindication and without an emergent need of ETI. NIV is a good choice of respiratory support in acute bronchiolitis, status asthmaticus, mild to moderate pneumonia, and possibly even early, mild ARDS (failure is likely in moderate to severe ARDS). After careful patient and interface selection, NIV requires close cardiorespiratory and blood gas monitoring over the first 2 hours. Failure to improve or any worsening of clinical status should prompt immediate consideration of escalation of care to ETI and IMV.

NIV has shown significant promise for the management of ARF in infants and children and may be used safely and effectively with careful patient selection, meticulous monitoring, and ongoing care by a well-trained multidisciplinary team. The authors eagerly await the results of several ongoing RCTs of NIV and HFNC to help better delineate the role of these modalities in the treatment of respiratory distress and ARF in infants and children.

REFERENCES

1. Antonelli M, Conti G, Rocco M, et al. A comparison of noninvasive positive-pressure ventilation and conventional mechanical ventilation in patients with acute respiratory failure. N Engl J Med 1998;339(7):429–35.

2. Akingbola OA, Hopkins RL. Pediatric noninvasive positive pressure ventilation. Pediatr Crit Care Med 2001;2(2):164–9.
3. Fanning JJ, Lee KJ, Bragg DS, et al. U.S. attitudes and perceived practice for noninvasive ventilation in pediatric acute respiratory failure. Pediatr Crit Care Med 2011;12(5):e187–94.
4. Ganu SS, Gautam A, Wilkins B, et al. Increase in use of non-invasive ventilation for infants with severe bronchiolitis is associated with decline in intubation rates over a decade. Intensive Care Med 2012;38(7):1177–83.
5. Wolfler A, Calderini E, Iannella E, et al. Evolution of noninvasive mechanical ventilation use: a cohort study among Italian PICUs. Pediatr Crit Care Med 2015;16(5):418–27.
6. Teague WG. Noninvasive ventilation in the pediatric intensive care unit for children with acute respiratory failure. Pediatr Pulmonol 2003;35(6):418–26.
7. Teague WG. Non-invasive positive pressure ventilation: current status in paediatric patients. Paediatr Respir Rev 2005;6(1):52–60.
8. Calderini E, Chidini G, Pelosi P. What are the current indications for noninvasive ventilation in children? Curr Opin Anaesthesiol 2010;23(3):368–74.
9. Pavone M, Verrillo E, Caldarelli V, et al. Non-invasive positive pressure ventilation in children. Early Hum Dev 2013;89(Suppl 3):S25–31.
10. Lee JH, Rehder KJ, Williford L, et al. Use of high flow nasal cannula in critically ill infants, children, and adults: a critical review of the literature. Intensive Care Med 2013;39(2):247–57.
11. Wing R, James C, Maranda LS, et al. Use of high-flow nasal cannula support in the emergency department reduces the need for intubation in pediatric acute respiratory insufficiency. Pediatr Emerg Care 2012;28(11):1117–23.
12. Spence KL, Murphy D, Kilian C, et al. High-flow nasal cannula as a device to provide continuous positive airway pressure in infants. J Perinatol 2007;27(12):772–5.
13. Spentzas T, Minarik M, Patters AB, et al. Children with respiratory distress treated with high-flow nasal cannula. J Intensive Care Med 2009;24(5):323–8.
14. Essouri S, Chevret L, Durand P, et al. Noninvasive positive pressure ventilation: five years of experience in a pediatric intensive care unit. Pediatr Crit Care Med 2006;7(4):329–34.
15. Mortamet G, Amaddeo A, Essouri S, et al. Interfaces for noninvasive ventilation in the acute setting in children. Paediatr Respir Rev 2017;23:84–8.
16. Thia LP, McKenzie SA, Blyth TP, et al. Randomized controlled trial of nasal continuous positive airways pressure (CPAP) in bronchiolitis. Arch Dis Child 2008;93(1):45–7.
17. Codazzi D, Nacoti M, Passoni M, et al. Continuous positive airway pressure with modified helmet for treatment of hypoxemic acute respiratory failure in infants and a preschool population: a feasibility study. Pediatr Crit Care Med 2006;7(5):455–60.
18. Chidini G, Calderini E, Cesana BM, et al. Noninvasive continuous positive airway pressure in acute respiratory failure: helmet versus facial mask. Pediatrics 2010;126(2):e330–6.
19. Chidini G, Calderini E, Pelosi P. Treatment of acute hypoxemic respiratory failure with continuous positive airway pressure delivered by a new pediatric helmet in comparison with a standard full face mask: a prospective pilot study. Pediatr Crit Care Med 2010;11(4):502–8.
20. Milési C, Boubal M, Jacquot A, et al. High-flow nasal cannula: recommendations for daily practice in pediatrics. Ann Intensive Care 2014;4:29, eCollection 2014.

21. Kesavan S, Ramachandran B. Humidified high-flow nasal cannula oxygen therapy in children-a narrative review. J Pediatr Crit Care 2016;3(4):29–34.
22. Essouri S, Durand P, Chevret L, et al. Physiological effects of noninvasive positive ventilation during acute moderate hypercapnic respiratory insufficiency in children. Intensive Care Med 2008;34(12):2248–55.
23. Cavari Y, Sofer S, Rozovski U, et al. Noninvasive positive pressure ventilation in infants with respiratory failure. Pediatr Pulmonol 2012;47(10):1019–25.
24. Yañez LJ, Yunge M, Emilfork M, et al. A prospective, randomized, controlled trial of noninvasive ventilation in pediatric acute respiratory failure. Pediatr Crit Care Med 2008;9(5):484–9.
25. Dohna-Schwake C, Stehling F, Tschiedel E, et al. Non-invasive ventilation on a pediatric intensive care unit: feasibility, efficacy, and predictors of success. Pediatr Pulmonol 2011;46(11):1114–20.
26. Larrar S, Essouri S, Durand P, et al. Effects of nasal continuous positive airway pressure ventilation in infants with severe acute bronchiolitis. Arch Pediatr 2006;13(11):1397–403 [in French].
27. Mayordomo-Colunga J, Medina A, Rey C, et al. Predictive factors of non invasive ventilation failure in critically ill children: a prospective epidemiological study. Intensive Care Med 2009;35(3):527–36.
28. James CS, Hallewell CP, James DP, et al. Predicting the success of non-invasive ventilation in preventing intubation and re-intubation in the paediatric intensive care unit. Intensive Care Med 2011;37(12):1994–2001.
29. Fortenberry JD, Del Toro J, Jefferson LS, et al. Management of pediatric acute hypoxemic respiratory insufficiency with bilevel positive pressure (BiPAP) nasal mask ventilation. Chest 1995;108(4):1059–64.
30. Padman R, Lawless ST, Kettrick RG. Noninvasive ventilation via bilevel positive airway pressure support in pediatric practice. Crit Care Med 1998;26(1):169–73.
31. Carroll CL, Sala KA. Pediatric status asthmaticus. Crit Care Clin 2013;29(2): 153–66.
32. Najaf-Zadeh A, Leclerc F. Noninvasive positive pressure ventilation for acute respiratory failure in children: a concise review. Ann Intensive Care 2011;1(1):15.
33. Sarnaik AA, Sarnaik AP. Noninvasive ventilation in pediatric status asthmaticus: sound physiologic rationale but is it really safe, effective, and cost-efficient? Pediatr Crit Care Med 2012;13(4):484–5.
34. Thill PJ, McGuire JK, Baden HP, et al. Noninvasive positive-pressure ventilation in children with lower airway obstruction. Pediatr Crit Care Med 2004;5(4):337–42.
35. Basnet S, Mander G, Andoh J, et al. Safety, efficacy, and tolerability of early initiation of noninvasive positive pressure ventilation in pediatric patients admitted with status asthmaticus: a pilot study. Pediatr Crit Care Med 2012;13(4):393–8.
36. Akingbola OA, Simakajornboon N, Hadley EF Jr, et al. Noninvasive positive-pressure ventilation in pediatric status asthmaticus. Pediatr Crit Care Med 2002;3(2):181–4.
37. Carroll CL, Schramm CM. Noninvasive positive pressure ventilation for the treatment of status asthmaticus in children. Ann Allergy Asthma Immunol 2006;96(3): 454–9.
38. Mayordomo-Colunga J, Medina A, Rey C, et al. Non-invasive ventilation in pediatric status asthmaticus: a prospective observational study. Pediatr Pulmonol 2011;46(10):949–55.
39. Korang SK, Feinberg J, Wetterslev J, et al. Non-invasive positive pressure ventilation for acute asthma in children. Cochrane Database Syst Rev 2016;(9):CD012067.

40. Silva Pde S, Barreto SS. Noninvasive ventilation in status asthmaticus in children: levels of evidence. Rev Bras Ter Intensiva 2015;27(4):390–6.
41. Baudin F, Buisson A, Vanel B, et al. Nasal high flow in management of children with status asthmaticus: a retrospective observational study. Ann Intensive Care 2017;7(1):55.
42. Hess DR. Aerosol therapy during noninvasive ventilation or high-flow nasal cannula. Respir Care 2015;60(6):880–91 [discussion: 891–3].
43. Jat KR, Mathew JL. Continuous positive airway pressure (CPAP) for acute bronchiolitis in children. Cochrane Database Syst Rev 2015;(1):CD010473.
44. Beggs S, Wong ZH, Kaul S, et al. High-flow nasal cannula therapy for infants with bronchiolitis. Cochrane Database Syst Rev 2014;(1):CD009609.
45. Donlan M, Fontela PS, Puligandla PS. Use of continuous positive airway pressure (CPAP) in acute viral bronchiolitis: a systematic review. Pediatr Pulmonol 2011; 46(8):736–46.
46. Turnham H, Agbeko RS, Furness J, et al. Non-invasive respiratory support for infants with bronchiolitis: a national survey of practice. BMC Pediatr 2017;17(1):20.
47. Javouhey E, Barats A, Richard N, et al. Non-invasive ventilation as primary ventilatory support for infants with severe bronchiolitis. Intensive Care Med 2008; 34(9):1608–14.
48. Milési C, Matecki S, Jaber S, et al. 6 cm H2O continuous positive airway pressure versus conventional oxygen therapy in severe viral bronchiolitis: a randomized trial. Pediatr Pulmonol 2013;48(1):45–51.
49. Borckink I, Essouri S, Laurent M, et al. Infants with severe respiratory syncytial virus needed less ventilator time with nasal continuous airways pressure then invasive mechanical ventilation. Acta Paediatr 2014;103(1):81–5.
50. Essouri S, Laurent M, Chevret L, et al. Improved clinical and economic outcomes in severe bronchiolitis with pre-emptive nCPAP ventilatory strategy. Intensive Care Med 2014;40(1):84–91.
51. McKiernan C, Chua LC, Visintainer PF, et al. High flow nasal cannulae therapy in infants with bronchiolitis. J Pediatr 2010;156(4):634–8.
52. Schibler A, Pham TM, Dunster KR, et al. Reduced intubation rates for infants after introduction of high-flow nasal prong oxygen delivery. Intensive Care Med 2011; 37(5):847–52.
53. Morgan SE, Mosakowski S, Solano P, et al. High-flow nasal cannula and aerosolized beta agonists for rescue therapy in children with bronchiolitis: a case series. Respir Care 2015;60(9):e161–5.
54. Ralston SL, Lieberthal AS, Meissner HC, et al. Clinical practice guideline: the diagnosis, management, and prevention of bronchiolitis. Pediatrics 2014; 134(5):e1474–502.
55. Milési C, Essouri S, Pouyau R, et al. High flow nasal cannula (HFNC) versus nasal continuous positive airway pressure (nCPAP) for the initial respiratory management of acute viral bronchiolitis in young infants: a multicenter randomized controlled trial (TRAMONTANE study). Intensive Care Med 2017;43(2):209–16.
56. Abboud PA, Roth PJ, Skiles CL, et al. Predictors of failure in infants with viral bronchiolitis treated with high-flow, high-humidity nasal cannula therapy*. Pediatr Crit Care Med 2012;13(6):e343–9.
57. Jouvet P, Thomas NJ, Wilson DF, et al, Pediatric Acute Lung Injury Consensus Conference Group. Pediatric acute respiratory distress syndrome: consensus recommendations from the Pediatric Acute Lung Injury Consensus Conference. Pediatr Crit Care Med 2015;16(5):428–39.

58. Essouri S, Carroll C. Noninvasive support and ventilation for pediatric acute respiratory distress syndrome: proceedings from the Pediatric Acute Lung Injury Consensus Conference. Pediatric Acute Lung Injury Consensus Conference Group. Pediatr Crit Care Med 2015;16(5 Suppl 1):S102–10.
59. Muñoz-Bonet JI, Flor-Macián EM, Brines J, et al. Predictive factors for the outcome of noninvasive ventilation in pediatric acute respiratory failure. Pediatr Crit Care Med 2010;11(6):675–80.
60. Abadesso C, Nunes P, Silvestre C, et al. Non-invasive ventilation in acute respiratory failure in children. Pediatr Rep 2012;4(2):e16.
61. Chisti MJ, Salam MA, Smith JH, et al. Bubble continuous positive airway pressure for children with severe pneumonia and hypoxaemia in Bangladesh: an open, randomised controlled trial. Lancet 2015;386(9998):1057–65.
62. Bernet V, Hug MI, Frey B. Predictive factors for the success of non-invasive mask ventilation in infants and children with acute respiratory failure. Pediatr Crit Care Med 2005;6(6):660–4.
63. Nava S, Hill N. Non-invasive ventilation in acute respiratory failure. Lancet 2009; 374(9685):250–9.
64. Kelly GS, Simon HK, Sturm JJ. High-flow nasal cannula use in children with respiratory distress in the emergency department: predicting the need for subsequent intubation. Pediatr Emerg Care 2013;29(8):888–92.

Pediatric Ventilator Management in the Emergency Department

Garrett S. Pacheco, MD[a,b,*], Jenny Mendelson, MD[a,b,c],
Mary Gaspers, MD[c]

KEYWORDS

- Mechanical ventilation • Airway • Pediatric • Blood gas analysis • Ventilator alarm
- Hemodynamic instability

KEY POINTS

- Pediatric mechanical ventilation often brings the emergency physician trepidation and hesitation.
- Common modes of pediatric invasive ventilation include pressure-assist control ventilation and pressure-regulated volume control ventilation.
- A methodic approach is needed when the emergency physician addresses ventilator alarms and the decompensating pediatric patient that is mechanically ventilated.

INTRODUCTION

There are few emergencies that are as anxiety provoking to the emergency physician (EP) as pediatric airway management. Pediatric intubation itself is relatively rare compared with adult intubations. The frequency of pediatric endotracheal intubation (ETI) is reported to occur 3 to 6 times less often per 1000 adult patients intubated.[1,2] Furthermore, once intubated, the EP usually has even less experience with pediatric ventilator management in the emergency department (ED). This article uses clinical cases to provide a reference for reviewing initiation of pediatric mechanical ventilation

Funding Sources/Disclosures: None.
[a] Department of Emergency Medicine, University of Arizona College of Medicine, Banner University Medical Center Tucson, 1501 North Campbell Avenue, PO Box 245057, Tucson, AZ 85724; [b] Department of Pediatrics, University of Arizona College of Medicine, Banner University Medical Center Tucson, 1501 North Campbell Avenue, PO Box 245057, Tucson, AZ 85724; [c] Pediatric Critical Care Medicine, Department of Pediatrics, University of Arizona College of Medicine, Banner University Medical Center Tucson, 1501 North Campbell Avenue, PO Box 245057, Tucson, AZ 85724
* Corresponding author. Department of Emergency Medicine, University of Arizona College of Medicine, Banner University Medical Center Tucson, 1501 North Campbell Avenue, PO Box 245057, Tucson, AZ 85724.
E-mail address: gpacheco@aemrc.arizona.edu

Emerg Med Clin N Am 36 (2018) 401–413
https://doi.org/10.1016/j.emc.2017.12.008

in the ED and adjusting the initial settings in response to blood gas analysis. The review also provides a reference for appropriately evaluating ventilator alarm triggers and accurately evaluating and managing the unstable ventilated pediatric patient. Common modes for emergency pediatric ventilation are discussed. These include pressure-assist control ventilation (PCV) and pressure-regulated volume control ventilation (PRVC).

CASES IN PEDIATRIC MECHANICAL VENTILATION MANAGEMENT
Case 1

A 7-year-old girl presented to the ED with massive hemoptysis and profound hypoxemia. The patient had signs of hemorrhagic shock and became apneic during the evaluation of her primary survey, subsequently requiring ETI and mechanical ventilation. A chest x-ray (CXR) study confirmed tube placement and showed significant bilateral opacification. She was placed on synchronized intermittent mandatory ventilation (SIMV) PCV. Her peak inspiratory pressure (PIP) was 18 cmH$_2$O above positive end-expiratory pressure (PEEP) of 10 cm H$_2$O, her respiratory rate (RR) was 24, and fraction of inspired oxygen (Fio$_2$) was 1.0. The patient remained hypoxic despite increases in PEEP and 100% Fio$_2$. What ventilator adjustments are necessary for this patient with refractory hypoxemia?

Case 2

A 4-year-old girl presented to the trauma center with traumatic brain injury (TBI). The patient was intubated for airway protection and for her anticipated clinical course. A venous blood gas level was obtained after intubation. The results were pH of 7.19 and partial pressure of carbon dioxide (Pco$_2$) of 52 mm Hg. Her weight was estimated to be 16 kg. The ventilator was set to the following parameters before intubation: SIMV PRVC; RR, 24; tidal volume (Vt), 96 mL; PEEP, 5; Fio$_2$, 1.0; and inspiratory time (Ti), 0.8 seconds. What ventilator setting adjustments should be made for this 4-year-old girl with TBI?

Case 3

A 3-year-old boy with a history of asthma presented with significant respiratory distress. He had a respiratory rate of 75 to 80 breaths per minute. Initial observation found that he was febrile and had subcostal, supraclavicular, intercostal retractions and tracheal tugging. On auscultation, there was biphasic wheezing in the upper lobes but very little aeration at the bases. He appeared somnolent and had very little crying with intravenous line placement. His peripheral capillary oxygen saturation (SpO$_2$) level was in the 80s despite being on 15-mg/h continuous albuterol facemask with a flow of 15 L/min and below that a humidified high-flow nasal cannula (HFNC) set at 8 L/min. The radiograph was concerning for multifocal pneumonia. He required intubation for acute respiratory failure and airway protection. He was placed on SIMV PRVC ventilation and started on a ketamine and epinephrine infusion for his airway obstruction component. His continuous albuterol was increased to 20-mg/h. He was pan cultured and started on empiric antibiotics. The ventilator triggered an alarm with peak airway pressures (PAP) of 49 cm H$_2$O. The oxygen saturation continued to decline. What is the next step to improve his respiratory status?

Case 4

A 6-month-old girl presented to the ED with 3 days of worsening respiratory distress. Her pediatrician recently diagnosed her with bronchiolitis. Despite nasal suctioning, she had little improvement in her work of breathing, and she had worsening hypoxia.

She was placed on HFNC with no improvement. A change to bi-level positive airway pressure RAM cannula did little to improve her condition. The patient was therefore intubated for hypoxic/hypercapnic respiratory failure. Shortly after intubation, while being mechanically ventilated, the patient became hemodynamically unstable with worsening hypoxia. What is the next intervention needed to stabilize the patient?

PEDIATRIC RESPIRATORY PHYSIOLOGY

Understanding the concepts of airway resistance and compliance are fundamental to approaching ventilator management. Respiratory failure includes an abnormality in one or all of the components of the pediatric respiratory triangle including increased respiratory rate, increased work of breathing, and hypoxia (**Fig. 1**). Decreased lung compliance or increased airway resistance or even both contribute to the triad of respiratory failure. Resistance to airway flow is governed by Poiseuille's law: $R = 8\eta L/\pi r^4$. This translates into significant airway compromise with even minor changes in airway radius caused by atelectasis, secretions, edema, and obstruction.[3] Children younger than 5 years have peripheral airway resistance 4 times higher compared with adults.[4]

Anatomically, children have pliable chest walls. This physical characteristic, along with the lung's natural elastic tendency to deflate, will predispose children to pulmonary atelectasis and decreased functional residual capacity (FRC).[3,4] Pulmonary compliance is defined by a given change in volume (ΔV) for every given change in pressure (ΔP). Compliance allows the alveoli to fill with air under a set pressure. If lung compliance is compromised, Vt decreases.[3] When lung compliance is affected to this extent, pediatric patients are unable to augment their Vt. They try to increase their minute ventilation (MV) by increasing their work of breathing, increasing their respiratory rate, which predisposes them to fatigue, hypoxia, and respiratory failure.[5]

Normal respiratory compliance for an infant or child ranges from 1.5 to 3.0 mL/cmH$_2$O/kg.[6] For example, a 3-year-old child that weighs 15 kg should have an approximate respiratory compliance of 22.5 to 45 mL/cmH$_2$O. This information is useful because during mechanical ventilation, the compliance can be calculated by dividing the Vt by the difference between the PAP and the PEEP, that is, $C = Vt/(PAP - PEEP)$. Checking this quick calculation helps providers assess the severity of the patient's lung disease. For the same 3-year-old child being ventilated with a Vt of 105 mL, PAP of 27, and PEEP of 10, their respiratory compliance on these settings is approximately 6 mL/cmH$_2$O ($\sim$0.4 mL/cmH$_2$O/kg)—significantly less compared with their predicted healthy state compliance.

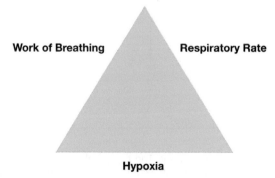

Fig. 1. Triad of pediatric respiratory failure. Specific anatomy and physiology unique to children contributes to the failure of one or all of the components. These should clue the provider that the child is at risk for respiratory insufficiency/failure.

MODES OF VENTILATION AND INITIAL SETTINGS

To understand invasive ventilation, there are 3 Ts that need to be recognized: the ventilator trigger, target, and termination. The trigger relates to whether the machine or patient initiates the breath or both are involved. Volume or pressure ventilation is the target. Assist control (AC), which is commonly used in adults, has a volume-targeted mode. SIMV has a pressure- or volume-targeted setting. Termination is the variable that ceases the breath given by the ventilator. When using a volume mode, a flow is prescribed to the patient. When the flow is given over a specific amount of time, a volume is achieved. In pressure mode, the breath terminates after an inspiratory time.

There are 2 mechanical ventilation modes primarily used in pediatric emergency medicine. Other ventilation modes exist, but their use is based on the EP's level of comfort, institutional availability, and preference. PCV is often selected for use in newborns and small infants. In adult studies, PCV has been associated with improved oxygenation at lower peak pressures and decreased work of breathing.[7,8] PCV delivers each breath at a set rate, and this positive pressure support is coupled with a decelerating flow pattern that is terminated when the PIP is reached during the set Ti. The PIP, the independent variable, determines the Vt that the patient receives, which is the dependent variable. In PCV, worsening compliance leads to decreased Vt and reduced MV. The EP should be able to look at the ventilator and identify mode and recognize parameters based on display ventilator waveforms (**Fig. 2**). PCV has a rectangular pressure curve compared with the exponential or "shark fin" pressure curve of volume control ventilation (VCV).

VCV ventilation is often used for the larger child. Adaptive pressure ventilation is a useful modality for the older child that combines features of both VCV and PCV. It has various names on different ventilator types: *PRVC, Volume Guarantee, Volume Control Plus+*. For this article, it will be further described as PRVC. The advantage

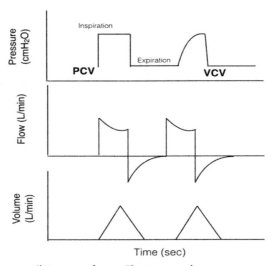

Fig. 2. Recognizing ventilator waveforms. The top graph compares a pressure (rectangle) waveform with a volume (exponential/shark fin) waveform. Typically, a ventilator display will show the flow below the pressure curve. A decelerating flow pattern is seen. VCV may show a rectangle shape that represents continuous flow. The bottom graph shows volume curves (typically an ascending pattern followed by a descending ramp).

of this modality is that there is still the decelerating flow pattern characteristic of the pressure-limited mode coupled with a set Vt.[9] This means that the preset Vt will be delivered to the patient while achieving the lowest possible PAP using the decelerating flow pattern. The ventilator is able to measure the plateau pressure (P_{PLAT}, discussed later in the review) intrinsically, and over the next few breaths, automatically adjusts the minimal inspiratory pressure required to obtain the desired Vt. If more Vt is achieved than the preset value, the ventilator will decrease the pressure with the next breath given.[10]

Initial settings for PCV include the age-appropriate RR, an appropriate Ti for the patient's age, and disease process (**Table 1**). The Ti is the length of the inspiratory phase of the breathing cycle. PCV also requires an applied PEEP. PEEP is the positive pressure maintained in the patient's airway during expiration. The addition of PEEP helps prevent alveolar collapse and thus prevents atelectasis that could cause alveolar trauma.[11] PEEP increases FRC, decreases shunt fraction, and improves oxygenation. In adults, PEEP can be set at 5 cmH_2O and increased if needed to improve mean airway pressure (P_{AW}) based on the patient's required Fio_2. The ARDSNET table was developed for adult patients, and unfortunately there is no pediatric equivalent.[12] The Pediatric Acute Lung Injury and Consensus Conference (PALICC) recommends "moderately" elevated levels of PEEP, defined as 10 to 15 cmH_2O, for patients with severe pediatric acute respiratory distress syndrome (ARDS), titrated to observed oxygenation and hemodynamic response.[13,14] When initiating PEEP in the ED, the EP should recognize that in the patient requiring increased Fio_2 and with more opacification on chest radiography, PEEP will need to be increased. It should not exceed 15 cmH_2O in the ED. The Fio_2 can be started at 1.0, but should be quickly titrated down to avoid hyperoxia and its associated complications.

PCV also requires a PIP. This is the maximum pressure delivered during inspiration. The PIP determines the patient's Vt. The PIP can start between 15 and 20 cmH_2O greater than PEEP.[15] The chest should be observed for equal rise, and the PIP may need to be adjusted to achieve this goal. The achieved Vt is usually calculated and displayed on the ventilator screen, and should be approximately 6 to 8 mL/kg ideal body weight. This goal range is based on lung protective ventilation and is found to be the only factor that may reduce mortality.[12] In PCV, the driving pressure ($\Delta P = PIP - PEEP$) is the primary determinant of Vt. The ΔP can be adjusted as needed to achieve the appropriate Vt. The PIP should not exceed a total pressure of 30 cmH_2O. High PAPs predispose the patient to barotrauma and ventilator-induced lung injury. These variables can be readily visualized on the ventilator display screen.

Initial settings for PRVC are similar to those for PCV except that instead of an assigned PIP, the EP will choose a Vt. The Vt should be set based on a lung protective strategy to avoid trauma to the alveoli caused by excess distention.[9] The goal for low Vts is extrapolated from adult data and recommended by PALICC.[13,15] The Vt is the

Table 1 Initial Mechanical Ventilation Settings			
Initial Ventilator Settings	**Neonate**	**Infant/Child**	**Adolescent**
Respiratory rate[a]	30–40	20–30	12–16
Inspiratory time (sec)[b]	0.3–0.5	0.5–0.7	0.7–1.0

[a] Consider the patient's MV before intubation. This should be matched unless the patient has obstructive disease in which a lower RR will be desired.
[b] These are reference starting Ti. Adjustments will likely be needed to achieve desired oxygenation and ventilation.

volume of gas that enters the patient's lung during inspiration. Adequate Vt occurs when good breath sounds are auscultated, and appropriate chest expansion is achieved. The remaining variables are similar to those of PCV and include Fio_2, PEEP, Ti, and RR.

PCV, VCV, and PRVC modes of ventilation are often paired with SIMV. Children often overbreathe the ventilator once their neuromuscular blockade agent wears off. If the patient receives AC/VCV after no longer being paralyzed, then each breath could be fully supported by the ventilator. This can cause patient-ventilator asynchrony, breath stacking, and respiratory alkalosis and is likely uncomfortable for the child. SIMV provides synchronized fully supported breaths for the set RR but additionally will allow the patient to receive at least partially supported breaths for every additional breath over and above the set RR. A pressure support is usually added to partially support the breaths not fully synchronized over the applied PEEP, and this is typically set at 5 to 10 cmH_2O. After initial settings are finalized, the patient should be assessed for ventilator synchrony, continuous pulse oximetry, and continuous capnography. An arterial/venous blood gas should be obtained, correlated with the end tidal CO_2, and adjustments to the initial settings should be made if needed.

CASE EXPLANATIONS
Case 1 Explanation

The patient has signs of type 1 respiratory failure. This entity is defined as a Pao_2 less than 55 mm Hg or SpO_2 less than 88%. Hypoxemia can be further classified into its 5 causes: decreased Po_2 caused by decreased inspired O_2 (eg, smoke inhalation, CO poisoning); diffusion abnormalities; hypoventilation; ventilation to perfusion (V/Q) mismatch (asthma, bronchiolitis); and shunt physiology (pneumonia, pulmonary edema, congenital heart disease). Pediatric patients with respiratory failure are particularly susceptible to V/Q mismatch and shunt physiology causes of hypoxemic respiratory failure.

This particular patient would later receive a diagnosis of idiopathic pulmonary hemosiderosis. She presented with massive hemoptysis secondary to alveolar hemorrhage. Despite securing her airway, she could not be successfully oxygenated secondary to her intrapulmonary shunt. The EP attempted to titrate Fio_2 and PEEP, but she still remained severely hypoxic. The EP was in the process of changing ventilator modes to airway pressure release ventilation; however, the pediatric intensivist noted that the Ti was not considered when troubleshooting her hypoxia. When the ventilator was inspected, the Ti was identified to be 0.3 seconds.

The Ti is not often thought of while initiating mechanical ventilation, but its role is vital. Ti directly affects P_{AW}, which has a powerful influence on oxygenation. For mechanical ventilation, the inspiratory/expiratory (I:E) ratio is typically set at 1:2 (1 second for inspiration and 2 seconds for expiration, which resembles physiologic breathing) but may need to be increased to 1:4 in obstructive lung disease. A longer Ti can be used cautiously to aid in improving oxygenation if there is no significant obstructive lung disease. This particular patient had an Ti that was set too low. An adequate P_{AW} could not be achieved to improve her oxygenation. While increasing the Ti, the patient had significant improvement in her oxygenation with the ability to decrease her Fio_2.

Case 2 Explanation

The first blood gas measurement is often obtained within 20 to 30 minutes of initiating mechanical ventilation. This often occurs while the patient is still in the ED. It is the EP's responsibility to obtain this vital laboratory study and adjust the ventilator as needed. By doing this, the patient does not have prolonged periods of inadequate ventilation before transfer to their definitive care destination. There should be a firm understanding of the variables that affect oxygenation and ventilation. This 4-year-old girl has significant TBI. Deficits in oxygenation and over- and underventilation contribute to poor outcomes in TBI. It is critical to assess these variables and make necessary adjustments before the patient is transferred.

This patient has increased P_{CO_2}. If the patient was being ventilated with PCV, adjustments that can be made include: the RR can be increased or the driving pressure can be increased. She was being ventilated in PRVC. In this modality, hypercapnia can be addressed by increasing the RR, or the Vt can be increased (preferably adjustments are made in the RR, as increases in Vt may compromise the lung protection strategy).

The 4-year-old girl's RR was increased. After this change, she became hypotensive. Whenever the RR is adjusted, the Ti should be rechecked to ensure there is no dynamic hyperinflation or intrinsic/auto-PEEP. A clue that this is occurring is that the flow wave does not return to baseline (**Fig. 3**).

In pediatrics, knowing the duration of the respiratory cycle is crucial and is often overlooked. This finding was overlooked for the 7-year-old girl with pulmonary hemorrhage in case 1 and the 4-year-old girl in case 2 after adjustments were made in her RR. The 4-year-old girl with TBI had a set RR of 24 breaths per minute. She has a respiratory cycle of 2.5 seconds (60 seconds ÷ 24 breaths per minute = 2.5 seconds). To achieve an I:E ratio of 1:2, her Ti should be 0.8 seconds. The maximum Ti at this set ventilator rate is 1.2 seconds (2.5 seconds ÷ 2 = 1.2 seconds). If not set correctly, the EP may unintentionally initiate inverse ratio ventilation. For example, the same 4-year-old with her RR increased to 35 breaths per minute to treat her hypercapnia on a blood gas now has a respiratory cycle of 1.7 seconds and a maximum Ti of 0.9 seconds. If there was no adjustment in the Ti of 0.8 seconds, the I:E ratio nears 1:1, which may not allow adequate time for exhalation. With inadequate time for exhalation, there is risk for dynamic hyperinflation, which may lead to air leak disease such as pneumothorax or, in her situation, increased intrathoracic volume causing decreased preload with subsequent hemodynamic collapse. Ensuring the volume curve returns to baseline ensures no dynamic hyperinflation and adequate time for exhalation.

The more appropriate adjustment for this 16-kg 4-year-old girl would be to adjust her Vt. Her Vt was set at 6 mL/kg; therefore, given her healthy lungs, this could be increased to treat her hypercapnia. However, the Vt should be increased to only what is necessary to prevent ventilator-induced lung injury (VILI).

Case 3 Explanation

The patient was in status asthmaticus complicated by multifocal pneumonia. He was intubated for both airway protection and management of his respiratory failure.

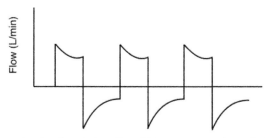

Fig. 3. Flow curve not returning to baseline. This represents dynamic hyperinflation and may lead to increased intrathoracic pressure leading to the consequence of decreased venous return and hypotension.

Despite this measure, the patient had no improvement in his oxygenation and ventilation. His ventilator continued to alarm to notify the EP of his steadily increasing PAPs.

When the ventilator alarm triggers, the EP should treat this warning as if it was announcing a code event. Increased PAP in VCV modes or reduced Vt alarm triggers in PCV modes should prompt the use of an algorithm to troubleshoot the patient's respiratory mechanics (**Fig. 4, Table 2**). Settings should be adjusted to ensure that a tidal volume is actually given while identifying the culprit for the alarm. Try and serially discard all etiologies of increased airway resistance versus decreased pulmonary compliance, and keep in mind what there is in the patient's clinical condition that may be contributing to the increased PAP alarm.

With worsening respiratory compliance, it should quickly be determined whether the patient is having issues with the airway, or if the problem is with the lungs (alveoli). The PAP represents the amount of positive pressure required to deliver a breath through the endotracheal tube (ETT), through the large conducting airways to get through the bronchioles, and ultimately arrive at the alveoli. The PAP includes the alveolar P_{PLAT}, which represents pulmonary compliance. As the P_{PLAT} increases, pulmonary compliance decreases. This can be readily measured in VCV modes by performing an inspiratory hold maneuver.[16] This is helpful when deciding if the issue is in the large conducting airways or the lungs (**Fig. 5**). When an inspiratory hold maneuver is performed in VCV, the difference between the PAP and P_{PLAT} is normally less than 5 cmH$_2$O. If there is an increase in PAP without an increase in P_{PLAT}, there is increased airway resistance (>5 cm H$_2$O difference between PAP and P_{PLAT}). Unfortunately, in PRVC and PCV, an inspiratory hold maneuver is not possible. The pressure modes with a deceleration flow pattern make it impossible to distinguish between airway

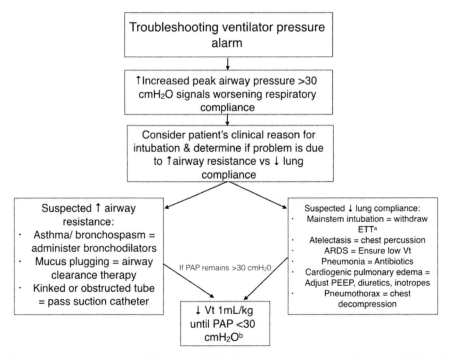

Fig. 4. Algorithm to approach increased PAP. [a]A very common cause of increased PAP and needs to be considered/addressed early. [b]May need to tolerate higher PAP if Vt and MV are inadequate for oxygenation and ventilation.

Table 2
Troubleshooting increased peak airway pressures

Cause of Increased PAP	Management
Mucus plugging	Obtain an immediate chest radiograph. Attempt to pass a suction catheter to retrieve tracheal secretions. Airway clearance therapy.
Kinked or obstructed ETT	Try to pass a suction catheter. Identify kink and address. May need increased sedation if patient is biting ETT.
Bronchospasm	Bronchodilators
Atelectasis	Chest physiotherapy
ARDS	Appropriate Vt (6–8 mL/kg). May even need to go lower.
Pneumonia	Appropriate antibiotics. Address parapneumonic effusion.
Cardiogenic pulmonary edema	Consider adjusting PEEP, add inotropes or diuretics.
Pneumothorax	Chest tube
Mainstem bronchus intubation	Pull the ETT back to appropriate depth

Data from Santanilla JI, Daniel B, Yeow ME. Mechanical ventilation. Emerg Med Clin North Am 2008;26(3):849–62.

resistance issues and pulmonary compliance. Both airway resistance and pulmonary compliance need to be considered and quickly eliminated as a cause of increased PAP.[17]

Causes of increased airway resistance include mucus plugging, a narrow ETT, a kinked or obstructed tube, or bronchospasm. If the patient is asthmatic, then the patient should quickly be assessed and treated for bronchospasm by giving bronchodilators through the ventilator circuit. Other medications should be used to minimize bronchospasm until the condition reverses (eg, magnesium, ipratropium, terbutaline, aminophylline, ketamine). If the patient has pneumonia or viral lower respiratory tract infection with associated thick secretions, increased airway resistance from possible mucus plugging should be suspected. Another clue for this process is auscultation of decreased breath sounds in the affected lung. A chest radiograph should be ordered immediately while resuscitating the patient. Although it may be delayed, the radiograph may aid in identifying a mucus plug/white out compromising ventilation while the patient is being evaluated, and in the interim a suction catheter should be passed through the ETT in attempt to remove obstructing secretions from the trachea. If tracheal suction is not effective, bronchoscopy may be required. As part of troubleshooting, the ETT should have already been inspected for obstruction or kinks. A suction catheter can be used for troubleshooting this condition and should pass easily.

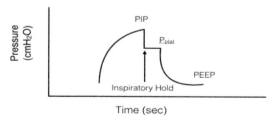

Fig. 5. Inspiratory hold maneuver is performed during VCV to determine the P_{PLAT}. Normally, the difference between the PIP and P_{PLAT} is less than 5 cmH$_2$O. Unfortunately, this maneuver is not possible with PRVC, and both etiologies need to be quickly considered.

A pediatric bougie is an alternative adjunct, as there are sizes as small as 10F that will fit through a 4.0-mm ETT. If the suction catheter or bougie does not pass easily, the patient will require reintubation.

Once an airway resistance issue has been eliminated, the EP should test pulmonary compliance. This may be obvious based on the patient's clinical condition and reason for initial intubation. Causes of increased PAP from decreased lung compliance include mainstem bronchus intubation (the most common culprit in pediatrics for increased PAP alarm), atelectasis, ARDS, pneumonia, cardiogenic pulmonary edema, and pneumothorax (see **Fig. 4, Table 2**).

A chest radiograph was immediately ordered for this 3-year-old boy. Bronchial breath sounds were appreciated on the left, and he had prolonged expiratory phase appreciated on the right. The cause of his increased PAP was multifactorial. A trial of bronchodilator was given considering the status asthmaticus. Point-of-care ultrasound scan (POCUS) was performed and showed no pneumothorax. Chest radiograph showed a large white out on the left side from a presumed mucus plug. Aggressive chest physiotherapy was started along with nebulized hypertonic saline to perform airway clearance. He was switched from PRVC to PCV and at a PIP of 37, a Vt of 6 mL/kg could be achieved. With ongoing therapy, the mucus plug resolved, and the PIP was decreased, reducing the risk of VILI.

Case 4 Explanation

Shortly after this 6-month-old girl was placed on mechanical ventilation, she became hemodynamically unstable. The decompensating ventilated pediatric patient should be assessed in a meticulous but rapid manner (**Fig. 6**).[17] Santanilla[17,18] published an algorithmic approach that can be followed and modified to address the decompensating ventilated pediatric patient. The patient should be immediately disconnected from the ventilator, and the DOPES mnemonic should be investigated. DOPES refers to the possibility of a Displaced endotracheal tube, Obstructed tube (mucus plug, kink), Pneumothorax, Equipment failure (disconnect ventilator and manually bag the patient, assess the tubing, assess settings), and Stacking/sedation (dynamic hyperinflation in the patient with obstructive lung disease/sedation should be considered last).

Shortly after this girl became unstable, the patient was taken off the ventilator and manually ventilated with a bag valve mask (BVM) attached to a 100% oxygen source. This eliminates equipment failure as the etiology of patient decompensation. If dynamic hyperinflation is the problem, removal from the ventilator and thus a decrease in the intrathoracic pressure should result in an immediate improvement in the patient's hemodynamics. While manually ventilating, the provider can assess the degree of airway resistance by the degree of difficulty squeezing the bag.

It is necessary to determine if the ETT is in the trachea.[18] Given the short tracheas and even shorter ETT lengths, even small movements can result in accidental extubation of the pediatric patient. To confirm placement, capnography, or alternately direct visualization or passing of a pediatric bougie/airway exchange catheter or suction catheter can aid in determining appropriate placement. Once the ETT is confirmed to be in place, and while the patient is being bagged, the patient is assessed for equal chest rise and the chest is felt for crepitus and auscultated to ensure no air leak or unequal breath sounds are present.[18] Unequal or unilateral bronchial breath sounds may indicate migration of the ETT into the right mainstem. This complication is a common etiology of increased PAP and significant hypoxia after intubation in children. This should be considered early when assessing the decompensated ventilated pediatric patient.

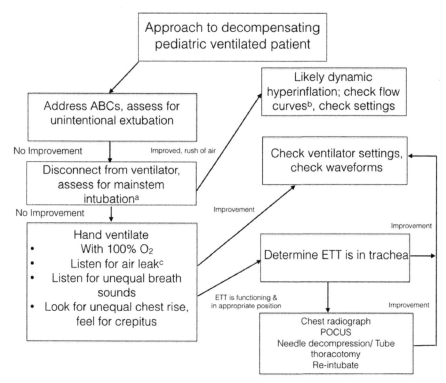

Fig. 6. Algorithm. Approach to the decompensating pediatric patient. [a]Right main stem intubation is a common complication in pediatric patients, thus should be considered and addressed early. [b]See **Fig. 2**; the flow waveform should return to baseline. [c]May be caused by damaged cuff or too narrow an ETT compromising ventilation. (*Courtesy of* ACEP; and *Modified from* Santanilla JI, Daniel B, Yeow ME. Mechanical ventilation. Emerg Med Clin North Am 2008;26(3):849–62; and Santanilla JI. The crashing ventilated patient. In: Winters ME, et al, editors. Emergency department resuscitation of the critically ill. 2nd edition. Dallas (TX): American College of Emergency Physicians; 2017. p. 17–26.)

Unequal breath sounds combined with crepitus is suggestive of pneumothorax. Air leak is highly suggestive of a cuff leak or an inadequately sized ETT. This can be detected by auscultating over the neck. With the presence of an air leak, air can be easily heard escaping when a stethoscope is used. The pilot balloon in a cuffed ETT can be felt for appropriate inflation. The ventilator display screen will also show a discrepancy between inspiratory tidal volume and expiratory tidal volume. If the air leak is too large, causing inadequate inspiratory pressures, the ETT may need to be replaced. After addressing these potential issues, the settings of the ventilator should be reassessed, ventilator waveforms observed, and gas exchange re-evaluated. Once stabilized and reconnected to the ventilator, the flow waveform should be scrutinized to ensure that dynamic hyperinflation is not occurring (see **Fig. 3**).[17,18] The flow waveform should completely return to baseline to complete exhalation before the next initiated ventilator breath.

If no improvement is achieved in the patient's clinical course, Santanilla[17,18] refers to special procedures that should be undertaken. It is helpful to order a chest radiograph immediately because of the inherent time delay that often occurs. POCUS can be used to identify pneumothorax, and, if found, immediate needle

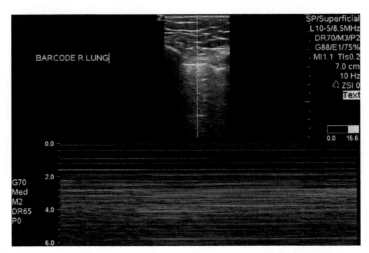

Fig. 7. Stratosphere sign/barcode sign indicates a pneumothorax is present.

decompression followed by tube thoracostomy can take place. POCUS for a well-appearing lung will show normal lung slide in the M-mode as the seashore sign. [19] With the presence of pneumothorax, the stratosphere sign/barcode sign will be present (**Fig. 7**). If the patient becomes more stable, but seems to be taking asynchronous breaths with the ventilator, sedation should be optimized. However, this should be a last measure to ensure no other abnormalities were missed that need to be addressed.

The algorithmic approach to management of the hemodynamically unstable 6-month-old girl was followed. She was found to have decreased breath sounds on the right associated with "stratosphere sign" with POCUS. She had a pneumothorax that developed tension in the setting of mechanical ventilation. She underwent needle decompression emergently followed by tube thoracostomy. Following these maneuvers, she had significant improvement in her hemodynamics.

SUMMARY

After pediatric intubation, ventilator management is often a secondary consideration to airway management in the ED. The EP is first to be asked to initiate ventilator settings, trouble shoot ventilator alarms, and evaluate and manage the unstable ventilated pediatric patient. A checklist can be used to identify and address causes of increased airway resistance or decreased pulmonary compliance leading to ventilator alarming. The EP should have a methodic, thorough, and rapid method to address the ventilated pediatric patient who is decompensating.

REFERENCES

1. Sakles JC, Laurin EG, Rantapaa AA, et al. Airway management in the emergency department: a one-year study of 610 tracheal intubations. Ann Emerg Med 1998; 31(3):325–32.
2. Losek JD, Olson LR, Dobson JV, et al. Tracheal intubation practice and maintaining skill competency: survey of pediatric emergency department directors. Pediatr Emerg Care 2008;24(5):294–9.
3. Reuter S, Moser C, Baack M. Respiratory distress in the newborn. Pediatr Rev 2014;35(10):417–28.

4. Morley SL. Non-invasive ventilation in paediatric critical care. Paediatr Respir Rev 2016;20:24–31.
5. Brambrink AM, Braun U. Airway management in infants and children. Best Pract Res Clin Anaesthesiol 2005;19(4):675–97.
6. Gregory GA, Andropoulo DB. Gregory's pediatric anesthesia. Hoboken (NJ): Wiley-Blackwell; 2011.
7. Campbell RS, Davis BR. Pressure-controlled versus volume- controlled ventilation: does it matter? Respir Care 2002;47:416–26.
8. Seet MM, Soliman KM, Sbeih ZF. Comparison of three modes of positive pressure mask ventilation during induction of anaesthesia: a prospective, randomized, crossover study. Eur J Anaesthesiol 2009;26:913–6.
9. Marraro GA. Innovative practices of ventilatory support with pediatric patients. Pediatr Crit Care Med 2003;4(1):8–20.
10. Kocis KC, Dekeon MK, Rosen HK, et al. Pressure-regulated volume control vs volume control ventilation in infants after surgery for congenital heart disease. Pediatr Cardiol 2001;22:233–7.
11. Ranieri VM, Suter PM, Tortorella C, et al. Effect of mechanical ventilation on inflammatory mediators in patients with acute respiratory distress syndrome: a randomized controlled trial. JAMA 1999;282(1):54–61.
12. The Acute Respiratory Distress Syndrome Network. Ventilation with lower tidal volumes as compared with traditional tidal volumes for acute lung injury and the acute respiratory distress syndrome. N Engl J Med 2000;342(18):1301–8.
13. Pediatric Acute Lung Injury Consensus Conference Group. Pediatric acute respiratory distress syndrome: consensus recommendations from the pediatric acute lung injury consensus conference. Pediatr Crit Care Med 2015;16(5):428–39.
14. Rimensberger PC, Cheifetz IM, Pediatric Acute Lung Injury Consensus Conference Group. Ventilatory support in children with pediatric acute respiratory distress syndrome: proceedings from the pediatric acute lung injury consensus conference. Pediatr Crit Care Med 2015;16(5 Suppl 1):S51–60.
15. Luten RC, Mick NW. Differentiating aspects of the pediatric airway. In: Walls RM, Murphy MF, editors. Manual of emergency airway management. 4th edition. Philadelphia: Lippincott, Williams & Wilkins; 2012. p. 276–92.
16. Weingart SD. Managing initial mechanical ventilation in the emergency department. Ann Emerg Med 2016;68(5):614–7.
17. Santanilla JI, Daniel B, Yeow ME. Mechanical ventilation. Emerg Med Clin North Am 2008;26(3):849–62.
18. Santanilla JI. The crashing ventilated patient. In: Winters ME, Bond MC, Marconi EG, et al, editors. Emergency department resuscitation of the critically ill. 2nd edition. Dallas (TX): American College of Emergency Physicians; 2017. p. 17–26.
19. Wilkerson RG, Stone MB. Sensitivity of bedside ultrasound and supine anteroposterior chest radiographs for the identification of pneumothorax after blunt trauma. Acad Emerg Med 2010;17:11–7.

Postoperative Tonsillectomy Hemorrhage

Jessica J. Wall, MD, MPH[a],*, Khoon-Yen Tay, MD[b]

KEYWORDS

- Tonsillectomy • Hemorrhage • Bleeding • Pediatric • Emergency medicine

KEY POINTS

- Tonsillectomy is a common surgery in pediatric patients for sleep-disordered breathing and recurrent throat infections.
- Postoperative bleeding is the leading cause of death in tonsillectomy patients.
- Any patient with bleeding, oozing, or clot formation requires observation, admission, or surgical intervention.
- Rapid, focused assessment is necessary to identify life-threatening hemorrhage.
- Management of severe bleeding includes direct pressure, intubation, blood volume replacement, and surgical intervention.

INTRODUCTION

Tonsillectomy is one of the most common surgeries performed in the field of otolaryngology, with greater than 500,000 performed in the pediatric population in the United States every year.[1] Most of these surgeries are now performed as same-day surgeries,[2] resulting in a shift in the management of postoperative complications from the inpatient setting to primary care clinics and emergency departments. Thus, every emergency physician should be familiar with the procedure, postoperative course and management of the life-threatening complications associated with tonsillectomy. Mortality associated with tonsillectomy is primarily related to anesthesia complications and postoperative hemorrhage.[3]

The two most common and accepted indications for tonsillectomy, with or without adenoidectomy, are recurrent throat infections and obstructive sleep disorders.[1] The American Academy of Otolaryngology-Head and Neck Surgery recommends

Disclosure Statement: The authors of this article have no commercial or financial conflicts of interest related to the content of this article.
^a Department of Emergency Medicine, Penn Presbyterian Medical Center, 51 North 39th Street, Philadelphia, PA 19104, USA; ^b Division of Emergency Medicine, Children's Hospital of Philadelphia, 3501 Civic Center Boulevard, Philadelphia, PA 19104, USA
* Corresponding author.
E-mail address: Jessica.j.wall@gmail.com

tonsillectomy in the setting of recurrent throat infections (characterized by temperature >38.3°C, cervical adenopathy, tonsillar exudate, or positive throat culture for group A β-hemolytic streptococci) to improve quality of life, reduce antibiotic usage, reduce health care provider visits, and reduce missed school days. Additionally, it recommends considering tonsillectomy in patients with sleep-disordered breathing to improve sleep patterns and vocal quality; however, the evidence is less compelling.[1] There are several controversial indications for tonsillectomy including peritonsillar cellulitis or abscess, pediatric autoimmune neuropsychiatric disorders associated with streptococcal infections (PANDAS),[4] cryptic tonsillitis, immunoglobulin A (IgA) nephropathy, hemorrhagic tonsillitis, or a chronic carrier state of group A β-hemolytic streptococci.[1,5,6]

TONSILLECTOMY: THE PROCEDURE

Familiarity with the anatomy of the peritonsillar space is necessary to understand the risk of postoperative hemorrhage. There are multiple arterial supplies to the palatine tonsils, originating from the external carotid artery and the tonsillar venous plexus, which are ligated or cauterized during surgery. It is this substantial vascular supply that predisposes the peritonsillar space to life-threatening arterial hemorrhage postoperatively.

A tonsillectomy involves the *en bloc* removal of the tonsil and its capsule from the peritonsillar space by dissecting it away from the muscular wall. Multiple techniques for tonsillectomy are in practice, including cold or traditional techniques, which utilize sharp instruments to incise and blunt instruments to dissect away the tonsil. Hemostasis is achieved by direct pressure, suture ligation, or chemical cautery. Hot techniques involve a variety of electrosurgical or thermal instruments to excise the tonsil and achieve hemostasis.[5,7] Debate continues within the literature regarding the ideal technique with regards to postoperative pain and complications, risk of regrowth, and efficacy with regards to indication. Cold techniques, however, are associated with a lower rate of postoperative bleeding when compared with hot techniques.[8–10]

Tonsillotomy, also known as an intracapsular tonsillectomy or partial tonsillectomy, is a newer technique that removes the majority of the tonsil while leaving a base of lymphoid tissue and the capsule.[11] Multiple studies have demonstrated varying degrees of benefit to this procedure including decreased pain and lower rates of postoperative bleeding. Tonsillotomy, however, is associated with higher rates of tonsillar regrowth and symptom recurrence, and thus is less widely utilized.[11–14]

POSTOPERATIVE RECOVERY

A tonsillectomy is a traumatic procedure with associated risks; thus understanding the normal postoperative course is useful in the identification of complications. Within several hours of the surgery, edema may develop on the uvula, tonsillar pillars, and tongue, resulting in discomfort and a globus sensation, yet this rarely results in clinically significant upper airway obstruction requiring admission for monitoring.[15]

The characteristic fibrin clot forms within the first 24 hours of surgery, coating the tonsillar fossa, and propagates into a thick cake over the next several days with a characteristic grey-white appearance.[16] Depending on technique, the fibrin clot typically separates from the tonsillar fossa between postoperative day 5 and 7, leaving a thin layer of new stroma and lining of epithelium in the peripheral fossa. This is the point when the vascular bed is relatively exposed and at highest risk for significant hemorrhage. By day 12 to 17, the tonsillar fossa is covered by a thickened layer of epithelium, and the risk of bleeding declines (**Fig. 1**).

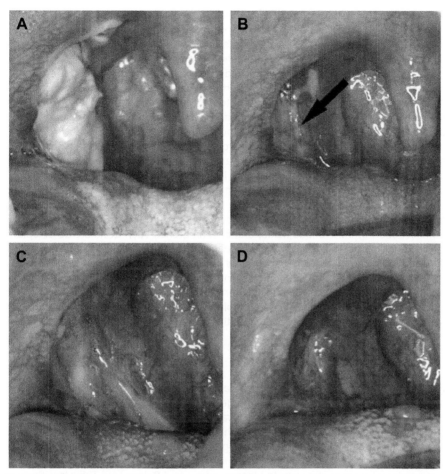

Fig. 1. Stages of post-tonsillectomy healing. (*A*) Postoperative day 5. Exudative fibrin clot fills tonsillar fossa, protruding beyond tonsillar pillars. (*B*) Postoperative day 7. Fibrin clot has separated from tonsillar fossa. New stroma lines tonsillar fossa. Initial ingrowth of posterior pillar epithelium is discernible (*arrow*). (*C*) Postoperative day 9. Bridge of epithelium has widened, advancing laterally across stromal bed. (*D*) Postoperative day 17. Tonsillar fossa is covered by layer of epithelium. Initial epithelial bridge has thickened and resembles normal mucosa. (*Data from* Isaacson G. Tonsillectomy healing. Ann Otol Rhinol Laryngol 2012;121(10):645–9.)

POSTOPERATIVE PAIN MANAGEMENT

Postoperative pain is a known and expected result of tonsillectomy, making pain management a crucial tenet of postoperative care to decrease readmission for pain control and dehydration.[17] Intraoperative dexamethasone is now routinely administered to improve postoperative nausea and vomiting, as well as reduce post-operative pain and swelling.[1] Post-tonsillectomy patients are also commonly discharged with opiate medications, such as oxycodone or acetaminophen-oxycodone, for pain control for the first week following surgery, although there are some data to suggest that management with nonopiate medications may be adequate.[1] Nonsteroidal anti-inflammatories, specifically ibuprofen, have been shown to improve pain control without increasing bleeding risk.[18,19] However, if nonopiate medications are not effective in managing pain putting the patient at risk for decreased oral intake and dehydration, then, families should be prescribed and instructed in the proper use of opiate medications, specifically dosage and timing of administration.

Poor post-tonsillectomy pain control and concern for dehydration are common reasons for presentation to emergency departments and readmission in the postoperative period.[17] Families should be instructed at discharge after surgery on general fluid intake goals in the postoperative period and to carefully pay attention to signs of dehydration, such as decreased urine output. When patients present with postoperative pain or poor oral intake, the emergency physician should assess for clinical signs of dehydration such as decreased urine output or concentrated urine, tachycardia, and dry mucous membranes. The home pain management strategies should be assessed, and if reasonable, a trial of an oral opiate medication could be indicated. However, if pain control is not attainable with oral medications, including correctly dosed opiate medications, consider placement of an intravenous catheter for the administration of intravenous fluids, anti-inflammatories such at ketorolac or opiate medications such as morphine, and a repeat dose of dexamethasone after consultation with the otolaryngologist. It is important to note that codeine is no longer recommended to pain control in pediatric patients given its variable metabolism, efficacy, and higher risk of complications in children.[20]

Patients who fail outpatient pain-control management and are unable to maintain their own hydration should be admitted to the hospital for intravenous pain medication administration and rehydration.

DEFINITIONS OF HEMORRHAGE

Postoperative hemorrhage is one of the leading causes of death associated with tonsillectomy.[3] Post-tonsillectomy hemorrhage is classified as primary or secondary. Primary hemorrhage is defined as postoperative bleeding within the first 24 hours of surgery. The incidence of primary hemorrhage is between 0.2% and 2.2%.[21,22] Secondary hemorrhage is defined as bleeding greater than 24 hours following surgery. The incidence of secondary hemorrhage is between 0.1% and 4.8%,[1,21,22] with an average time from tonsillectomy to bleeding of 5.7 to 7.8 days.[23,24] This classification system is used for tracking of postoperative complications and does not relate to the severity of bleeding. It is important to realize that while traditional teaching has focused on the peak incidence of bleeding between 5 to 7 days, patients can have significant hemorrhage at any point during the postoperative period.

RISK FACTORS FOR HEMORRHAGE

Age is the most well documented risk factor of post-tonsillectomy hemorrhage.[25,26] Higher rates of post-tonsillectomy hemorrhage are associated with older age, specifically the 11- to 17-year-old age group.[2] Furthermore, age greater than 6 years old is associated with a higher need for interventions to achieve hemorrhage control.[27] The indication of chronic/recurrent infections for tonsillectomy has also been shown to be associated with higher risk of hemorrhage.[26,28] Interestingly, the various types of hot surgical technique are not an independent risk factor for hemorrhage, but cold techniques are associated with a lower incidence of bleeding.[7,12,29] Increased experience level of the surgeon is associated with lower rates of both primary and secondary hemorrhage.[10,29] Bleeding has also been associated with various coagulopathies, most commonly both treated and undiagnosed von Willebrand disease.[30,31] Thus, the emergency clinician should focus on a personal and family history of bleeding disorders or prior history of abnormal or excessive hemorrhage and send appropriate testing when indicated. In patients with a history concerning for von Willebrand disease or other coagulopathy, consider the administration von Willebrand factor and desmopressin, or the replacement of additional blood products such as platelets and fresh frozen plasma.

ASSESSMENT OF THE POST-TONSILLECTOMY PATIENT

Given the high rates of bleeding and risk of life-threatening hemorrhage, a focused emergency department assessment is crucial in post-tonsillectomy patients to identify those patients actively bleeding and at higher risk of severe hemorrhage. One study found that among post-tonsillectomy patients presenting to the emergency department with concern for secondary bleeding, 22.8% were actively bleeding; 9.5% were anemic, and 3.3% were hypotensive.[27] The initial assessment should focus on active bleeding and hemodynamic stability. The presence of active bleeding, oozing, or clot in the oropharynx generally requires surgical management and should be transferred to a center with otolaryngology and operative capabilities.[5]

A focused history should include the volume of blood visualized by the parents or patient, duration of bleeding, number of episodes of bleeding, and time since the last episode of bleeding. Additional information including the child's medical history, family or personal history of bleeding diathesis, date of surgery and time of last oral intake are also useful in determining the need for adjunctive therapy and timing of urgent surgical intervention.

In a stable patient, careful inspection of the oropharynx with a good light source is warranted to assess for small clot formation and oozing in the fossa (**Figs. 2** and **3**). A complete view of the tonsillar fossa may be difficult due to patient discomfort and inadequate light. If the otoscope does not provide appropriate visualization, consider using a headlamp with the gentle assistance of a tongue depressor, using caution to not induce coughing or contact the surgical site. In older patients, allowing them to hold the light source may be effective. Consider using an age-appropriate Macintosh laryngoscope held by the patient to prevent oral trauma. In this technique, the patient is seated holding the laryngoscope in their hand and inserts the blade along the tongue to gently depress the tongue and provide light to the oropharynx. Finally, a video

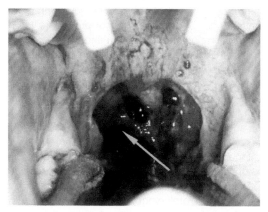

Fig. 2. Post-tonsillectomy hemorrhage. *Arrow* indicates clot with continued bleeding. (*Courtesy of* Dr Christopher Chang, Fauquier ENT, 550 Hospital Drive, Warrentown, VA 20186, USA.)

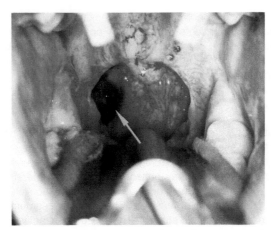

Fig. 3. Post-tonsillectomy hemorrhage with clot formation. *Arrow* indicates clot without continued bleeding. (*Courtesy of* Dr Christopher Chang, Fauquier ENT, 550 Hospital Drive, Warrentown, VA 20186.)

laryngoscope can be used with a similar technique, allowing for better direct visualization of the tonsillar fossa and the ability to capture images, which can be electronically shared with the consulting otolaryngologist. If there is difficulty visualizing the source of bleeding due to blood in the oropharynx, having the patient lean forward will help quantify the rate of bleeding while not obstructing the airway. Patients can also be asked to swish and spit to remove excessive clots and allow for improved visualization of the oropharynx.

MANAGEMENT OF MINOR BLEEDING

When evaluating minor bleeding, it is important to keep in mind that even in episodes that resolve or have a notable clot, there is a continued risk of severe bleeding. In fact, 41% of severe bleeding episodes have been shown to be preceded by a light bleeding episode, and 10.2% of all minor bleeding patients developing severe bleeding.[32] Patients and families will often report minor bleeding that has stopped at the time of presentation to the emergency department. While not requiring emergent intervention, up to 34% of these patients will undergo a surgical procedure for post-tonsillectomy bleeding,[24] and thus observation and admission should be considered. The decision to observe, admit, or transfer the patient should be made in consultation with an otolaryngologist when possible given the high risk of recurrent bleeding. When communicating with a surgical consult, several historical elements and physical examination findings are imperative to determine and help stratify their risk of further bleeding and need of further intervention. These factors are listed in **Box 1**.

Older children and adults can be cauterized at bedside for minor bleeding with silver nitrate or electrocautery by the emergency physician when allowed by institutional policy; however, younger children are more likely to require management in the operating room.[24] Occasionally, the bleeding source will be the nares or emesis of ingested blood from the procedure; however, when in doubt, observation in the emergency department, consultation with otolaryngology, and possible admission should be considered. While in the emergency department, the patient should remain nil per os (NPO) in case of recurrent bleeding. Intravenous access and laboratory evaluation, including a complete blood count, PT/PTT and type and screen, should be considered

---

Box 1
Historical and physical examination findings for the assessment of post-tonsillectomy bleeding

History

Patient age

Date of surgery

Type of surgery (tonsillectomy or tonsillotomy)

Volume of blood visualized

Duration of bleeding

Number of episodes of bleeding

Timing of last episode of bleeding

Past medical history, specifically bleeding disorders

NPO time

Physical examination findings

Vital signs

General appearance and signs of anemia or airway compromise

Tonsillar fossa
    Presence of clot
    Presence of fibrin clot
    Active bleeding

---

in these patients. Obtaining a complete blood count may further assist the clinician in quantifying blood loss; however, clinicians should not be overly reassured by normal values.

MANAGEMENT OF LIFE-THREATENING BLEEDING

The patient who presents with active bleeding should be considered a surgical emergency. At the time of presentation, assessment of the patient should be completed while notifying the operating room and otolaryngologist. In emergency departments without access to an otolaryngologist, contacting the nearest pediatric center with surgical capabilities should be initiated immediately while attempting to stabilize the patient.

The initial assessment and primary survey should focus on the airway and hemodynamic stability. Initial management includes immediate intravenous access and volume resuscitation with isotonic saline. Severe bleeding may warrant blood transfusion in the emergency department for hypovolemia and severe anemia; thus complete blood count, PT/PTT, and type and cross should be obtained.[24] In the case of an unstable patient with difficult intravenous access, consider placing one or more intraosseous lines for volume resuscitation. Additionally, blood work can be sent from an arterial puncture if functional access is obtained but unable to provide blood return.

Most of the blood lost from the bleeding site is swallowed; therefore, pediatric patients rarely have difficulty with aspiration or breathing while their mentation is intact.[33] Initially, placing the awake patient in an upright position, leaning forward will assist in management of the blood in the oropharynx, alternatively patients may be placed in the lateral decubitus position for comfort. If the patient is able to tolerate direct pressure while awake without emesis, this is the best initial option for management of severe hemorrhage.

Techniques to apply direct pressure and achieve adequate hemostasis should be attempted immediately after initial assessment. Any clot or blood in the oropharynx should be evacuated with suction or gauze to allow for adequate visualization and application of pressure. Direct pressure can be applied with gauze and the clinician's fingers, but there is a risk of losing control of the gauze and inadvertently causing an airway foreign body. Thus, securing the gauze with an instrument is a safer option. Magill forceps with a folded gauze pack may be used to first clear the clot, and then apply direct pressure laterally into the tonsillar fossa with counterpressure using the clinician's fingers placed inferior to the mandible and directed upward. Counterpressure may compress the external carotid artery; thus, it is crucial to closely monitor the mental status of the patient. Soaking the gauze in epinephrine, lidocaine with epinephrine, topical thrombin, tranexamic acid (TXA), or other hemostatic agent will assist with bleeding control.[24,34–39] See **Box 2** for details of topical agents.

In patients who have difficulty tolerating this procedure or whose mentation begins to decline, judicious use of sedation or rapid sequence intubation should be considered. Assessment of airway patency and consideration of sedation or intubation remain challenging for the emergency medicine provider in patients with post-tonsillectomy hemorrhage. The decision to sedate or intubate depends on the skill level of the provider, access to rescue airway equipment, stability for transport, and condition of the patient.

Sedation with medications like ketamine to facilitate tolerance of direct pressure requires vigilance and preparation. Complete monitoring equipment including end tidal capnography, appropriately sized intubation equipment, and adequate suction, should be at the bedside. Rapid-sequence intubation medications should be available in the case of laryngospasm or aspiration, and a highly experienced emergency provider and/or anesthesiologist should be at the bedside. During the sedation, care should be made to not obstruct the airway with the gauze used to tamponade the bleeding and to provide continuous suction to prevent aspiration of blood.

Airway management with intubation in patients with post-tonsillectomy hemorrhage is complicated by the risks of emesis, hypoxia, aspiration, hypovolemia, decompensated shock, and the potential for a difficult airway. Intubation in the operating room has been shown to have a 3.3% incidence of hypoxia and 2.7% incidence of difficult

---

Box 2
Topical hemostatic agents

Epinephrine 1:10,000

Lidocaine 1% with epinephrine 1:100,000

Topical thrombin
    Multiple formulations: human and recombinant
    Consider combining solution with an absorbable hemostatic agent

Absorbable hemostatic agents[37]
    Gelatin sponges: Gelfoam, Surgifoam
    Thrombin/gelatin solution: Floseal
    Oxidized regenerated cellulose: Surgicel

Tranexamic acid-soaked gauze[38,39]
    Oral formulation: crush a 500 mg tablet and dissolve in 10 mL of sterile water
    Intravenous formulation: use 500 mg in 5 mL solution

intubation,[33] with the majority of cases using intravenous sedation and succinylcholine for paralysis. If intubation is to occur in the emergency department, rapid-sequence intubation should be utilized with adjuncts such additional suction catheters and video laryngoscopy. When available, consider anesthesia backup or activation of a difficult airway protocol if it exists. When sedating or intubating these patients, multiple suction apparatuses should be available with large-bore catheters, such as the Yankauer catheter. Difficult airway adjuncts should be readily available, and back-up devices should be prepared. An appropriately sized laryngeal mask airway (LMA) may be used temporarily if the practitioner is unable to intubate the patient.[40]

The choice of medications for rapid-sequence intubation in the pediatric patient is often institution specific and based on provider comfort level. The authors recommend selecting sedation agents with hemodynamic stability, such as ketamine or etomidate, as post-tonsillectomy hemorrhage can rapidly lead to hypovolemia and the risk of hypotension.[41] Paralysis may be achieved with succinylcholine or rocuronium, depending on providers' comfort and institutional policy. Succinylcholine has fallen out of favor in several pediatric institutions because of the multiple contraindications including the theoretic risk of undiagnosed myopathy or malignant hypothermia. When appropriate, volume resuscitate the patient prior to rapid-sequence intubation to prevent post-intubation hypotension.

After intubation, it is important to maintain direct pressure on the bleeding tonsillar fossa for hemostasis. Surgical packing such as sterile vaginal packing is useful because of its bulk and radiopaque properties, which assist in complete removal once the patient is taken to the operating room for definitive management. Placement of a throat pack is intended to use the substantial bulk of the material to maintain pressure on the bleeding site; thus multiple packs may need to be placed after intubation to achieve hemostasis. Once the airway is secure and/or the bleeding has been controlled, care should be taken to ensure euvolemia with appropriate blood volume replacement, especially if the patient requires transfer or there is a delay to surgical intervention. For unstable patients uncrossmatched blood should be initiated until crossmatched blood is available. In the exsanguinating patient, consider activating the institution's massive transfusion protocol early to assist in the replacement of blood products.[42]

Currently, operative management is the definitive treatment for life-threatening bleeding in post-tonsillectomy patients. However, there are emerging data to support endovascular treatment with embolization in the setting of recurrent bleeding following surgery or as an alternative to surgical intervention.[43] Thus, the emergency provider should be familiar with institutional protocols for this common form of hemorrhage prior to presentation.

SPECIAL CONSIDERATIONS FOR TRANSFER

Patients who present to hospitals without a pediatric otolaryngologist on-call present a challenging case for the emergency provider. Many community emergency departments have anesthesia on call and/or a general otolaryngologist. When the patient is unstable or the transport time and risk of decomposition are substantial, discussion with these resources may be beneficial in assisting with airway management and temporizing measures. For patients who will likely require transfer, early consultation with the receiving institution may assist in guiding management of the patient and expedite transfer.

Intubation prior to transfer is a difficult decision for the emergency care provider. Stable patients without active bleeding do not typically require airway management prior to transfer. Patients who are either unstable or actively bleeding, however, may require intubation for stabilization and hemorrhage control prior to transfer. Active bleeding, transfusion requirement, travel time, capabilities of the transporting agency, hospital resources such as anesthesiology, provider skill level, and the availability of appropriate equipment for intubation are all factors that should be considered in making the decision to intubate a patient prior to transfer.

SUMMARY

Post-tonsillectomy hemorrhage in pediatric patients represent a potentially complicated presentation because of the risk of significant blood loss, difficulty achieving hemostasis, and challenging airway. The savvy emergency provider should be cognizant that post-tonsillectomy hemorrhage is potentially a life-threatening condition that occurs in up to 5% of patients, with an average time of presentation of between 5 and 7 days postoperatively. Minor bleeding episodes often precede severe tonsillar hemorrhage; thus careful inspection of the tonsillar fossa to assess for small areas of oozing or clot is a key portion of evaluation of these patients. For patients with minor and self-resolving bleeding, observation in the emergency department and/or admission for monitoring should be considered given the high rate of recurrent bleeding. Further, consultation with an otolaryngologist is crucial, as often patients with signs of prior bleeding will be managed operatively at the discretion of the surgeon.

Severe bleeding or active bleeding is considered a life-threatening emergency that warrants immediate evaluation. Management of severe bleeding includes immediate surgical consultation or initiation of the transfer process to a center with surgical capabilities, direct pressure to the site of hemorrhage with or without the addition of a hemostatic agent, possible intubation using rapid sequence induction medications, and management of hemodynamic instability with blood product replacement. With this potentially life-threatening condition, it is imperative that the emergency medicine provider be familiar with the tenets of its management.

REFERENCES

1. Baugh RF, Archer SM, Mitchell RB. Clinical practice guideline: tonsillectomy in children. Otolaryngol Head Neck Surg 2011. https://doi.org/10.1177/0194599810389949.
2. Harounian JA, Schaefer E, Schubart J, et al. Pediatric adenotonsillectomy and postoperative hemorrhage: demographic and geographic variation in the US. Int J Pediatr Otorhinolaryngol 2016;87(C):50–4.
3. Morris LGT, Lieberman SM, Reitzen SD, et al. Characteristics and outcomes of malpractice claims after tonsillectomy. Otolaryngol Head Neck Surg 2008; 138(3):315–20.
4. Windfuhr JP. Tonsillectomy remains a questionable option for pediatric autoimmune neuropsychiatric disorders associated with streptococcal infections (PANDAS). GMS Curr Top Otorhinolaryngol Head Neck Surg 2016;15:Doc07.
5. Isaacson G. Tonsillectomy care for the pediatrician. Pediatrics 2012;130(2): 324–34.
6. Windfuhr JP. Indications for tonsillectomy stratified by the level of evidence. GMS Curr Top Otorhinolaryngol Head Neck Surg 2016;15:Doc09.
7. Noordzij JP, Affleck BD. Coblation versus unipolar electrocautery tonsillectomy: a prospective, randomized, single-blind study in adult patients. Laryngoscope 2006;116(8):1303–9.

8. Magdalena ML, Solé A, Blanco V, et al. Histological analysis of tonsillectomies: relationship with surgical technique, post-operative pain and haemorrhage. J Laryngol Otol 2016;130(12):1142–6.
9. Metcalfe C, Muzaffar J, Daultrey C, et al. Coblation tonsillectomy: a systematic review and descriptive analysis. Eur Arch Otorhinolaryngol 2017;274(6):2637–47.
10. Hinton-Bayre AD, Noonan K, Ling S, et al. Experience is more important than technology in paediatric post-tonsillectomy bleeding. J Laryngol Otol 2017; 131(S2):S35–40.
11. Koltai PJ, Solares CA, Mascha EJ, et al. Intracapsular partial tonsillectomy for tonsillar hypertrophy in children. Laryngoscope 2002;112(8 Pt 2 Suppl 100):17–9.
12. Papaspyrou G, Linxweiler M, Knöbber D, et al. Laser CO2 tonsillotomy versus argon plasma coagulation (APC) tonsillotomy: a retrospective study with 10-year follow-up. Int J Pediatr Otorhinolaryngol 2017;92(C):56–60.
13. Sathe N, Chinnadurai S, McPheeters M, et al. Comparative effectiveness of partial versus total tonsillectomy in children: a systematic review. Otolaryngol Head Neck Surg 2017;156(3):456–63.
14. Wood JM, Cho M, Carney AS. Role of subtotal tonsillectomy ("tonsillotomy") in children with sleep disordered breathing. J Laryngol Otol 2014;128(Suppl 1): S3–7.
15. Isaacson G. Avoiding airway obstruction after pediatric adenotonsillectomy. Int J Pediatr Otorhinolaryngol 2009;73(6):803–6.
16. Isaacson G. Tonsillectomy healing. Ann Otol Rhinol Laryngol 2012;121(10): 645–9.
17. Curtis JL, Harvey DB, Willie S, et al. Causes and costs for ED visits after pediatric adenotonsillectomy. Otolaryngol Head Neck Surg 2015;152(4):691–6.
18. Lewis SR, Nicholson A, Cardwell ME, et al. Nonsteroidal anti-inflammatory drugs and perioperative bleeding in paediatric tonsillectomy. Cochrane Database of Syst Rev 2013;7:CD003591.
19. Pfaff JA, Hsu K, Chennupati SK. The use of ibuprofen in posttonsillectomy analgesia and its effect on posttonsillectomy hemorrhage rate. Otolaryngol Head Neck Surg 2016;155(3):508–13.
20. Tobias JD, Green TP, Coté CJ, Section on Anesthesiology and Pain Medicine, Committee on Drugs. Codeine: time to say "no". Pediatrics 2016;138(4). https://doi.org/10.1542/peds.2016-2396.
21. Francis DO, Fonnesbeck C, Sathe N, et al. Postoperative bleeding and associated utilization following tonsillectomy in children: a systematic review and meta-analysis. Otolaryngol Head Neck Surg 2017;156(3):442–55.
22. Windfuhr JP, Chen YS, Remmert S. Hemorrhage following tonsillectomy and adenoidectomy in 15,218 patients. Otolaryngol Head Neck Surg 2005;132(2): 281–6.
23. Windfuhr JP, Schloendorff G, Baburi D, et al. Serious post-tonsillectomy hemorrhage with and without lethal outcome in children and adolescents. Int J Pediatr Otorhinolaryngol 2008;72(7):1029–40.
24. Steketee KG, Reisdorff EJ. Emergency care for posttonsillectomy and postadenoidectomy hemorrhage. Am J Emerg Med 1995;13(5):518–23.
25. Lee WT, Witsell DL, Parham K, et al. Tonsillectomy bleed rates across the CHEER Practice Research Network. Otolaryngol Head Neck Surg 2016;155(1):28–32.
26. Spektor Z, Saint-Victor S, Kay DJ, et al. Risk factors for pediatric post-tonsillectomy hemorrhage. Int J Pediatr Otorhinolaryngol 2016;84:151–5.
27. Arora R, Saraiya S, Niu X, et al. Post tonsillectomy hemorrhage: who needs intervention? Int J Pediatr Otorhinolaryngol 2015;79(2):165–9.

28. Myssiorek D, Alvi A. Post-tonsillectomy hemorrhage: an assessment of risk factors. Int J Pediatr Otorhinolaryngol 1996;37(1):35–43.
29. Tomkinson A, Harrison W, Owens D, et al. Risk factors for postoperative hemorrhage following tonsillectomy. Laryngoscope 2011;121(2):279–88.
30. Witmer CM, Elden L, Butler RB, et al. Incidence of bleeding complications in pediatric patients with type 1 von Willebrand disease undergoing adenotonsillar procedures. J Pediatr 2009;155(1):68–72.
31. Prim MP, De Diego JI, Jimenez-Yuste V. Analysis of the causes of immediate unanticipated bleeding after pediatric adenotonsillectomy. Int J Pediatr Otorhinolaryngol 2003. https://doi.org/10.1016/S0165-5876(02)00396-8.
32. Sarny S, Ossimitz G, Habermann W, et al. Hemorrhage following tonsil surgery: a multicenter prospective study. Laryngoscope 2011;121(12):2553–60.
33. Fields RG, Gencorelli FJ, Litman RS. Anesthetic management of the pediatric bleeding tonsil. Paediatr Anaesth 2010;20(11):982–6.
34. Riviello RJ, Brown NA. Otolaryngologic procedures. In: Roberts JR, Hedges JR, editors. Clinical procedures in emergency medicine. 5 edition. Philadelphia: Elsevier Saunders p. 1215–6.
35. Hinder D, Tschopp K. Topical application of tranexamic acid to prevent post-tonsillectomy haemorrhage. Laryngorhinootologie 2015;94(2):86–90 [in German].
36. Chan CC, Chan YY, Tanweer F. Systematic review and meta-analysis of the use of tranexamic acid in tonsillectomy. Eur Arch Otorhinolaryngol 2012;270(2):735–48.
37. Lew WK, Weaver FA. Clinical use of topical thrombin as a surgical hemostat. Biologics 2008;2(4):593–9.
38. Nuvvula S, Gaddam K, Kamatham R. Efficacy of tranexamic acid mouthwash as an alternative for factor replacement in gingival bleeding during dental scaling in cases of hemophilia: a randomized clinical trial. Contemp Clin Dent 2014;5(1):49.
39. Zahed R, Moharamzadeh P, Alizadeharasi S, et al. A new and rapid method for epistaxis treatment using injectable form of tranexamic acid topically: a randomized controlled trial. Am J Emerg Med 2013;31(9):1389–92.
40. Walls RM, Murphy MF. Manual of emergency airway management. 3rd edition. Philadelphia: Lippincott, Williams & Wilkins; 2008.
41. Gerardi MJ, Sacchetti AD, Cantor RM, et al. Rapid-sequence intubation of the pediatric patient. Pediatric Emergency Medicine Committee of the American College of Emergency Physicians. Ann Emerg Med 1996;28(1):55–74.
42. Nystrup KB, Stensballe J, Bøttger M, et al. Transfusion therapy in paediatric trauma patients: a review of the literature. Scand J Trauma Resusc Emerg Med 2015;23(1):21.
43. Gratacap M, Couloigner V, Boulouis G, et al. Embolization in the management of recurrent secondary post-tonsillectomy haemorrhage in children. Eur Radiol 2014;25(1):239–45.

Emergency Department Management of Pediatric Shock

Jenny Mendelson, MD[a,b,*]

KEYWORDS

- Pediatric • Children • Shock • Hypotension • Sepsis • Vasopressors
- Emergency department

KEY POINTS

- Clinical history and physical examination findings are crucial for the early recognition and classification of shock in the pediatric patient.
- Hypotension is a late and ominous finding in the pediatric patient in shock.
- Rapid fluid resuscitation is the first line of treatment in most forms of shock.
- Three 20 mL/kg isotonic crystalloid boluses should be given within the first 20 to 60 minutes after shock is identified.
- Epinephrine is usually the preferred vasopressor in pediatric shock and should be started peripherally if central access is not present.

INTRODUCTION

Shock is a state of acute energy failure stemming from a decrease in adenosine triphosphate production and subsequent failure to meet the acute metabolic demands of the body. More simply put, it is a state of inadequate oxygen supply to meet the body's cellular demands. Hypoxemia or decreased perfusion results in decreased oxygen delivery to the tissues, causing a shift from more efficient aerobic pathways to anaerobic metabolism, resulting in the production of lactic acid. As oxygen deprivation persists, cellular hypoxia leads to the disruption of critical biochemical processes, eventually resulting in cell membrane ion pump dysfunction, intracellular edema, inadequate regulation of intracellular pH, and cell death.

Disclosures: None.
[a] Pediatrics, Division of Pediatric Critical Care Medicine, University of Arizona College of Medicine, Banner-University Medical Center, 1501 North Campbell Avenue, PO Box 245073, Tucson, AZ 85724-5073, USA; [b] Emergency Medicine, University of Arizona College of Medicine, Banner-University Medical Center, 1501 North Campbell Avenue, Tucson, AZ 85724-5073, USA
* Pediatrics, Division of Pediatric Critical Care Medicine, University of Arizona College of Medicine, Banner-University Medical Center, 1501 North Campbell Avenue, PO Box 245073, Tucson, AZ 85724-5073.
E-mail address: jmendelson@peds.arizona.edu

Emerg Med Clin N Am 36 (2018) 427–440
https://doi.org/10.1016/j.emc.2017.12.010
emed.theclinics.com
0733-8627/18/© 2018 Elsevier Inc. All rights reserved.

Oxygen delivery to the tissues is determined by cardiac output and arterial oxygen content. Cardiac output depends on heart rate and stroke volume. Stroke volume is determined by preload (the amount of filling of the ventricle at end-diastole), afterload (the force against which the ventricle must work to eject blood during systole, which is greatly affected by systemic vascular resistance [SVR]); contractility (the force generated by the ventricle during systole), and lusitropy (the degree of myocardial relaxation during diastole). In children, compared with adults, cardiac output is more dependent on heart rate than stroke volume owing to myocardial immaturity, which limits the ability to increase contractility. Arterial oxygen content depends on hemoglobin concentration, arterial oxygen saturation, and the arterial partial pressure of oxygen, with most oxygen being carried on hemoglobin and a small portion delivered as dissolved O_2.[1]

Under normal conditions of increased oxygen demand, such as exercise, oxygen delivery must increase by redistribution of blood flow. Similarly, in pathologic instances of increased oxygen demand or decreased oxygen delivery (shock), initial compensatory mechanisms occur to preserve tissue perfusion. In compensated shock, vital organ function is maintained and blood pressure remains normal. In uncompensated shock, hypotension develops and organ and cellular function deteriorate. Left untreated, uncompensated shock progresses to irreversible shock, characterized by irreversible organ failure, cardiovascular collapse, cardiac arrest, and death.

Pediatric shock results in a significant amount of morbidity and mortality worldwide. Sepsis and hypovolemia owing to infectious gastroenteritis are leading causes of child mortality worldwide, with an estimated 3 to 5 billion cases of acute gastroenteritis and nearly 2 million deaths occurring each year in children under 5 years of age, with 98% of those deaths occurring developing countries.[2] In developed countries like the United States, shock is also a common occurrence in the emergency department (ED). These children have a higher mortality rate compared with patients not in shock (11.4% vs 2.6%). The presence of shock is also associated with worse outcomes in a variety of emergency conditions, including traumatic brain injury and cardiac arrest.[3,4]

CLASSIFICATIONS OF SHOCK

Several classifications of shock exist (**Table 1**). Rapid identification of the etiology may help to guide specific therapies.

Table 1
Categories of shock

Category	Hemodynamics	Causes
Hypovolemic	↓Preload, ↑SVR, ↓CO	Gastrointestinal loses, renal loses, hemorrhage, third spacing, burns
Distributive	↓Preload, ↓↓SVR, ↓↑CO	Sepsis, anaphylaxis, neurogenic shock
Cardiogenic	↑Preload, ↑SVR, ↓CO	Congenital heart disease, arrhythmia, cardiomyopathy, myocarditis, severe anemia
Obstructive	↓↑Preload, ↑SVR, ↓CO	Pulmonary embolus, pericardial tamponade, tension pneumothorax, certain congenital heart lesions

Abbreviations: CO, cardiac output; SVR, systemic vascular resistance.

Hypovolemic Shock

Hypovolemia is the most common cause of shock in children[5] and is a leading cause of child mortality worldwide. Hypovolemic shock occurs owing to inappropriately low intravascular blood volume (either owing to intravascular volume loss or hemorrhage), leading to decreased cardiac output. Additionally, hemorrhagic shock decreases oxygen-carrying capacity secondary to direct loss of available hemoglobin.

Intravascular volume loss can occur owing to gastrointestinal, renal, skin (ie, burns), or interstitial (ie, third spacing) losses. Hypovolemia can develop rapidly! Children with gastroenteritis can lose a significant percentage of their circulating volume within a few hours. Even if there is ongoing vomiting or diarrhea, it is usually preferable to attempt oral rehydration if dehydration is mild to moderate. Several studies including large metaanalyses have shown oral rehydration to be highly successful (<5% failure rate) and resulting in shorter ED stays and fewer adverse events compared with intravenous (IV) hydration.[6] If a patient shows signs of decreased end-organ function, however, forego attempts at oral rehydration and proceed to IV resuscitation. Capillary leak syndrome owing to sepsis, burns, or other systemic inflammatory diseases can result in profound intravascular volume loss in patients that may otherwise seem to be edematous and volume overloaded.

Hemorrhage may occur from traumatic or nontraumatic bleeding. Hemorrhagic shock can be further broken down into stages of severity based on percent volume loss and physical examination findings (**Table 2**). In an infant/toddler in shock with unclear etiology, consider occult hemorrhage owing to nonaccidental trauma.

Distributive Shock

In distributive shock, normal peripheral vascular tone becomes inappropriately relaxed. In this state, vasodilation results in effective hypovolemia, although a net fluid loss may not have actually occurred. Common causes of distributive shock include sepsis, anaphylaxis, neurologic injury (ie, spinal shock), or drug-related causes. In

Table 2				
Classification of pediatric hemorrhagic shock by clinical signs				
	Class I Very Mild Blood Loss (<15%)	Class II Mild Blood Loss (15%–30%)	Class III Moderate Blood Loss (30%–40%)	Class IV Severe Blood Loss (>40%)
HR	Normal to mildly increased	Tachycardic	Tachycardic	Severely tachycardic
Pulse quality	Normal	Peripheral pulses decreased	Peripheral pulses decreased	Central pulses decreased
Respiratory rate	Normal	Tachypneic	Tachypneic	Severely tachypneic
Mental status	Normal/ slightly anxious	Anxious/irritable	Irritable/confused	Confused/lethargic/ obtunded
Urine output	Normal	Decreased	Decreased	Anuric
Skin	Warm/pink	Cool/mottled	Cool/mottled/pallor	Cold/pallor/cyanotic

Adapted from American College of Surgeons. Advanced trauma life support (ATLS) study guide. Chicago (IL): American College of Surgeon; 2012; with permission.

sepsis, massive inflammatory response along with nitric oxide and cytokine release lead to peripheral vasodilation. In anaphylaxis, mast cell degranulation leads to vasodilatory cytokine release. In spinal shock, injury to the cranial portion of the spinal cord disrupts the sympathetic chain of the autonomic nervous system, resulting in unopposed parasympathetic vasodilation. Spinal shock, unlike most types of shock, often presents with bradycardia owing to unopposed vagal effects.

Sepsis is a common clinical syndrome that complicates severe infection and is characterized by immune dysregulation, systemic inflammation, microcirculatory derangements, and end-organ dysfunction. Sepsis is 10 times more common in children under 1 year than in older children and adolescents.[7] Pediatric sepsis is commonly encountered in the ED, and is a major cause of morbidity, mortality, and health care use costs worldwide. The American College of Critical Care Medicine (ACCM) defines septic shock as a clinical diagnosis made when children have suspected infection manifested by hypothermia or hyperthermia and clinical signs of inadequate tissue perfusion including any of the following: decreased/altered mental status, abnormal capillary refill time (CRT) or pulse characteristic, or decreased urine output (<1 mL/kg/h). Hypotension is not required for the clinical diagnosis of septic shock.[8]

Septic shock can present in one of two ways: cold shock or warm shock. Cold shock is characterized by high SVR resulting in cool/cold extremities, delayed CRT (<2 seconds), diminished peripheral pulses or differential between peripheral and central pulses, and narrow pulse pressure. Warm shock is characterized by low SVR, with warm/dry extremities with brisk ("flash") CRT, tachycardia, and bounding pulses with a wide pulse pressure.

Cardiogenic Shock

Cardiogenic shock can result from a variety of conditions that impair cardiac output. In children, cardiac failure is most commonly due to congenital heart disease, cardiomyopathies, or myocarditis. Additionally, arrhythmias can result in decreased cardiac output and shock.

Categories of heart failure and cardiogenic shock can be classified according to the presence/absence of 2 traits: venous congestion (owing to increased filling pressures) and hypoperfusion (owing to decreased cardiac output or myocardial contractility). This concept is summarized in **Box 1**. The presence of venous congestion is considered "wet" and the absence is described as "dry," and hypoperfusion is "cold" and normal perfusion is "warm." The wet patient may have findings including edema, hepatomegaly, ascites, jugular venous distension, S3 gallop, or crackles on lung auscultation owing to pulmonary edema. The cold patient may have cool extremities, weak pulses with narrow pulse pressure, delayed CRT, altered mental status, or hypotension.[9,10]

Obstructive Shock

Obstructive shock occurs when either pulmonary or systemic blood flow is impaired, resulting in impaired cardiac output. Causes of obstruction to heart function may be intracardiac or extracardiac and may be congenital or acquired. Examples include obstructive congenital heart lesions, cardiac tamponade, tension pneumothorax, massive pulmonary embolism, severe pulmonary hypertension, and hypertrophic cardiomyopathy. Obstructive shock in infants occurs when congenital lesions interfere with the outflow of blood from the heart, requiring the systemic output to be supplied by the pulmonary artery system via the ductus arteriosus. When the ductus closes within the first few days or weeks after birth, these infants present with severe shock. Obstructive shock generally requires prompt recognition with medical management

---

Box 1
Hemodynamic profiles in pediatric heart failure, classified by presence of hypoperfusion and/ or venous congestion (increased filling pressures)

Warm and dry:

Normal perfusion and no congestion.

Well-compensated but may have significant cardiac dysfunction.

Cold and dry:

Poor perfusion without venous congestion. Decompensating. Sick appearing.

Increased peripheral vascular resistance.

May have oliguria and altered mental status.

Warm and wet:

Normal perfusion with venous congestion.

Still partially compensated.

May benefit from diuretics or inodilators.

Cold and wet:

Poor perfusion with venous congestion.

The sickest group of all.

Usually requires inotropes.

May require mechanical support.

(eg, initiation of prostaglandin therapy for a ductal-dependent lesion) and/or procedural management (eg, pericardiocentesis for tamponade or tube thoracostomy for tension pneumothorax).

RECOGNITION

Clinical history is important in children presenting to the ED in shock, and it may help to classify the etiology of shock and help direct therapies. Attention should be paid to past medical history and medication use (especially immunosuppression or steroid use). All infants under 3 months of age presenting in shock should be considered septic until proven otherwise. A history of fever or trauma may be particularly elucidative; however, often the history of a child in shock is often nonspecific with symptoms such as lethargy, fussiness, poor feeding, or decreased urine output.

Children are usually able to compensate for shock with tachycardia and increased SVR to maintain cardiac output and critical organ perfusion. Tachycardia is the most common presenting physical examination finding in pediatric shock. Persistent tachycardia in a calm, afebrile child should be concerning to the emergency provider and should prompt further investigation. For normal heart rates and blood pressure by age, see **Table 3**.[11] Increased SVR manifests as delayed CRT and diminished peripheral pulses. A recent metaanalysis showed that children with prolonged CRT have a 4-fold greater risk of dying compared with children with normal CRT. They found CRT to be highly specific, but not sensitive, for mortality.[12] Another study showed the combination of prolonged CRT and hypotension has a staggering mortality rate of 26.9%.[13]

When compensatory mechanisms fail, hypotension occurs. Guidelines define hypotension as a systolic blood pressure of less than the 5th percentile for age.[5] In addition

Table 3
Pediatric heart rate ranges and hypotensive systolic blood pressure levels by age

Age	HR (bpm)	Hypotensive SBP (mm Hg)
<1 mo	110–180	<60
1–12 mo	100–170	<70
1–2 y	85–150	<70 + (2 × age in y)
3–5 y	70–140	<70 + (2 × age in y)
6–10 y	60–110	<70 + (2 × age in y)
>10	50–100	<90

to hypotension, a child with decompensated shock will present with signs of inadequate end-organ perfusion, including depressed mental status, decreased urine output, metabolic acidosis, tachypnea, weak central pulses, and worsening peripheral perfusion. These signs of hypoperfusion are highly specific for the development of organ dysfunction, even in the absence of hypotension.[14]

ULTRASOUND EXAMINATION

Another useful tool increasingly used for the assessment of children in shock is point-of-care ultrasound (POCUS) examination.[15] The focused assessment with sonography for trauma (FAST) examination is used routinely in both pediatric and adult trauma to identify hemoperitoneum, hemopericardium, and hemothorax (plus pneumothorax in the extended e-FAST). One small study found that, when combined with increased liver transaminases of greater than 100 IU/L, the specificity of the FAST examination was 98%, suggesting a negative FAST and transaminases of less than 100 IU/L have a low likelihood of significant intraabdominal injury and should prompt patient observation instead of abdominal computed tomography scanning.[16] Although standard measurements of the inferior vena cava and aorta are not established in children (as they are in adults), in the evaluation of pediatric hypovolemic shock, both the ratio of the aorta to inferior vena cava and the dynamic assessment of inferior vena cava collapsibility have been studied and both metrics may correlate with hydration status.[17–19]

In the adult emergency medicine/critical care literature, several POCUS algorithms for the assessment of shock exist, and may dramatically affect treatment decisions and improve survival.[20–24] Evidence for the use of POCUS for the assessment of pediatric cardiac function, volume status, and shock management has lagged behind that for adult patients, yet the concepts remain similar. Clearly, further studies are needed in this area.

TREATMENT

Because shock is a problem of inadequate oxygen delivery, every child in shock should be given supplemental oxygen. Place the child on continuous cardiorespiratory and pulse oximetry monitors and obtain peripheral IV access as soon as possible. Check blood sugar and correct hypoglycemia if present. Hypocalcemia (ionized calcium <1.1 mmol/L) may contribute to cardiac dysfunction and should also be corrected.

Fluid Resuscitation

Isotonic crystalloid solutions are the fluid of choice for resuscitation of a child in shock. Crystalloids are preferred because of their safety, effectiveness, low cost, and wide availability.[25] In less common circumstances, such as in resource-limited settings in developing countries with a high incidence of malaria, anemia, and malnutrition, take caution with IV fluid resuscitation and consider use of colloid (5% albumin) or early transfusion for suspected anemia.[26,27] Treat signs of shock with a fluid bolus of 20 mL/kg, even if blood pressure is normal, and give additional boluses if systemic perfusion fails to improve. In neonates or children with suspected cardiogenic shock, use 10 mL/kg boluses and reassess the patient frequently for signs of volume overload, including hepatomegaly, S3 gallop, or pulmonary rales/crackles. Volume resuscitation in hypovolemia and sepsis commonly requires 40 to 60 mL/kg, but may require as much as 200 mL/kg. POCUS may be useful to help determine if shock is still volume responsive. It is generally accepted that children remaining in shock after 60 mL/kg of IV fluid should be started on vasopressors.

Fluid administration in shock should be as rapid as possible. In infants and children with smaller gauge IVs, a "push/pull" method should be used. Push/pull uses a 3-way stopcock to manually draw a large syringe of fluid from the IV bag (pull) and then rapidly deliver it to the patient (push), and then repeat this process until the full volume is delivered. In 1 trial, fluid administration rates were equivalent in children using a pressure bag versus push/pull system, and both were faster than gravity or an IV infusion pump. Investigators have shown that 20 mL/kg of fluid can be delivered in 5 minutes or less via pressure bag or push methods.[28]

Although placement of a central venous line (CVL) is common in resuscitation in adults, this is unnecessary in children, at least in the initial stages. For the management of a child in shock, the goal should be placement of PIVs of the largest bore possible. If the child is in extremis and without access, intraosseous access should be placed without delay.

Vasoactive Medications

When shock remains refractory to fluid resuscitation, vasoactive infusions should be initiated (**Box 2**). Although infusion of vasoactive medications through a CVL is preferred, placement may be difficult in children. If the child is in fluid-refractory shock,

---

Box 2
Usual dosing ranges for vasoactive medications

Inotropes

Epinephrine 0.05 to 1.00 (or more) μg/kg/min

Dopamine: 5 to 20 μg/kg/min

Dobutamine 5 to 20 μg/kg/min

Vasopressors

Norepinephrine 0.05 to 0.50 (or more) μg/kg/min

Dopamine 10 to 20 μg/kg/min

Vasopressin 0.0005 to 0.0100 U/kg/min

Inotropes increase cardiac contractility. Vasopressors cause vasoconstriction, increasing systemic vascular resistance. Some medications fit into both categories. Start at the low end of the range and titrate rapidly until shock reversal is achieved. If administering via peripheral an intravenous line, dilute the solution (usually 10× the usual central concentration). Additional "driver" fluid (3–5 mL/h of saline) may be needed if the infusion rate is very low (<1 mL/h).

start vasopressors through whatever line is available (peripheral IV access, intraosseous access, or a CVL). A recent small study of peripheral vasoactive medication use in children in a pediatric intensive care unit found IV infiltration and extravasation to occur in only 2% of patients, with none requiring medical or surgical intervention.[29] Another larger study in adults found similarly low rates of complications with the peripheral administration of vasoactive medications, including norepinephrine, dopamine, and phenylephrine.[30] If a peripheral IV is used for vasopressor administration, the medication solution should be diluted and the IV site should be assessed frequently for problems. The use of peripheral vasopressors may be particularly relevant in children requiring transport to a higher level of care. Transport should not be delayed for CVL placement.[31]

The choice of which vasoactive medication to use depends on the clinical picture. Dopamine has long been the initial medication of choice in pediatric shock; however, several recent studies in both adults and children have challenged this dogma.[32–34] In adults, dopamine is associated with increased mortality and occurrence of arrhythmias compared with norepinephrine.[32] Two recent pediatric studies randomized epinephrine versus dopamine use in septic shock. One showed children receiving epinephrine versus dopamine for fluid-refractory septic shock had a lower mortality rate (7% vs 20%). Both groups used peripheral IVs for the initiation of vasoactive medications until central lines could be placed.[33] The other study did not show a difference in mortality, but children in the epinephrine group had faster resolution of shock and less organ dysfunction than those receiving dopamine.[34] In response to this study and other data, the newest ACCM guidelines recommend epinephrine as first-line treatment for cold fluid-refractory shock, with dopamine use (5–10 µg/kg/min) reserved for when epinephrine is unavailable.[8]

Warm shock is seen much less commonly in children than adults (for whom warm shock predominates). For children in warm shock, norepinephrine is recommended as first-line therapy. Dopamine may be used if norepinephrine is unavailable, and generally requires higher doses than in cold shock (10–20 µg/kg/min). In adults with septic shock, vasopressin levels are frequently low and this finding is thought to contribute to vasodilation. This state has not been found consistently in children, and trials of vasopressin for shock have failed to show benefit.[35] However, vasopressin remains available as an adjunctive therapy for refractory vasodilatory shock not responsive to norepinephrine.

Intubation

Airway management and ventilatory support is often necessary in children in shock. Often underrecognized, intubation of a child in shock may be indicated for hemodynamic instability alone. A significant portion of a child's oxygen consumption (up to 40%) goes into the work of breathing. Support with mechanical ventilation can reduce this oxygen consumption and divert critical cardiac output to vital organs. Care must be taken to fluid resuscitate (and sometimes even start on peripheral vasoactive medication) as best as possible before intubation because initiation of positive-pressure ventilation will decrease venous return and exacerbate hypotension. In a child with decreased cardiac function, the increased intrathoracic pressure associated with mechanical ventilation will afterload reduce the left ventricle and improve cardiac output.

Consider the etiology of shock when choosing intubation medications. Although etomidate has been shown to facilitate endotracheal intubation in infants and children with minimal hemodynamic effect, it is not recommended for use in patients with suspected sepsis owing to its adrenal-suppressive effects. In children and adults with septic shock, use of etomidate is associated with increased mortality.[36,37] Ketamine has a favorable hemodynamic profile, but without the adrenal suppression, and is the recommended choice for children in septic shock. For shock without sepsis, such as in trauma, the choice of either medication is reasonable.

Antibiotics

When sepsis is suspected, administer broad-spectrum antibiotics within the first hour of presentation. In a study examining adult patients with sepsis, each hour of delay in antibiotic administration was associated with a mean decrease in survival of 7.6%.[38] If possible, obtain cultures to identify the source of infection before antibiotic delivery. Antibiotics should not be delayed if there is difficulty obtaining specimens. Factors such as local antibiotic resistance patterns, recent antibiotic use, existing immunosuppression, drug allergies, and suspected source of infection may influence what antibiotic is chosen.

Steroids

If shock persists despite escalating vasoactive medication doses (catecholamine-resistant shock), consider the adjunctive use of stress-dose corticosteroids. Patients with known or suspected adrenal insufficiency (ie, steroid use within the last 6 months, known pituitary or adrenal abnormalities, or sepsis with purpura fulminans) should receive stress-dose hydrocortisone as soon as possible after shock is identified. Evidence for the use of steroids in pediatric shock is limited and demonstrates conflicting results. In 1 study, children with sepsis who received corticosteroids had no improvement in mortality, days of vasoactive infusion, or hospital duration of stay.[39] A recent metaanalysis showed no difference in mortality rates between those who did and did not receive steroids.[40] For catecholamine-resistant shock, hydrocortisone dosing of 50 to 100 mg/m^2/d or 2 to 4 mg/kg/d is generally used, although some investigators advocate for doses as high as 50 mg/kg/d in refractory shock.[8] Ideally, a baseline cortisol level should be drawn before hydrocortisone dosing.

RESUSCITATION ENDPOINTS

Reversal of shock depends on the reestablishment of sufficient oxygen delivery to the body. The Surviving Sepsis Campaign identifies these therapeutic endpoints for resuscitation of pediatric shock: restoration of a CRT of less than 2 seconds, normal blood pressure for age, normal pulses, warm extremities, normal urine output, and normal mental status.

Goal-Directed Therapy

In addition to clinical resuscitation endpoints, the Surviving Sepsis Campaign and ACCM recommend that resuscitation of children in septic shock should target a mixed venous saturation (SvO$_2$) of 70% or greater, a perfusion pressure (mean arterial pressure – central venous pressure) of 55 + 1.5 × age in years, and cardiac index between 3.3 and 6.0 L/min/m^2. Low cardiac output is associated with increased mortality in children with septic shock; a cardiac index between 3.3 and 6.0 is associated with the best outcomes in pediatric septic shock patients compared with patients without shock for whom a cardiac index above 2.0 L/min/m^2 is sufficient. Cardiac output measurement can be measured invasively or noninvasively with a variety of devices. Additionally, to maximize oxygen and glucose delivery to help reverse

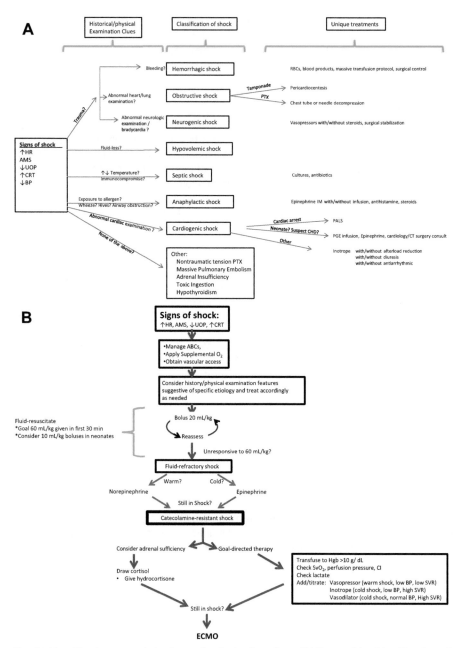

Fig. 1. Algorithmic approach to the pediatric shock patient. (A) Recognition/classification of pediatric shock. (B) Treatment of pediatric shock. For all patients, (1) Manage ABC's. (2) Apply supplemental O2 & obtain vascular access. (3) Use history/physical exam +/- POCUS to classify shock and guide treatment. (4) Frequently reassess response to treatment. (5) Clinical goals = normalization of heart rate, mental status, perfusion, blood pressure, urine output. Signs of shock: ↑HR = tachycardia; ↓UOP = decreased urine output; ↑CRT = delayed capillary refill time; ↓BP = hypotension; ABCs, airway, breathing, circulation; AMS, altered mental status; BP, blood pressure; CHD, congenital heart disease; CI, cardiac index; CT, computed

shock, the ACCM recommends transfusion to a hemoglobin concentration of greater than 10 g/dL and the administration of maintenance fluids containing D10 (D10 normal saline or D10 ½ normal saline).[8,41] In the Surviving Sepsis Campaign's nonpediatric recommendations, a lactate concentration 4 mmol/L or greater is identified as a key marker of tissue hypoperfusion, and normalization of lactate is a key resuscitation goal. Several pediatric studies have shown that increased lactate levels and failure to clear lactate correlate with mortality and organ dysfunction.[42,43] Lactate clearance, however, was notably excluded from the pediatric guidelines as a resuscitation endpoint based on the observation that many children in shock have normal lactate levels as well as the fact that lactate may be increased for many reasons other than cellular hypoxia.[8]

Targeted resuscitation has its foundation in the classic Rivers' early goal-directed therapy (EGDT) trial, which showed a significant mortality benefit when specific resuscitation goals were used in the ED management of adults with septic shock.[44] A pediatric trial of EGDT found significant mortality reduction and decreased organ dysfunction when resuscitation was titrated using SvO_2 goals.[45] However, EGDT (particularly the requirement for invasive CVP measurement and continuous SvO_2 monitoring) has lost some support after 3 recent large methodologically robust trials in adults with septic shock comparing EGDT with usual care showed no benefit in either mortality or secondary clinical and economic outcomes.[46]

Resuscitation to specific EGDT goals may eventually go by the wayside in pediatric algorithms, but for now the ACCM continues to advocate for the titration of therapies to SVO_2, perfusion pressure, and cardiac index goals. In the initial ED management, if invasive monitoring is not used, then usual care must mean vigilant, attentive care. Early recognition with prompt delivery of IV fluids and antibiotics and frequent reassessment is critical. Consider trending lactate levels and using noninvasive methods such as POCUS to assess the adequacy of resuscitation.

PUTTING IT ALL TOGETHER

When a child presents to the ED with tachycardia and signs/symptoms of shock, the most immediate concern should be stabilization of the airway, breathing, and circulation, followed by a rapid assessment of historical clues, physical examination findings, and laboratory studies that may aid classification and help to guide treatment. Refer to **Fig. 1** for an algorithmic approach to pediatric shock management. Some types of shock require specific therapies. Most shock requires some degree of fluid resuscitation, but be cautious if there is concern for a cardiogenic etiology. If shock remains refractory to fluids, add inotropes and/or vasopressors. If catecholamine-resistant shock occurs, advanced hemodynamic monitoring may be required to help to titrate therapies. Consider hydrocortisone supplementation. At multiple points along the way, POCUS may assist diagnosis and help to guide therapies including assessment of preload, fluid responsiveness, and cardiac function. At each step, reassess for response to treatment.

---

tomography; ECMO, extracorporeal membrane oxygenation; Hgb, hemoglobin concentration; IM, intramuscular; PALS, pediatric advanced life support guidelines; PGE, prostaglandin E infusion; POCUS, point of care ultrasound examination (used to help diagnose reasons for shock and assess volume responsiveness and cardiac function); PTX, tension pneumothorax; RBCs, red blood cells; SvO_2, venous oxygen saturation; SVR, systemic vascular resistance.

SUMMARY

Shock is an unstable pathophysiologic state of inadequate tissue perfusion that must be identified and treated promptly. Failure to recognize and reverse shock can have catastrophic results. In the ED, initial therapies should be titrated to normalize vital signs and physical examination abnormalities. If initial resuscitation with fluids and vasoactive medications do not reverse the shock state, advanced hemodynamic monitoring may be required to guide treatment (goal-directed therapy). Early recognition and resuscitation can improve mortality and outcomes for pediatric shock patients.

REFERENCES

1. Sinha R, Nadel S, Kisson N, et al. Recognition and initial management of shock. In: Nichols DG, Shaffner DH, editors. Rogers' textbook of pediatric intensive care. 5th edition. Philadelphia: Wolters Kluwer; 2016. p. 380–93.
2. King CK, Glass R, Bresee JS, et al, Centers for Disease Control and Prevention. Managing acute gastroenteritis among children: oral rehydration, maintenance, and nutritional therapy. MMWR Recomm Rep 2003;52(RR16):1–16.
3. Kannan N, Wang J, Mink RB, et al. Timely hemodynamic resuscitation and outcomes in severe pediatric traumatic brain injury: preliminary findings. Pediatr Emerg Care 2016. [Epub ahead of print].
4. Topjian AA, French B, Sutton RM, et al. Early postresuscitation hypotension is associated with increased mortality after pediatric cardiac arrest. Crit Care Med 2014;42(6):1518–23.
5. Kleinman ME, Chameides L, Schexnayder SM, et al. Part 14: pediatric advanced life support: 2010 American Heart Association guidelines for cardiopulmonary resuscitation and emergency cardiovascular care. Circulation 2010; 122:S876–908.
6. Bellemare S, Hartling L, Wiebe N, et al. Oral rehydration versus intravenous therapy for treating dehydration due to gastroenteritis in children: a meta-analysis of randomised controlled trials. BMC Med 2004;2:11.
7. Watson RS, Carcillo JA, Linde-Zwirble WT, et al. The epidemiology of severe sepsis in children in the United States. Am J Respir Crit Care Med 2003;167: 695–701.
8. Davis AL, Carcillo JA, Aneja RK, et al. American College of Critical Care Medicine clinical practice parameters for hemodynamic support of pediatric and neonatal septic shock. Crit Care Med 2017;45:1061–93.
9. Nohria A, Tsang SW, Fang JC, et al. Clinical assessment identifies hemodynamic profiles that predict outcomes in patients admitted with heart failure. J Am Coll Cardiol 2003;41:1797–804.
10. Brissaud O, Botte A, Cambonie G, et al. Experts' recommendations for the management of cardiogenic shock in children. Ann Intensive Care 2016;6:14.
11. Fleming S, Thomson M, Stevens R, et al. Normal ranges of heart rate and respiratory rate in children from birth to 18 years of age: a systematic review of observational studies. Lancet 2011;377:1011.
12. Fleming S, Gill P, Jones C, et al. The diagnostic value of capillary refill time for detecting serious illness in children: a systematic review and meta-analysis. PLoS One 2015;10(9):e0138155.
13. Carcillo JA. Capillary refill time is a very useful clinical sign in early recognition and treatment of very sick children. Pediatr Crit Care Med 2012;13(2):211–2.

14. Scott HF, Donoghue AJ, Gaieski DF, et al. Effectiveness of physical exam signs for early detection of critical illness in pediatric systemic inflammatory response syndrome. BMC Emerg Med 2014;14:24.

15. Marin JR, Abo AM, Arroyo AC, et al. Pediatric emergency medicine point-of-care ultrasound: summary of the evidence. Crit Ultrasound J 2016;8:16.

16. Sola JE, Cheung MC, Yang R, et al. Pediatric FAST and elevated liver transaminases: an effective screening tool in blunt abdominal trauma. J Surg Res 2009; 157(1):103–7.

17. Chen L, Kim Y, Stantucci KA. Use of ultrasound measurement of the inferior vena cava diameter as an objective tool in the assessment of children with clinical dehydration. Acad Emerg Med 2007;14:841–5.

18. Chen L, Hsiao A, Langhan M, et al. Use of bedside ultrasound to assess degree of dehydration in children with gastroenteritis. Acad Emerg Med 2010;17:1042–7.

19. Levine AC, Shah SP, Umulisa I, et al. Ultrasound assessment of severe dehydration in children with diarrhea and vomiting. Acad Emerg Med 2010;17:1035–41.

20. Perera P, Mailhot T, Riley D, et al. The RUSH exam: rapid ultrasound in shock in the evaluation of the critically ill. Emerg Med Clin North Am 2010;28(1):29–56.

21. Labovitz AJ, Noble VE, Bierig M, et al. Focused cardiac ultrasound in the emergent setting: a consensus statement of the American Society of Echocardiography and American College of Emergency Physicians. J Am Soc Echocardiogr 2010;23(12):1225–30.

22. Atkinson PR, McAuley DJ, Kendall RJ, et al. Abdominal and cardiac evaluation with sonography in shock (ACES): an approach by emergency physicians for the use of ultrasound in patients with undifferentiated hypotension. Emerg Med J 2009;26(2):87–91.

23. Shokoohi H, Boniface KS, Pourmand A, et al. Bedside ultrasound reduces diagnostic uncertainty and guides resuscitation in patients with undifferentiated hypotension. Crit Care Med 2015;34(12):2562–9.

24. Kanji HD, McCallum J, Sirounis D, et al. Limited echocardiography-guided therapy in sub-acute shock is associated with change in management and improved outcomes. J Crit Care 2014;29(5):700–5.

25. Medeiros DN, Ferranti JF, Delgado AF, et al. Colloids for the initial management of severe sepsis and septic shock in pediatric patients: a systematic review. Pediatr Emerg Care 2015;31(11):e11–16.

26. Maitland K, Kiguli S, Opoka RO, et al. Mortality after fluid bolus in African children with severe infection. N Engl J Med 2011;364:2483–95.

27. de Caen AR, Berg MD, Chameides L, et al. Part 12: pediatric advanced life support: 2015 American Heart Association guidelines update for cardiopulmonary resuscitation and advanced emergency cardiovascular care. Circulation 2015; 132:S526–42.

28. Stoner MJ, Goodman DG, Cohen DM, et al. Rapid fluid resuscitation in pediatrics: testing the American College of Critical Care Medicine guideline. Ann Emerg Med 2007;50(5):601–7.

29. Patregnani JT, Sochet AA, Klugman D. Short-term peripheral vasoactive infusions in pediatrics: where is the harm? Pediatr Crit Care Med 2017;18(8):e378–81.

30. Cardenas-Garcia J, Schaub KF, Belchikov YG, et al. Safety of peripheral intravenous administration of vasoactive medication. J Hosp Med 2015;10(9):581–5.

31. Turner DA, Kleinman ME. The use of vasoactive agents via peripheral intravenous access during the transport of critically ill infants and children. Pediatr Emerg Care 2010;26(8):563–6.

32. De Backer D, Biston P, Devriendt J, et al, SOAP II Investigators. Comparison of dopamine and norepinephrine in the treatment of shock. N Engl J Med 2010; 362:779–89.
33. Ventura AM, Shieh HH, Bousso A, et al. Double-blind prospective randomized controlled trial of dopamine versus epinephrine as first-line vasoactive drugs in pediatric septic shock. Crit Care Med 2015;43:2292–302.
34. Ramaswamy KN, Singhi S, Jayashree M, et al. Double-blind randomized clinical trial comparing dopamine and epinephrine in pediatric fluid-refractory hypotensive septic shock. Pediatr Crit Care Med 2016;17:e502–512.
35. Choong K, Bohn D, Fraser DD, et al, Canadian Critical Care Trials Group. Vasopressin in pediatric vasodilatory shock: a multicenter randomized controlled trial. Am J Respir Crit Care Med 2009;180:632–9.
36. den Brinker M, Hokken-Koelega AC, Hazelzet JA, et al. One single dose of etomidate negatively influences adrenocortical performance for at least 24h in children with meningococcal sepsis. Intensive Care Med 2008;24(1):163–8.
37. Sprung CL, Annane D, Keh D, et al. Hydrocortisone therapy for patients with septic shock. N Engl J Med 2008;258(2):111–24.
38. Kumar A, Roberts D, Wood KE, et al. Duration of hypotension before initiation of effective antimicrobial therapy is the critical determinant of survival in human septic shock. Crit Care Med 2006;34:1589–96.
39. Zimmerman JJ, Williams MD. Adjunctive corticosteroid therapy in pediatric severe sepsis: observations from the RESOLVE study. Pediatr Crit Care Med 2011;12:2–8.
40. Menon K, McNally D, Choong K, et al. A systematic review and meta-analysis on the effect of steroids in pediatric shock. Pediatr Crit Care Med 2013;14(5): 474–80.
41. Dellinger RP, Levy MM, Rhodes A, et al. Surviving sepsis campaign: International guidelines for management of severe sepsis and septic shock: 2012. Crit Care Med 2013;41:580–637.
42. Choudhary R, Sitaraman S, Choudhary A. Lactate clearance as a predictor of outcome in pediatric septic shock. J Emerg Trauma Shock 2017;10(2):55–9.
43. Scott HF, Brou L, Deakyn SJ, et al. 30-day mortality in clinically suspected sepsis in children. JAMA Pediatr 2017;171(3):249–55.
44. Rivers E, Nguyen B, Havstad S, et al. Early goal-directed therapy in the treatment of severe sepsis and septic shock. N Engl J Med 2001;345:1368–77.
45. deOliveira CF, deOliveira DS, Gottschald AF, et al. ACCM/PALS haemodynamic support guidelines for paediatric septic shock: an outcomes comparison with and without monitoring central venous oxygen saturation. Intensive Care Med 2008;34:1065–75.
46. The PRISM Investigators. Early, goal-directed therapy for septic shock—a patient-level meta-analysis. N Engl J Med 2017;376:2223–34.

Emergency Care of Pediatric Burns

Ashley M. Strobel, MD[a],*, Ryan Fey, MD[b]

KEYWORDS

- Burn • Inhalation injury • Resuscitation • Total body surface area • Abuse
- Emergency • Scald

KEY POINTS

- The emergency department fundamentals of pediatric burn resuscitation are early airway management, accurately calculating the total body surface area (TBSA) involved, fluid resuscitation, evaluating the patient for concomitant trauma or toxicity, and appropriate disposition.
- Airway management should be considered in younger children (<2 years old) with larger (>20% TBSA) scald injuries, as well as in children with flame or inhalational injury.
- Intravenous fluid resuscitation should be initiated for children with greater than or equal to 15% TBSA affected by partial-thickness or full-thickness burn within 2 hours of injury.
- Risk factors for mortality in burned children are a larger TBSA, inhalation injury, multiorgan failure, age less than 4 years old, and nonaccidental burn.

In the United States, injuries continue to be the leading cause of death among children. Of these deaths, 0.7% are caused by fire or burns, which is similar in prevalence to deaths from poisoning.[1,2] From the 1970s to the 2000s, the reported number of burn-related injuries trended downward 30% to 50%.[2–4]

Approximately 90% of pediatric burns occur at home,[2–8] whereas adolescents are about 3 times more likely to get burned outside the home.[3] The type of burn injury is related to the child's age and developmental stage.[2] Toddlers and preschool children sustain majority of scalds, intraoral burns, and electrical injuries.[5,6,8–21] Boys are burned more often than girls.[2,3,5–13,17–20,22–25] Scalds are more common in younger children and flame burns are more common in older children.[8,13,22]

The overall mortality rate is 0.4% to 2.8% among burned children.[8,16,22,23,26,27] Death is very rare in children who have been scalded; however, mortality increases

Neither A. Strobel nor R. Fey has any financial disclosures.

[a] Department of Emergency Medicine, University of Minnesota School of Medicine, Hennepin County Medical Center, University of Minnesota Masonic Children's Hospital, 701 South Park Avenue R2.123, Minneapolis, MN 55414, USA; [b] Department of Surgery, University of Minnesota School of Medicine, Hennepin County Medical Center, 701 South Park Avenue, Minneapolis, MN 55414, USA
* Corresponding author.
E-mail address: Ashley.strobel@gmail.com

Emerg Med Clin N Am 36 (2018) 441–458
https://doi.org/10.1016/j.emc.2017.12.011   emed.theclinics.com
0733-8627/18/© 2017 Elsevier Inc. All rights reserved.

significantly in cases of pediatric abuse, possibly because of concomitant injuries.[25,28] Fire and flame-induced burns account for most of the fatalities.[2,23] Larger total body surface area (TBSA) burns tend to be due to injuries related to exposure to flames.[23,29] Multiorgan failure increases mortality, with 3 failed organs being nearly universally fatal[30] (**Box 1**). Despite these mortality risk factors, long-term outcomes are optimistic provided the child has access to multidisciplinary specialty care.[31,32]

DEPTH OF THE BURN

Burns are categorized as superficial (first degree), partial-thickness (second degree), full-thickness (third degree), or those involving deeper tissues or structures (fourth degree) (**Table 1**). Most of the burns in children are classified as partial-thickness.[2,9] A burn may have multiple-thickness components, with the deepest part of the burn typically in the center. The burn depth is proportional to the source temperature, consistency, and duration of contact. Thicker, sticky substances (eg, noodles, oatmeal) stay in contact with the skin longer, causing deeper burns. The depth of the burn might evolve and deepen in the first 24 to 48 hours and requires reevaluation.

TYPES OF BURNS
Scalds

In 1977, tap water scald burns constituted half of scald burns.[33] Recommended bath water temperature is 37.8°C; however, 80% of homes tested in Seattle had unsafe hot water temperature (>54°C). For children less than 6 years old, full-thickness epidermal burns can occur within 60 seconds of exposure to water higher than 53°C and within 1 second if the water is hotter than 70°C.[2,33] Standards changed such that new hot water heaters have a maximum temperature preset of 49°C.[34] Currently, hot beverages are the most common cause of scalds.[3,5,7,8,13,16,19,35] In younger children, a bib pattern distribution is sustained when the child pulls a container of hot liquid down from a higher surface (**Fig. 1**).[14]

Contact Burns

Contact with hot surfaces is another common cause of burns among children, especially those younger than 5 years old. Contact burns are often on the upper extremity, specifically the hand.[20] Common sources of contact burns are glass-front fireplaces, oven doors, hair iron products, and irons.[9,20]

Box 1
Factors that increase mortality risk in burned children

- Presence of inhalation injury
- Larger TBSA burned (≥60% signifies a poor prognosis)
- Age less than 4 years
- Burn injury caused by nonaccidental trauma
- Multiorgan failure (especially liver and renal)
- Emerging multidrug-resistant organism sepsis

Data from Refs.[4,8,16,22,23,28,30]

Table 1
Burn depth classification and documentation with prognosis to aid in patient education

Classification	Depth	Examination Description	Healing Time	Risk for Scar	Pain Control	Wound Care
Superficial (1st degree)[a]	Epidermis	• Erythematous • No blister • Painful	4–5 d	None	• Ibuprofen • Acetaminophen	• Aloe vera • Emollient moisturizers
Superficial partial-thickness (2nd degree)	Epidermis and dermis	• Pink, moist, blanching with intact capillary refill • Blister • Painful when blister deroofed and open to air	7–10 d	• Minimal • Dark-skinned individuals may lose melanin and be hypopigmented during healing	• Narcotic 30 min before dressing change	• Soap and water twice daily dressing change with bacitracin or petroleum jelly and non-adherent gauze • Commercial long-term dressings Mepilex Ag (Molnlycke, Norcross, GA, USA) or Aquacel Ag (ConvaTec, Princeton, NJ, USA) • SSD has fallen out of favor because it has more adverse effects (ie, sulfa allergy, kernicterus in neonates, anemia G-6-PD) without proof of superiority
Deep partial-thickness (2nd degree) and indeterminate-thickness	Deeper dermis	• Erythematous or yellow, nonblanching • Dry to waxy • Blister easily unroofs • Possibly not painful if nerve fibers involved. • Presence of hair follicles. • Capillary burst with red punctum of bleeding at times	2–3 wk	Probable	• Narcotics 30 min before dressing changes • Acetaminophen • Ibuprofen	• Acticoat (Smith & Nephew, Canada) • Surgical consultation for early excision and grafting of indeterminate-thickness and full-thickness burns decreases infection, cost, and mortality rates • Physical therapy and occupational therapy
Full-thickness (3rd degree)	Dermis	• White, waxy, and leathery • Lack hair follicles • Insensate	Weeks	Definite	—	Surgical consultation for early excision and grafting.
4th degree	Subcutaneous tissues into the fascia, muscle, tendon, bone	• Deep structures visualized	Months	Definite	• Narcotics • Ibuprofen • Acetaminophen	Surgical consultation

Abbreviations: bid, twice a day; G-6-PD, glucose-6-phosephate deficiency; SSD, silver sulfadiazine.
[a] Not included in TBSA estimation.

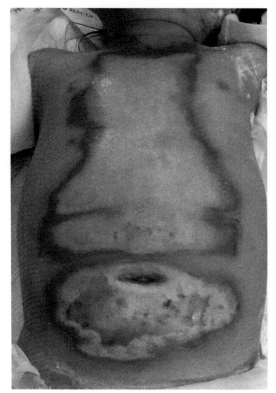

Fig. 1. After emergency department (ED) debridement, a 12% TBSA bib pattern scald burn from a onesie on a toddler. Note the deeper (*yellow*) full-thickness burn in the center, a middle (*white*) deep partial-thickness burn, and an outer (*red*) superficial partial-thickness burn.

Electrical Burns

Most household exposures are low-voltage and alternating current from exposed wiring, putting objects in outlets, or biting on cords (**Fig. 2**).[6] The leading causes of death from electrical injury are cardiac or respiratory arrest. Patients with high-voltage or lightning injury should also be evaluated for cardiac injury, rhabdomyolysis, and renal failure.

Oral electrical injuries, typically from biting an electrical cord, are a unique entity and require a surgical evaluation because the burn is often full-thickness. Eschars should not be debrided because the circumoral artery can become exposed and bleed. Hemorrhage most commonly occurs 10 days after the burn. The parents should be advised to keep the area moist with an agent such as petroleum jelly. Education on achieve hemostasis by applying direct digital pressure (eg, pinching the lip just below the commissure) should be given to families.[36,37]

Chemical Burns

The most common agents causing chemical burn are oven cleaners, aerosols, drain cleaners, bleach, acetone, strong acids, hair dye, airbags, laxatives, and concrete.[38] Exposures in toddlers tend to occur in the home.[38] Exposures in teenage can be related to suicide attempts.[38] Most chemical burns were found to involve less than or equal to 2% TBSA; however, 16% required skin grafting.[38]

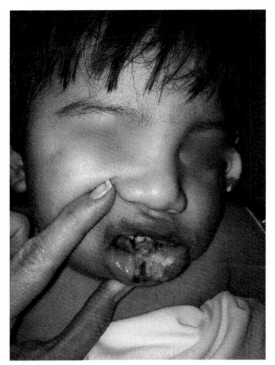

Fig. 2. A toddler with a lip full-thickness burn after biting an electrical cord. The electrocardiogram was normal. Burn consultation was obtained in the ED, and this family went home with good anticipatory guidance once pain control and the child's ability to tolerate oral fluids were achieved.

Treadmill Friction Burns

Treadmill friction burns often cause full-thickness injury, and many required skin grafting.[21] A child's slow withdrawal reflex and thin volar epidermis are likely why this injury pattern is most common on the hands of toddlers.[21]

INITIAL CARE

The goal of initial first aid is to reduce pain, minimize the extent of the burn, and not to interfere with advanced care evaluation and management. Prehospital first aid is often inadequate; only 13% to 20% of children receive analgesia.[4,5,14,35,38,39] Pain control should not be withheld and can be achieved with a variety of medications and routes (**Box 2**). Simply covering the burn with wet gauze may also reduce pain. If available, a petroleum-based dressing, nonadherent gauze, or cling film can be used as a nonadherent dressing.[40]

Following the mantra to "cool the burn and warm the patient" is essential to avoid hypothermia. Clothing should be removed to stop continued thermal exposure. The wound should be rinsed under lukewarm water (2°–15°C) for 20 minutes or until pain is relieved.[35,40] Ice can worsen the damage and cause hypothermia, thus it should not be used. Similarly, heavy creams and ointments should be avoided because they interfere with evaluation of the burn. The use of oils or honey has not been shown to reduce scarring, and may be a hindrance.[35]

Box 2
Dosing for pain medication commonly used in pediatric burn care

- Acetaminophen
  - Orally (PO) or rectally: 15 mg/kg every 4 to 6 hours (max dose 1000 mg)
- Ibuprofen
  - Orally: 10 mg/kg every 6 to 8 hours (max dose 800 mg)
- Ketorolac
  - Intramuscular (IM): 1 mg/kg (max dose 30 mg)
  - Intravenous (IV): 0.5 mg/kg (max dose 15 mg)
- Diphenhydramine
  - Orally, IM, IV: 1.25 mg/kg every 6 hours (max dose 50 mg)
- Hydroxyzine
  - Orally: 0.5 mg/kg every 6 hours (max dose 25 mg)
- Oxycodone
  - Orally: 0.1 mg/kg orally every 4 to 6 hours
- Fentanyl
  - IN or Intranasal: 2 μg/kg
  - IV or intraosseous (IO): 1 to 4 μg/kg
- Morphine
  - IM, IV, or IO: 0.1 mg/kg
- Ketamine
  - IM: 4 mg/kg
  - IV or IO: 1 to 2 mg/kg
- Propofol
  - IV or IO: 1 mg/kg

Codeine-containing analgesics should be avoided in pediatric pain management.
From Tobias JD, Green TP, Cote CJ. Codeine: time to say "no". Pediatrics 2016;138:e1–7; with permission.

Most burned children receive initial care and stabilization away from a burn center due to regional variation in availability.[41] Critically burned children, especially those with larger TBSA and full-thickness burns, should be referred and admitted to an American Burn Association center because survival may be improved.[16,23,27,42]

Indications for pediatric burn referral to an American Burn Association center can be found at http://ameriburn.org/public-resources/burn-center-referral-criteria/. Referral includes both outpatient and inpatient burn center evaluation. Children with partial-thickness burns <10% TBSA can often be managed in the outpatient setting if resources are available and the family is reliable.

RESUSCITATION

The goal of resuscitation is to maximize perfusion and oxygenation to tissues to promote healing, minimize wound conversion, decrease bacterial colonization, and prepare the tissue for early excision and grafting. The fundamentals of burn resuscitation are managing the airway, accurately calculating TBSA, hemodynamic stabilization, evaluating the patient for concomitant trauma or toxicity, and appropriate disposition.

AIRWAY

The airway should be secured if the patient exhibits any of the following conditions: hoarseness, stridor, drooling, respiratory distress, or altered mental status. Fear of unnecessary intubation should not cause hesitation for emergency care providers when deciding to secure the airway.[43] There is no adequate evidence to determine who does or does not require endotracheal intubation after smoke exposure. When in doubt about the presence or absence of inhalation injury, nasopharyngoscopy can be used to directly visualize the upper airway; however, edema might not be clinically apparent for up to 48 hours.

The upper airway dissipates heat; therefore, supraglottic edema is caused by direct thermal injury, whereas tracheal edema and subsequent respiratory failure is secondary to damage as a consequence of inhaled smoke, chemicals, or toxins. Children have smaller diameter airways, so even a small amount of edema induced by an inflammatory or inhalational mechanism can cause exponential airway narrowing compared with adults with respiratory impairment (**Fig. 3**).[44] Early intubation is imperative before edema narrows the upper airway, so the physician should err on the side of caution. Early airway management should also be considered in younger children (<2 years old) with larger (>20% TBSA) scald injuries.[45,46] Although scalds rarely require intubation (including scalds on the face), administration of large volumes for fluid resuscitation could lead to respiratory failure or acute respiratory distress syndrome.

Although inhalation injury is uncommon, with an incidence of 4.5% in burned children younger than 12 years of age,[28] it is associated with a 3 times higher risk for

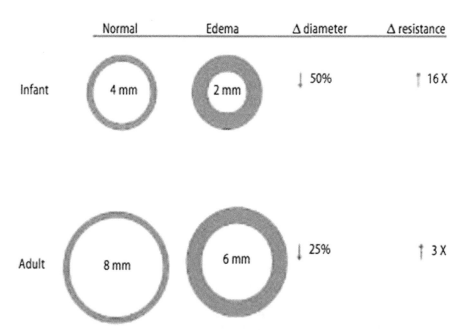

Fig. 3. Age-dependent effects of reduction in airway caliber on airway resistance and air flow to demonstrate the effect of airway edema, secondary to inhalation injury, on the respiratory mechanics in children compared with adults. A millimeter of circumferential edema will reduce the diameter of the airway by 2 mm, resulting in a 16-fold increase in airway resistance for the pediatric airway versus a 3-fold increase for the adult airway. It is even possible the resistance will increase by 32-fold when a child is crying in the resuscitation room. (*From* Wheeler DS, Spaeth JP, Mehta R, et al. Assessment and management of the pediatric airway. In: Wheeler DS, Wong HR, Shanley TP, editors. Resuscitation and stabilization of the critically ill child. New York: Springer; 2008. p. 224; with permission.)

death.[23] Acute inhalational lung injury is due to a combination of direct mucosal injury from particulate debris and a secondary inflammatory cascade.[30,47] Inhaled particulate debris cause local mucosal hyperemia, increasing microvascular permeability, exfoliating the epithelial lining, and increasing mucous secretion. A cascade of inflammatory mediators leads to airway obstruction 24 to 72 hours after injury.[48] Early use (within 2–4 hours) of an inhaled anticoagulant (eg, tissue plasminogen activator, heparin) may prevent some of this obstructive fibrin formation.[47,48] Beta-agonists have been used; however, large trials assessing their efficacy are lacking.[49]

If the child was involved in a fire in an enclosed space or a house fire, additional concerns involving oxygenation and ventilation include consideration for possible carbon monoxide and cyanide poisoning should be considered. Appropriate therapy (ie, hyperoxygenation and hydroxycobalamin) may be required empirically.[50]

TOTAL BODY SURFACE AREA CALCULATION

Accurate calculation of the TBSA is fundamental to guide resuscitation, prognosis, and disposition. Large TBSA involvement correlates with increased mortality, surgeries, and infection risk. Most pediatric burns affect less than 10% of the TBSA.[15,24,39,51,52] Overestimation is common, especially when evaluating the TBSA of smaller (<20%) noncontiguous burns and leads to excessive intravenous (IV) fluid resuscitation.[39,53–56]

A simple, quick, reproducible method that does not interfere with resuscitation is essential for calculation of the TBSA affected. A relatively accurate method for TBSA calculation in pediatric patients is to use the patient's hand (palm plus the adducted fingers) as an estimation of 1% of the TBSA.[57,58] The Lund and Browder chart (**Fig. 4**) is most accurate; however, it is cumbersome to use in the emergency department while leading a resuscitation.[59–61] The Wallace rule of nines requires modification for children to account for their disproportionately large head and smaller legs. Because the rule of nines can overestimate pediatric burns, it is not recommended for pediatric TBSA calculations. Three-dimensional photography is an emerging modality and telemedicine may help with TBSA estimation, fluid resuscitation, and disposition.[36,62–64]

Regardless of the method used to estimate the TBSA, calculations should only include partial-thickness and full-thickness burns.

FLUIDS

A massive hypermetabolic response occurs in children after burn injury and affects all organs. Cytokines are elevated and a release of inflammatory mediators (eg, interleukin-6, C-reactive protein, and tumor necrosis factor-α) contributes to multiorgan failure.[23,30,65] Major fluid loss from increased capillary permeability and loss of evaporative protection from the skin require fluid resuscitation aimed to restore microvascular cellular perfusion and hemodynamic stability.

Until 1952, inadequate IV fluids were recommended for burned children.[66] Currently, fluid resuscitation calculations are based on formulas (**Box 3**) that account for the child's weight and the percent of TBSA burned; however, none is considered a gold standard. Therefore, burn centers differ regarding resuscitation parameters, so it is imperative to communicate with the burn center.[29,67] Securing IV, and other devices, can be challenging in burn victims; however, various modalities can be used for effective securement, including staples, sutures, and specialized adhesive foam dressing such as Mepilex Ag (Mölnlycke, Norcross, Georgia, USA).[69]

Lund and Browder Charts for area of body burnt

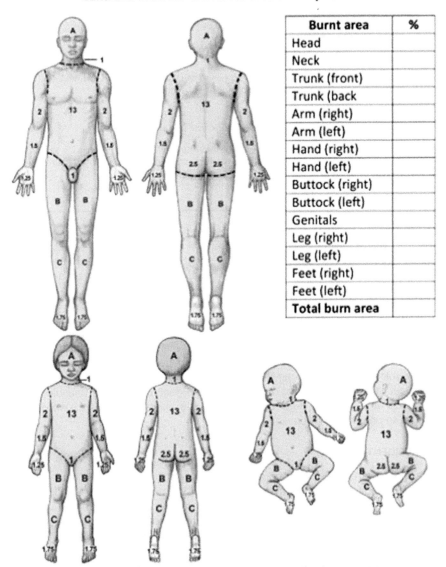

Burnt area	%
Head	
Neck	
Trunk (front)	
Trunk (back	
Arm (right)	
Arm (left)	
Hand (right)	
Hand (left)	
Buttock (right)	
Buttock (left)	
Genitals	
Leg (right)	
Leg (left)	
Feet (right)	
Feet (left)	
Total burn area	

Age (years)	Under 1	2–4	5–9	10–14	15	Adult
A — ½ of head	9½	8½	6½	5½	4½	3½
B — ½ of one thigh	2¾	3¼	4	4½	4½	4¾
C — ½ of one leg	2½	2½	2¾	3	3¼	3

Fig. 4. Lund and Browder chart. (*From* the American Burn Association; and *Reprinted from* the Journal of the American College of Surgeons, formerly Surgery Gynecology & Obstetrics, with permission; and Nagel TR, Schunk JE. Using the hand to estimate the surface area of a burn in children. Pediatr Emerg Care 1997;13:254–5.)

Box 3
Formulas for fluid resuscitation after total body surface area calculation

(1500 mL × body surface area [BSA]) + (35 + %TBSA) × (BSA × 2) = 24-hour fluid and goal urine output 1 to 2 mL/kg/h

The Galveston formula:

5000 mL/m^2 TBSA/24 h + 2000 mL/m^2 TBSA/24 h of D5LR with 12.5 g albumin/L with half given in the first 8 hours and half during the subsequent 16 hours

The Parkland formula:

4 mL/kg × weight in kg × %TBSA = 24-hour crystalloid requirements

For young children weighing less than 30 kg, maintenance fluids containing D5 should be added to resuscitation calculations while enteral feedings are increased to goal to prevent hypoglycemia.
Abbreviations: D5, 5% dextrose; D5LR, lactated ringers with 5% dextrose.
Data from Refs.[65–68]

IV fluid resuscitation should be initiated for children with partial-thickness or full-thickness burns involving greater than or equal to 15% of the TBSA.[68] Fluid resuscitation can be started with lactated Ringer solution or normal saline as a 20 mL/kg crystalloid bolus. For children younger than 5 years old, maintenance fluids containing dextrose should be added to the determined resuscitation fluid volume. There is no strong evidence to support any resuscitation fluid versus another.[67,68,70]

The paradigm of fluid resuscitation for burned children has shifted from an absolute volume determined by the Parkland formula to a dynamic process involving frequent reassessment of the patient's hemodynamic parameters. Current practice is to titrate the fluid volume according to the individual's urine output (goal of 0.5–1 mL/kg/h) combined with other hemodynamic monitoring.[70] The goal of titration is to avoid overresuscitation and edema, both of which lead to multiorgan failure, while being cautious to prevent underresuscitation.[67,68,70–72]

NONACCIDENTAL BURNS

Nonaccidental trauma is an important consideration to help prevent future injury or death (**Box 4**). It is estimated that up to 20% of burn injuries are the result of child abuse or neglect, with highest incidence among young children (0–4 years of age).[22,26,28,73–78] The likelihood of death is 4 times greater among those with suspected abuse.[22,26,28,77] The anatomic location of the injury is affecting unreliable in differentiating nonaccidental and accidental burns; however, burns on both legs convey a 3 times greater likelihood of being abusive injury.[22,26,28,74,76]

Emergency physicians are mandatory reporters and do not need to definitively diagnose abuse but rather to reasonable cause to suspect abuse. Obtaining collateral information from social workers is beneficial because previous child protective services involvement is documented in 15% to 90% of reported nonaccidental burn cases.[19,26,42,73,74] If there is any suspicion of nonaccidental trauma, the child should be admitted so that collateral information can be obtained while the child is safe.

SECONDARY SURVEY

Patients with circumferential partial-thickness or full-thickness burns may require escharotomy due to restrictive compartment syndrome. Extremities with circumferential

---

Box 4
Factors that raise concern for abuse or neglect in burned children

History:

1. Delay in presentation and lack of first aid

2. Inconsistent history with either burn mechanism or developmental stage of the child

3. Presentation for treatment with someone other than the parent

4. Age less than 4 years

5. Lack of parental willingness to participate in follow-up care

Physical examination:

1. Injury not compatible with developmental stage

2. Injury not consistent with history provided

3. Concomitant fractures or bruising

4. Burns appear older than history provided

5. Symmetric distribution

6. Bilateral lower extremity burns

7. Pattern burns (eg, cigarette, iron, stocking and glove, sharp demarcation lines, buttock doughnut–sparing, flexor crease–sparing)

8. Deeper burn or burns requiring skin grafting

Data from Refs.[19,22,26,28,73,74]

---

burns should be assessed frequently for signs of compartment syndrome. It is important that jewelry and clothing be removed to avoid a tourniquet effect.

Completing the 4 Cs of burn care; that is, cooling, clothing, cleaning, and chemoprophylaxis (tetanus immunization status), is necessary and should be done before the child proceeds to disposition.

INFECTION

Prophylactic antibiotics are not indicated and may cause harm by selecting multidrug-resistant organisms.[79,80] Close follow-up and good anticipatory guidance about infectious complications are paramount.[79,80] In the first 48 to 72 hours following a burn, the hypermetabolic phase may lead to fever; however, after 72 hours, a fever should provoke concern for a developing infection. Risk factors for infection are greater than 30% TBSA involvement, flame burns, inhalation injury, and deeper burns.[80,81] Use of optimal topical therapy with burn wound monitoring, aggressive surgical debridement, and nutritional support is the best prophylaxis for burn wound infection.[82] Finally, the patient's tetanus immunization status should be addressed. Those who have not received booster dosing within the past 5 years should do so and those who are unimmunized or under-immunized with less than 3 doses should receive initial dosing along with tetanus immunoglobulin.[80]

NUTRITION

Children are more susceptible to hypoglycemia and serial glucose assessments can prevent unrecognized hypoglycemia. Within 12 to 24 hours after injury, initiation of enteral nutrition is essential to burn care because it alleviates the catabolism of the hypermetabolic response, reduces the risk of gastrointestinal bleeding, and improves outcomes.[83,84]

DEBRIDEMENT

The management of partial-thickness burns is within the purview of emergency medicine. Management of blisters is a source of much controversy in the burn care community because randomized controlled trials are lacking.[85,86] Debridement and further assessment may require procedural sedation, which can be accomplished with several agents (see **Box 2**).[87,88] Loose tissue and blisters can be debrided with coarse gauze, soap, and warm water. There is no added benefit to povidone-iodine solution.[89]

The goals of blister management are to prevent infection, reduce timing to reepithelialization, improve functional and aesthetic outcome, increase patient comfort, provide ease of dressing care, and contain the cost of care.[13] The current trend of burn center protocols is to debride partial-thickness burns and apply a long-term burn dressing, which has shown to reduce costs.[90–95] These silver-impregnated fabric and foam dressings have largely replaced silver sulfadiazine as the initial dressings. They are best suited for superficial partial-thickness burns of less than 10% of the TBSA and can be changed every 3 to 7 days or until reepithelialization of the burn. This often only requires 1 to 2 dressing changes.[96,97] These dressings can be applied to give comfort, protect the wound, and start healing while awaiting follow-up. Specialized dressings also mitigate parental concern about needing to change dressings at home.

DISPOSITION

Training varies among providers so it is important to ensure adequate follow-up with providers familiar in burn care. One outpatient option is an ambulatory burn clinic.[93,96] This outpatient approach, including emergency department sedated burn debridement and dressing, with ambulatory burn clinic referral, is cost-effective for families and hospitals, reduces psychological stress and pain, and improves resource utilization, without sacrificing infection rates or time to wound healing.[10,11,13,15,96] For outpatient burn care to be effective, however, emergency physicians must be skilled in evaluation, initial management, and outpatient anticipatory guidance until follow-up can be achieved. Criteria to consider for inpatient or critical care admission are in **Box 5**.

Box 5	
Disposition decision aid for outpatient, admission, or critical level of care for pediatric burns	
ADMIT	**ICU**
5–10% peds, 10–20% adult	>15% peds, >20% adult
2–5% FT	>5% FT
High voltage injury	Voltage burn (cardiac dysrrhythmia 72 hr post obs until no ST/T wave nonspecific changes)
Suspect inhalation (12–24 hr obs, check COHb >10% → HBO)	Known inhalation
Circumferential PT/FT	Face, eyes, ears, genitalia, joints
PMH predisposes to infection. DM, HbSS, CF, etc	

Box 6
An ounce of prevention is worth a pound of cure

- No irons on the floor and keep curling irons and clothes irons out of reach of children.
- Keep matches out of reach of children.
- Decrease smoking in the home.
- Use childproof lighters and do not remove the safety mechanisms.
- Monitor for exposed wires on cords and keep outlets covered.
- Teach children a home fire evacuation plan.
- Smoke detectors should be in each bedroom, outside each living quarter, and on every floor.
- Keep cooking pots to the back of the stove with the handle turned inward.
- Keep the hot water heater less than 120°F and test bath water before allowing children to enter the bath.
- Never use gasoline to start or enhance a fire.

Remind families about burn prevention, and use this emergency department visit as a teachable moment to prevent future harm.

ANTICIPATORY GUIDANCE

At home, pain control is best accomplished by using a combination of oral acetaminophen and ibuprofen with oxycodone 30 minutes before dressing changes. Parents can be advised that the pain caused by dressing changes can be diminished by performing them in the bathtub. Burns may become pruritic, which is an indication of epithelialization and healing. Diphenhydramine or hydroxyzine can be used to mitigate itch. Newly epithelialized skin is very thin and friable therefore, it bleeds easily when scratched. The healing wound should be moisturized regularly. The scar should be protected from sun for 12 months after the injury with at least sun protection factor 25. Burn prevention strategies should also be discussed (**Box 6**).

SUMMARY

Burns remain a significant source of morbidity and mortality in children. Fortunately, most burns are minor and can often be managed in the primary care setting. Children with major burns require resuscitation and their care should differ only slightly from that for adults, with administration of IV fluid for burns involving greater than or equal to 15% of the TBSA and different admission criteria. The calculation of the TBSA burned is crucial to determine resuscitation parameters, prognosis, and disposition. Risk factors for death should prompt early burn center transfer. Whether a minor burn or a major burn, disposition to multidisciplinary burn specialty care is imperative to excellent psychological and functional outcome for burned children.

ACKNOWLEDGMENTS

This article was copy edited by Linda J. Kesselring, MS, ELS. Special thanks to Rachel Nygaard, PhD, for her assistance preparing this article.

REFERENCES

1. Borse NN, Gilchrist J, Dellinger AM, et al. CDC childhood injury report: patterns of unintentional injuries among 0-19 year olds in the United States,

2000-2006. Atlanta (GA): US Department of Health and Human Services; 2008.

2. Shields BJ, Comstock RD, Fernandez SA, et al. Healthcare resource utilization and epidemiology of pediatric burn-associated hospitalizations, United States, 2000. J Burn Care Res 2007;28:811–26.

3. D'Souza AL, Nelson NG, McKenzie LB. Pediatric burn injuries treated in US emergency departments between 1990 and 2006. Pediatrics 2009;124:1424–30.

4. Blaisdell LL, Chace R, Halagan LD, et al. A half-century of burn epidemiology and burn care in a rural state. J Burn Care Res 2012;33:347–53.

5. Riedlinger DI, Jennings PA, Edgar DW, et al. Scald burns in children aged 14 and younger in Australia and New Zealand—an analysis based on the Burn Registry of Australia and New Zealand (BRANZ). Burns 2015;41:462–8.

6. Garcia CT, Smith GA, Cohen DM, et al. Electrical injuries in a pediatric emergency department. Ann Emerg Med 1995;26:604–8.

7. Rimmer RB, Weigand S, Foster KN, et al. Scald burns in young children—a review of Arizona Burn Center pediatric patients and a proposal for prevention in the Hispanic community. J Burn Care Res 2008;29:595–605.

8. Lee CJ, Mahendraraj K, Houng A, et al. Pediatric burns: a single institution retrospective review of incidence, etiology, and outcomes in 2273 burn patients (1995-2013). J Burn Care Res 2016;37:e579–85.

9. Rawlins JM, Khan AA, Shenton AF, et al. Epidemiology and outcome analysis of 208 children with burns attending an emergency department. Pediatr Emerg Care 2007;23:289–93.

10. Johnson SA, Shi J, Groner JI, et al. Inter-facility transfer of pediatric burn patients from U.S. emergency departments. Burns 2016;42:1413–22.

11. Rose AM, Hassan Z, Davenport K, et al. Adherence to national burn care review referral criteria in a paediatric emergency department. Burns 2010;36:1165–71.

12. Hartstein B. Burn injuries in children and the use of biological dressings. Pediatr Emerg Care 2013;29:939–45.

13. Brown M, Coffee T, Adenuga P, et al. Outcomes of outpatient management of pediatric burns. J Burn Care Res 2014;35:388–94.

14. Sahu SA, Agrawal K, Patel PK. Scald burn, a preventable injury: analysis of 4306 patients from a major tertiary care center. Burns 2016;42:1844–9.

15. Ewings EL, Pollack J. Pediatric upper extremity burns: outcome of emergency department triage and outpatient management. J Burn Care Res 2008;29:77–81.

16. Hodgman EI, Saeman MR, Subramanian M, et al. The effect of burn center volume on mortality in a pediatric population: an analysis of the national burn repository. J Burn Care Res 2016;37:32–7.

17. Cowan D, Ho B, Sykes KJ, et al. Pediatric oral burns: a ten-year review of patient characteristics, etiologies, and treatment outcomes. Int J Pediatr Otorhinolaryngol 2013;77:1325–8.

18. Glatstein MM, Ayalon I, Miller E, et al. Pediatric electrical burn injuries. experience of a large tertiary care hospital and a review of electrical injury. Pediatr Emerg Care 2013;29:737–40.

19. Campos JK, Wong YM, Hasty BN, et al. The effect of socioeconomic status and parental demographics on activation of department of child and family services in pediatric burn injury. J Burn Care Res 2017;38:e722–33.

20. Toor J, Crain J, Kelly C, et al. Pediatric burns from glass-fronted fireplaces in Canada: a growing issue over the past 20 years. J Burn Care Res 2016;37:e438–88.

21. Juang D, Fike FB, Laituri CA, et al. Treadmill injuries in the pediatric population. J Surg Res 2011;170:139–42.
22. Thombs BD, Singh VA, Milner SM. Children under 4 years are at greater risk of mortality following acute burn injury: evidence from a national sample of 12,902 pediatric admissions. Shock 2006;26:348–52.
23. Kraft R, Herndon DN, Al-Mousawi AM, et al. Burn size and survival probability in paediatric patients in modern burn care: a prospective observational cohort study. Lancet 2012;379:1013–21.
24. Kishikova L, Smith MD, Cubison TCS. Evidence based management for pediatric burn: new approaches and improved scar outcomes. Burns 2014;40:1530–7.
25. Klein MB, Nathens AB, Heimbach DM, et al. An outcome analysis of patients transferred to a regional burn center: transfer status does not impact survival. Burns 2006;32:940–5.
26. Andronicus M, Oates RK, Peat J, et al. Non-accidental burns in children. Burns 1998;24:552–8.
27. Palmieri TL, Taylor S, Lawless M, et al. Burn center volume makes a difference for burned children. Pediatr Crit Care Med 2015;16:319–24.
28. Thombs BD. Patient and injury characteristics, mortality risk, and length of stay related to child abuse by burning. Ann Surg 2008;247:519–23.
29. Barrow RE, Jeschke MG, Herndon DN. Early fluid resuscitation improves outcomes in severely burned children. Resuscitation 2000;45:91–6.
30. Kraft R, Herndon DN, Finnerty CC, et al. Occurrence of multiorgan dysfunction in pediatric burn patients. Ann Surg 2014;259:381–7.
31. Sheridan RL, Hinson MI, Liang MH, et al. Long-term outcomes of children surviving massive burns. JAMA 2000;283:69–73.
32. Jeschke MG, Herndon DN. Burns in children: standard and new treatments. Lancet 2014;383:1168–78.
33. Feldman KW, Schaller RT, Feldman JA, et al. Tap water scald burns in children. Pediatrics 1977;62:1–7.
34. Erdmann TC, Feldman KW, Rivara FP, et al. Tap water burn prevention: the effect of legislation. Pediatrics 1991;88:572–7.
35. Cuttle L, Pearn J, McMillan JR, et al. A review of first aid treatments for burn injuries. Burns 2009;35:768–75.
36. Roberts S, Meltzer JA. An evidence-based approach to electrical injuries in children. Pediatr Emerg Med Pract 2013;10:1–20.
37. Chen EH, Sareen A. Do children require ECG evaluation and inpatient telemetry after household electrical exposures? Ann Emerg Med 2005;49:64–7.
38. D'Cruz RD, Pang TC, Harvey JG, et al. Chemical burns in children: aetiology and prevention. Burns 2015;41:764–9.
39. Goverman J, Bittner EA, Friedstat JS, et al. Discrepancy in initial pediatric burn estimation and its impact on fluid resuscitation. J Burn Care Res 2015;36:574–9.
40. Varley A, Sarginson J, Young A. Evidence-based first aid advice for paediatric burns in the United Kingdom. Burns 2016;42:571–7.
41. Klein MB, Kramer B, Nelson J, et al. Geographic access to burn center hospitals. JAMA 2009;302:1774–81.
42. Sheridan R, Weber J, Prelack K, et al. Early burn center transfer shortens the length of hospitalization and reduces complications in children with serious burn injuries. J Burn Care Rehabil 1999;20:347–50.
43. Romanowski KS, Palmieri TL, Sen S, et al. More than one third of intubation in patients transferred to burn centers are unnecessary: proposed guidelines for appropriate intubation in the burn patient. J Burn Care Res 2016;37:e409–14.

44. Wheeler DS, Spaeth JP, Mehta R, et al. Assessment and management of the pediatric airway. In: Wheeler DS, Wong HR, Shanley TP, editors. Resuscitation and stabilization of the critically ill child. New York: Springer; 2008. p. 1–30.

45. Zak AL, Harrington DT, Barillo DJ, et al. Acute respiratory failure that complicates the resuscitation of pediatric patients with scald injuries. J Burn Care Rehabil 1999;20:391–9.

46. Mosier MJ, Peter T, Gamelli RL. Need for mechanical ventilation in pediatric scald burns: why it happens and why it matters. J Burn Care Res 2016;37:e1–6.

47. Enkhbaatar P, Cox RA, Traber LD, et al. Aerosolized anticoagulants ameliorate acute lung injury in sheep after exposure to burn and smoke inhalation. Crit Care Med 2007;35:2805–10.

48. Miller AC, Elamin EM, Suffredini AF. Inhaled anticoagulation regimens for the treatment of smoke inhalation associated acute lung injury: a systematic review. Crit Care Med 2014;42:413–9.

49. Palmieri TL. Use of β-agonists in inhalation injury. J Burn Care Res 2009;30: 156–8.

50. Baud FJ, Borron SW, Megarbane B, et al. Value of lactic acidosis in the assessment of the severity of acute cyanide poisoning. Crit Care Med 2002;30:2044–50.

51. Tobias JD, Green TP, Cote CJ. Codeine: time to say "no". Pediatrics 2016;138: e1–7.

52. Baartmans MGA, de Jong AEE, van Baar ME, et al. Early management in children with burns: cooling, wound care, and pain management. Burns 2016;42:777–82.

53. Freiburg C, Igneri P, Sartorelli K, et al. Effects of differences in percent total body surface area estimation on fluid resuscitation of transferred burn patients. J Burn Care Res 2007;28:42–8.

54. Hammond JS, Ward CG. Transfers from emergency to burn center: errors in burn size estimate. J Trauma 1987;27:1161–5.

55. Giretzlehner M, Dimberger J, Owen R, et al. The determination of total burn surface area: how much difference? Burns 2013;39:1107–13.

56. Chan QE, Barzi F, Cheney L, et al. Burn size estimation in children: still a problem. Emerg Med Australas 2012;24:181–6.

57. Haycock GB, Schwartz GJ, Wisotsky DH. Geometric method for measuring body surface area: a height weight formula validated in infants, children and adults. J Pediatr 1978;1:62–6.

58. Boyd E. The growth of the surface area of the human body. Minneapolis (MN): University of Minnesota Press; 1935.

59. Nagel TR, Schunk JE. Using the hand to estimate the surface area of a burn in children. Pediatr Emerg Care 1997;13:254–5.

60. Rhodes J, Clay C, Phillips M. The surface area of the hand and the palm for estimating percentage of total body surface area: results of a meta-analysis. Br J Dermatol 2013;169:76–84.

61. Lund C, Browder NC. The estimation of areas of burns. Surg Gynecol Obstet 1944;79:352–8.

62. Nichter LS, Bryant CA, Edlich RF. Efficacy of burned surface area estimates calculated from charts—the need for a computer-based model. J Trauma 1985; 25:477–81.

63. Wurzer P, Parvizi D, Lumenta DB, et al. Smartphone applications in burn. Burns 2015;41:977–89.

64. Gee Kee EL, Kimble RM, Stockton KA. 3D photography is a reliable burn wound area assessment tool compared to digital planimetry in very young children. Burns 2015;41:1286–90.

65. Parvizi D, Giretzlehner M, Dirnberger J, et al. The use of telemedicine in burn care: development of a mobile system for TBSA documentation and remote assessment. Ann Burns Fire Disasters 2014;27:94–100.

66. Wibbenmeyer L, Kluesner K, Wu H, et al. Video-enhanced telemedicine improves the care of acutely injured burn patients in a rural state. J Burn Care Res 2016;37: e531–8.

67. Kraft R, Herndon DN, Branski LK, et al. Optimized fluid management improves outcomes of pediatric burn patients. J Surg Res 2013;181:121–8.

68. Carvajal HF. Fluid resuscitation of pediatric burn victims: a critical appraisal. Pediatr Nephrol 1994;8:357–66.

69. El Hachem M, Zambruno G, Bourdon-Lanoy E, et al. Multicentre consensus recommendations for skin care in inherited epidermolysis bullosa. Orphanet J Rare Dis 2014;9:76.

70. Rogers AD, Karpelowsky J, Millar AJW, et al. Fluid creep in major pediatric burns. Eur J Pediatr Surg 2010;20:133–8.

71. Faraklas I, Lam U, Cochran A, et al. Colloid normalizes resuscitation ratio in pediatric burns. J Burn Care Res 2011;32:91–7.

72. Cocks AJ, O'Connell A, Martin H. Crystalloids, colloids and kids: a review of paediatric burns in intensive care. Burns 1998;24:717–24.

73. Saffle JR. The phenomenon of "fluid creep" in acute burn resuscitation. J Burn Care Res 2007;28:382–95.

74. Arlati S, Storti E, Pradella V, et al. Decreased fluid volume to reduce organ damage: a new approach to burn shock resuscitation? A preliminary study. Resuscitation 2007;72:371–8.

75. Peck MD, Priolo-Kapel D. Child abuse by burning: a review of the literature and an algorithm for medical investigations. J Trauma 2002;53:1013–22.

76. Chester DL, Jose RM, Aldlyami E, et al. Non-accidental burns in children—are we neglecting neglect? Burns 2006;32:222–8.

77. Greenbaum AR, Donne J, Wilson D, et al. Intentional burn injury: an evidence-based, clinical forensic review. Burns 2004;30:628–42.

78. Daria S, Sugar NF, Feldman KW, et al. Into hot water head first: distribution of intentional and unintentional immersion burns. Pediatr Emerg Care 2004;20: 302–10.

79. Purdue GF, Hunt JL, Prescott PR. Child abuse by burning—an index of suspicion. J Trauma 1988;28:221–4.

80. American Academy of Pediatrics Committee on Infectious Diseases, Kimberlin DW, Brady MT, Jackson MA, et al. Red book section 3: tetanus. 2015.

81. Ergun O, Celik A, Ergun G, et al. Prophylactic ntibiotic use in pediatric burn units. Eur J Pediatr Surg 2004;14:422–6.

82. Church D, Elsayed S, Lindsay R, et al. Burn wound infections. Clin Microbiol Rev 2006;2:403–34.

83. Rodgers GL, Mortensen J, Fisher MC, et al. Predictors of infectious complications after burn injuries in children. Pediatr Infect Dis J 2000;19:990–5.

84. Vyles D, Sinha M, Rosenberg DI, et al. Predictors of serious bacterial infections in pediatric burn patients with fever. J Burn Care Res 2014;35:291–5.

85. Gottschlich MM, Jenkins ME, Mayes T, et al. The 2002 Clinical Research Award: An evaluation of the safety of early vs delayed enteral support and effects on clinical, nutritional, and endocrine outcomes after severe burns. J Burn Care Res 2002;23:401–15.

86. Mosier MJ, Pham TN, Klein MB, et al. Early enteral nutrition in burns: compliance with guidelines and associated outcomes in a multicenter study. J Burn Care Res 2011;32:104–9.
87. Shaw J, Dibble C. Management of burns blisters. Emerg Med J 2006;23:648–9.
88. Sargent RL. Management of blisters in the partial-thickness burn: an integrative research review. J Burn Care Res 2006;27:66–81.
89. Canpolat DG, Esmaoglu A, Tosun Z, et al. Ketamine-propofol vs ketamine-dexmedetomidine combinations in pediatric patients undergoing burn dressing changes. J Burn Care Res 2012;33:718–22.
90. Miner JR, Moore JC, Austad EJ, et al. Randomized, double-blinded, clinical trial of propofol, 1:1 propofol/ketamine, and 4:1 propofol/ketamine for deep procedural sedation in the emergency department. Ann Emerg Med 2015;65:479–88.
91. Coetzee E, Rode H, Kahn D. *Pseudomonas aeruginosa* burn wound infection in a dedicated paediatric burns unit. S Afr J Surg 2013;51:50–3.
92. Paddock HN, Fabia R, Giles S, et al. A silver-impregnated antimicrobial dressing reduces hospital costs for pediatric burn patients. J Pediatr Surg 2007;42:211–3.
93. Gotschall CS, Morrison MIS, Eichelberger MR. Prospective, randomized study of the efficacy of mepitel on children with partial thickness scalds. J Burn Care Rehabil 1998;19:279–83.
94. Verbelen J, Hoeksema H, Heyneman A, et al. Aquacel(®) Ag dressing versus Activcoat™ dressing in partial thickness burns: a prospective, randomized, controlled study in 100 patients. Part 1: burn wound healing. Burns 2014;40:416–27.
95. Foglia RP, Moushey R, Meadows L, et al. Evolving treatment in a decade of pediatric burn care. J Pediatr Surg 2004;39:957–60.
96. Brown M, Dalziel SR, Herd E, et al. Randomized, controlled study of silver-based dressing in a pediatric emergency department. J Burn Care Res 2016;37:e340–7.
97. Gee Kee EL, Kimble RM, Cuttle L, et al. Randomized controlled trial of three burn dressings for partial thickness burns in children. Burns 2015;41:946–55.

Pediatric Major Head Injury

Not a Minor Problem

Aaron N. Leetch, MD[a,b,]*, Bryan Wilson, MD[a,b]

KEYWORDS

- Traumatic brain injury • Intracranial hemorrhage • Blunt head injury
- Abusive head trauma

KEY POINTS

- Emergency department management should focus on identifying the primary brain injury and preventing secondary brain injury. Secondary injury is multifactorial but most pronounced with hypotension and hypoxia.
- Hyperventilation should be avoided except as a temporizing measure for symptoms of acute herniation.
- Goals for preventing secondary injury include maintenance of physiologic normalcy, prevention of ischemia, and reduction of increased intracranial pressure.
- Induced hypothermia and decompressive craniotomy have not shown to lead to neurologically favorable outcomes in large recent studies.
- Abusive head trauma should always be considered in younger children with traumatic brain injury.

INTRODUCTION

Head injury is an increasingly common cause of emergency department (ED) visits for pediatric patients.[1] In 1 year in the United States, pediatric traumatic brain injury (TBI) led to more than 2.5 million encounters and 50,000 hospitalizations, accruing more than $1 billion in hospital charges.[2] Deaths from pediatric TBI are most common in the adolescent/young adult (from motor vehicle collisions) and in those younger than 4 year of age (from falls).[1,3] In 2013, pediatric trauma contributed to more than 40,000 hospitalizations and 7000 deaths. Nonaccidental trauma or inflicted trauma is an unfortunately common cause of TBI in the very young. Male infants, those

Disclosure Statement: The authors have no significant financial disclosures to make.
[a] Department of Emergency Medicine, The University of Arizona, PO Box 245057, Tucson, AZ 85724-5057, USA; [b] Department of Pediatrics, The University of Arizona, PO Box 245057, Tucson, AZ 85724-5057, USA
* Corresponding author. Department of Emergency Medicine, The University of Arizona, PO Box 245057, Tucson, AZ 85724-5057.
E-mail address: aleetch@aemrc.arizona.edu

Emerg Med Clin N Am 36 (2018) 459–472
https://doi.org/10.1016/j.emc.2017.12.012
0733-8627/18/© 2017 Elsevier Inc. All rights reserved.
emed.theclinics.com

younger than 6 months of age, and those with mothers less than 21 years of age seem to be at the greatest risk.[4,5]

Much work has been done to risk stratify head-injured children with decision rules to be discussed elsewhere. Recently, the goal of the ED evaluation seems to be shifting toward a patient-oriented outcome measure rather than a disease-oriented outcome.[6–9] The idea of a clinically important TBI (ciTBI) separates those patients with intracranial hemorrhage requiring immediate intervention from those managed similar to a severe concussion. There is no consensus on what constitutes a ciTBI for pediatric patients, but the inclusion criteria from the 4 largest trials provide an excellent framework for discussion[10,11] (**Table 1**). The evaluation and management of ciTBI focuses on 2 goals:

1. Identification of the primary injury, and
2. Prevention of secondary injury.

Table 1
"Clinically important" traumatic brain injury definitions

Study	Clinical Outcome	CT Findings
PECARN	Death from head injury Neurosurgical intervention Intubation for >24 h Hospital admission >2 nights for persistent neurologic symptoms	Intracranial hemorrhage or contusion Cerebral edema Traumatic infarction Diffuse axonal injury Shearing injury Sigmoid sinus thrombosis Midline shift or herniation Diastasis of skull Pneumocephalus Skull fracture depressed by more than the width of the skull table
CHALICE	Death from head injury Neurosurgical intervention	Any new, acute traumatic intracranial pathology Intracranial hematomas of any size Cerebral contusion Diffuse cerebral edema Depressed skull fracture
CATCH	Within 7 d: death from head injury Neurosurgical intervention Intubation	Any acute intracranial finding attributable to acute injury
NEXUS II	Neurosurgical intervention Likely to have significant long term impairment	EDH/SDH >1 cm or causing mass effect Cerebral contusion >1 cm or multiple Extensive SAH Mass effect or sulcal effacement Herniation Basal cistern compression or midline shift Posterior fossa hemorrhage Bilateral hemorrhage Depressed/diastatic skull fracture Pneumocephalus Diffuse cerebral edema Diffuse axonal injury

Abbreviations: CT, computed tomography; EDH/SDH, epidural hematomas/subdural hematomas; SAH, subarachnoid hemorrhage.
Data from Refs.[6–9]

PATHOPHYSIOLOGY
Identification of the Primary Injury

Prevention of the primary injury is clearly the most important step in ciTBI management. Primary injury occurs from blunt trauma, penetrating trauma, or blast injury.[12] This article focuses mainly on blunt trauma, which makes up the majority of pediatric ciTBI. The acceleration-deceleration injury that results from blunt trauma can cause a seemingly endless spectrum of clinical sequelae; however, only a small number of identifiable lesions can be seen on computed tomography or MRI (**Table 2**). Despite the radiation risk, computed tomography is ubiquitous in EDs around the country and provides high diagnostic accuracy for emergent conditions with rapid results.[13] Once identified, the location, size, and progression of injury dictates clinical management and often the clinical outcome. Lesions ranging from parenchymal damage to vessel injury to axonal shearing can be multiple and coexistent. Even before the primary injury is identified, prevention of secondary injury should begin immediately upon suspicion of a ciTBI.

Prevention of Secondary Injury

Secondary injury involves progression of cerebral ischemia and neuronal death from other clinical conditions.[14] Hypoxia and hypotension have long been implicated as the most prominent causes of secondary injury.[12,15–18] The injured brain is physiologically fragile and susceptible to both hypoxia and hypotension. The combination of both is an especially potent risk factor for mortality. This physiologic susceptibility is further complicated by rapid desaturation times in children with lower lung reserve capacity and higher metabolic rates.[19] Hyperthermia, hypocapnea, hypoglycemia, and intracranial hypertension have also been implicated as independent predictors of mortality.[15] Hyperoxia and hyperglycemia also seem to be detrimental, indicating that a therapeutic balance must be maintained for optimal outcome.[20,21] Maintenance of this balance is based on the Monro-Kellie doctrine:

Cerebral perfusion pressure (CPP) = mean arterial pressure – intracranial pressure (ICP)

Mass effect from primary injury increases the ICP and decreases the CPP. Current methods are directed at either ICP, CPP, or microvascular management with

Table 2
Clinically important traumatic brain injuries and their managements

Lesion	Pathophysiology	Mechanism	CT Findings
Epidural hematoma	Injury to large arteries or veins	Direct blow to the head, same side as injury	Lenticular shape Does not cross suture lines
Subdural hematoma	Injury to small bridging veins	Acceleration-deceleration injury	Crescent shaped Crosses suture lines
Subarachnoid hemorrhage	Injury to tiny pial veins	Direct blow and/or acceleration-deceleration injury	Gathered along sulci/fissures Can be diffuse
Parenchymal contusion	Injury to brain capillaries	Direct blow to the head, coup/contrecoup injury	May have delayed appearance on CT
Diffuse axonal injury	Shearing injury of axons	Acceleration-deceleration injury	Rarely seen on CT MRI often necessary to visualize

Abbreviation: CT, computed tomography.

CPP-directed management being the most common. In 2012, a consensus group convened to author the second edition of the Guidelines for the Acute Management of Severe Traumatic Brian Injury in Infants, Children and Adolescents with an aim to produce evidence-based guidelines from high-quality sources.[22] Much of the previous guidelines were dependent on adult studies given the dearth of data on the management of pediatric ciTBI.[16] These guidelines establish 3 main goals of resuscitation and stabilization (**Table 3**):

- Maintain physiologic normalcy,
- Prevent cerebral ischemia, and
- Treat elevated intracranial hypertension.

Normal ranges of Po_2, Pco_2, temperature, and mean arterial pressure seem to provide the best outcome, or at least prevent a worse outcome. Decreasing ICP is a widely accepted goal, although few studies have shown a positive patient-centered outcome with this strategy. ED management should focus on the optimization of physiologic parameters with the beginnings of critical care management in ICP reduction.

THE APPROACH TO THE HEAD-INJURED CHILD

The initial approach to the child with suspected or obvious TBI is well-described in the Advanced Trauma Life Support and Advanced Pediatric Life Support programs.[23–25] A suggested stepwise approach based on these 2 programs is presented herein.

Recognition

The Pediatric Assessment Triangle can provide crucial evidence of a sick child.[26] A brief consideration of a child's appearance, work of breathing, and color can reveal much of their underlying pathology. Appearance should be assessed based on their

Table 3
Goals of traumatic brain injury management

	Maintain Physiologic Normalcy	Prevent Cerebral Ischemia	Treat Intracranial Hypertension
First-tier interventions	Normal oxygen (saturation >90%; Pao_2 60–470 mm Hg) Avoid prolonged hyperventilation ($Paco_2$ 35–45 mm Hg; $EtCO_2$ 30–40 mm Hg) Normal systolic blood pressure (50%–75% for age)		Elevate head of bed at 30° Hyperosmolar infusion
	Normal temperature (35.5°C – 37.0°C) Euvolemia	Neutral head position	
Second-tier interventions		Adequate sedation Seizure prophylaxis	Intracranial pressure monitor Extraventricular drain Decompressive craniotomy

Abbreviations: $EtCO_2$, end-tidal carbon dioxide; $Paco_2$, partial pressure of carbon dioxide in arterial blood; Pao_2, partial pressure of oxygen in arterial blood.

Data from Carney N, Totten AM, O'reilly C, et al. Guidelines for the management of severe traumatic brain injury. Neurosurgery 2017;80(1):6–15; and Kochanek P, Carney N, Adelson P. Guidelines for the acute medical management of severe traumatic brain injury in infants, children, and adolescents. Pediatr Crit Care Med 2012;13(2):252. [Pediatr Crit Care Med 2012;13(1 Suppl):S1–82].

level of alertness, response to stimulation and age-appropriate interaction with care providers. Children do an excellent job of protecting their injuries so a still or quiet child is an ominous sign.

Primary Survey

Primary survey of airway, breathing, circulation, disability, and exposure should be performed rapidly with appropriate inventions for life-threatening airway and/or other polytrauma issues. A brief history should be obtained simultaneously from emergency medical services or caregivers/witnesses, although a caregiver history may not be reliable in abusive cases.

Disability assessment generally uses the Glasgow Coma Score (GCS) to risk stratify into mild (13–15), moderate (9–12), and severe (3–8) neurologic injury.[14] In verbal children, the initial GCS has excellent prognostic value for identifying ciTBI and its subsequent outcomes.[27] A modified Infant GCS can have variable interpretation, but still has general acceptance as an reliable assessment method.[28,29] The assessment of verbal response and the child's cooperation can often vary between providers and change with situations (pain control, parental presence, etc). Newer literature suggests that the motor score of the GCS the portion most predictive of overall mortality.[30,31] This would streamline the assessment and bring it closer to the AVPU scale suggested by Pediatric Advanced Life Support algorithm[32] (**Table 4**).

Secondary Survey

After the primary examination, a more thorough history and physical should be performed. Glucose should also be checked during the primary survey and hyperglycemia can be indicative of ciTBI in those younger than 3 years of age.[33] Mechanism of injury, seatbelt use, helmet use, and condition of other passengers can help to guide diagnostics. Verbal, cooperative children should be asked about loss of consciousness. A complete, age-appropriate neurologic examination should be performed. Head examination should include palpation for hematomas, bulging fontanelles, or skull fractures. Secondary signs of basilar skull fracture include mastoid bruising (Battle's sign), hemotympanum, ear bleeding, periorbital bruising (raccoon eyes), or persistent rhinorrhea/otorrhea. Pupillary size, activity, and symmetry are excellent markers of focal neurologic status. When possible, a fundoscopic examination may reveal retinal hemorrhages. The digital rectal examination is unlikely to yield any pertinent information without other obvious signs of paralysis or injury.[34] A head-to-toe examination should also evaluate

Table 4
Infant GCS and AVPU scale

AVPU Scale		Motor GCS		Verbal GCS		Eye GCS
Alert	6	Spontaneous movement	5	Normal interaction for age	4	Eyes open spontaneously
Verbal	5	Withdraws to voice/touch	4	Crying, consolable	3	Eyes open to voice
Pain	4	Withdraws to pain	3	Cries to pain	2	Eyes open to pain
Unresponsive	3	Decerebrate flexion	2	Moans to pain	1	No response
	2	Decorticate extension	1	No response	—	
	1	No response	—		—	

Abbreviations: AVPU, alert verbal painful unresponsive; GCS, Glasgow Coma Scale.

for concomitant injury, which can contribute to a higher mortality in patients with ciTBI.[35]

IMMEDIATE MANAGEMENT AND RESUSCITATION
Airway Management and Oxygenation

The multifactorial difficulty of pediatric traumatic airway management warrants careful preparation, judicious intubation decisions, and performance by the most experienced provider. Known or suspected cervical spine injury require precautions that limit patient positioning. Patients with a GCS of less than 8 are at risk for aspiration and disordered breathing from their neurologic insult. Rapid sequence intubation (RSI) with midline cervical immobilization is the ideal approach in ciTBI. Young children have proportionally larger heads and may require extra padding under the torso to maintain proper cervical spine alignment. Preoxygenation and apneic oxygenation improve intubating conditions for adult ciTBI by preventing hypoxemia.[36] Data suggest that preoxygenation and apneic oxygenation provide a safe apnea time of 2 minutes in infants and 10 minutes in children.[19,37] Although not studied in children with ciTBI, apneic oxygenation could prevent periintubation hypoxemia.

Classically, pretreatment with fentanyl, lidocaine, and other adjuncts have been used to blunt the sympathetic surge and potential increase in ICP during laryngoscopy. Recent research has shown little to no effect from lidocaine, but a modest effect from fentanyl.[38,39] When used for pretreatment, the dose of fentanyl should be increased to doses of 2 to 5 μg/kg for optimal effect.[40]

The pediatric ciTBI guidelines do not make recommendations on RSI induction agents.[16,22] An ideal agent would be hemodynamically neutral with a rapid onset and adequate analgesia, anesthesia, and amnesia. Such a drug exists in ketamine, although its use has been discouraged based on a few case studies inappropriately extrapolated to ciTBI.[41–43] Multiple studies have debunked the notion that ketamine increases ICP in patients with ciTBI[44,45] and 1 pediatric study actually showed decreased ICP with hemodynamic neutrality.[46] Ketamine is, therefore, a reasonable choice for a first-line induction agent. Etomidate is another hemodynamically neutral induction agent used successfully in pediatric ciTBI.[47] One small study has demonstrated decreased ICP with a single dose of etomidate.[48] Etomidate is more accepted for RSI in children, although some still postulate whether it leads to subsequent adrenal suppression.

Neuromuscular blockade agents include rapid, brief-acting succinylcholine or delayed, sustained-acting rocuronium. Succinylcholine's rapid onset and resolution allows for quick reassessment of the neurologic examination and sedation needs. It does, however, carry the risk of increased ICP and an overall increased in-hospital mortality for adult patients with ciTBI compared with rocuronium.[49] Conversely, rocuronium's long duration of action precludes serial neurologic examinations and can lead to delayed anesthesia and increased ICP. Given the options, providers should choose the agent best suited for their patient's needs. Patients who are spontaneously breathing with adequate airway protection may not warrant intubation, although they should be monitored closely for mental status changes requiring further intervention.

Breathing and Ventilation

Once intubated, the partial pressure of carbon dioxide in arterial blood ($Paco_2$) should be maintained within an appropriate window. Hyperventilation is a potent vasoconstrictor and can briefly reduce ICP by reducing cerebral blood flow.[50] However, it can also worsen secondary injury through resultant cerebral hypoxemia and ischemia.[50,51] Although hyperventilation may temporarily abort clinical signs of herniation, it should generally be avoided. End-tidal carbon dioxide measurement is becoming more readily available and can serve as a fair surrogate for $Paco_2$ until the latter can be measured.

Circulation and Fluid Resuscitation

Hypotension is a major contributor to ischemic damage, especially when complicated by hemorrhagic shock.[12,52] Judicious fluid types, volumes, and concentrations should be used to minimize secondary injury. Hypotonic fluids should be avoided to prevent osmolar shifts and worsening cerebral edema.[53] Systolic blood pressure goals can be estimated with 90 mm Hg + (age $\times$ 2). Isotonic fluids should be used to maintain euvolemia and a systolic blood pressure of 50% to 75% for age.[22,54,55] There is some growing literature supporting hypertonic saline for volume resuscitation in hypotensive patients with ciTBI.[56] Any patient with significant hemorrhage should be transfused to increase oxygen-carrying capacity.

NONPHARMACOLOGIC THERAPIES
Head Position

Head position seems to augment secondary injury with a higher head position producing a lower ICP.[57,58] Maintenance of neutral head position and 30° elevation can improve venous drainage and further lower the ICP. Clinical outcome and CPP have been variably correlated, although the intervention is simple and without much risk for harm.

Targeted Temperature Regulation

Temperature regulation is important for all trauma patients, and hyperthermia after ciTBI is associated with increased morbidity and mortality.[59,60] Initial studies on induced hypothermia after TBI hypothesized that progression of secondary injury could be slowed. Subsequent studies in pediatric patients have shown equivocal outcomes with similar mortality and neurologic outcomes regardless of temperature.[61,62] One large randomized controlled trial (Cool Kids) ended early citing futility, although a recent metaanalysis showed therapeutic hypothermia to infer a 66% increased risk in mortality and a 10% increase in poor neurologic outcome.[63] This suggests that targeted temperature management between 35.5°C and 37.0°C is likely an appropriate goal.

SURGICAL THERAPY

Early neurosurgical involvement is important for the subset of patients with a surgically amenable lesion. Surgical management of ciTBI is directed by the type, size, and location of the lesion found on neuroimaging, the degree of midline shift, clinical status, and GCS. Epidural hematomas and subdural hematomas may be surgically decompressed in the setting of increased ICP, midline shift, or herniation.[64] An extraventricular drain may be placed by a neurosurgeon to both measure and reduce ICP. Decompressive craniotomy has been used to decrease ICP through removing the volume restrictions of the skull. Recently, 2 large clinical trials have shown a decrease in mortality with craniotomy, but also an overall increase in unfavorable neurologic outcome.[65,66] Currently, guidelines do not recommend decompressive craniotomy as an early intervention strategy.

PHARMACOLOGIC THERAPY
Sedation, Analgesia, and Neuromuscular Blockade

Pain, stress, and agitation can increase mean arterial pressure, which in turn affects the CPP. Adequate sedation can mitigate the pain of injury, invasive monitoring, and interventions. The 2012 pediatric consensus guidelines do not recommend specific sedative infusions during initial management.[22] The adult guidelines recommend propofol to decrease ICP,[67] but prolonged infusion in children carries the risk of propofol-related infusion syndrome.[68] Without solid recommendations, the goal should be adequate sedation while avoiding hypotension from overadministration. Sustained neuromuscular blockade after RSI can mask extubation and seizures, and should be avoided initially.

Seizure Prophylaxis

Posttraumatic seizures occur in about 10% of patients with TBIs, increasing metabolic demand and further compromising cerebral metabolism.[69,70] Seizures are more common in patients with a GCS of less than 8, age less than 2 years, and nonaccidental trauma. Phenytoin prophylaxis can significantly reduce the early posttraumatic seizure rate.[71] However, no studies have shown improved patient-centered outcomes with early posttraumatic seizure prophylaxis. Levetiracetam has shown similar rates of early seizure prevention though at a much higher cost.[72] Current pediatric and adult guidelines suggest phenytoin for prophylaxis.

Hyperosmolar Therapy

Mannitol and hypertonic saline are common adjuncts to decrease ICP through osmotic pathways.[73] Mannitol reduces cerebral edema through osmotic diuresis, whereas hypertonic saline directly increases osmolality by increasing serum sodium. The 2012 pediatric guidelines revealed little evidence to recommend either, although studies in adults show increased benefit from hypertonic saline over mannitol.[74,75] Concentrations between 1.7% and 23.4% have been used, although the best evidence supports the use of 3% normal saline, 6 to 10 mL/kg over 10 to 30 minutes.[22,76]

Currently, no other medications have improved patient-oriented outcomes. Progesterone and tranexamic acid have not shown harm nor efficacy.[77,78] Corticosteroids have shown increased mortality in adults and are unlikely to be studied in children.[79]

ABUSIVE HEAD TRAUMA

Patients with abusive head trauma (AHT) are twice as likely to die compared with accidental injury.[80] Infants less than 1 year of age are at increased risk and survivors often have significant neurologic morbidity. The triad of retinal hemorrhages, subdural hematomas, and diffuse brain injury is commonly described as AHT.[81,82] The injury to the retina, brain, and subdural vessels occur from a combination of shaking and blunt trauma. Rapid acceleration/deceleration causes shearing injury to fragile vessels resulting in hemorrhage. Skull fractures can occur from accidental trauma, although bilateral, nonlinear, and depressed fracture or those crossing suture lines are suspicious for abuse. Subdural hematomas are more likely to be abusive than epidural hematomas.[83] Of those found on imaging, multiple lesions, posterior fossa location, and the coincidence of cerebral edema were highly correlated with abuse.

The history is often given by the perpetrator and should always be scrutinized in light of the patient's developmental level and the severity of trauma. Chief complaints are not always related to trauma and may instead include apnea, breathing difficulty, vomiting, seizures, or difficulty arousing the child from sleep.[84–86] A 2011 study showed 6 findings to be associated with AHT[85]:

- Rib fractures,
- Retinal hemorrhages,
- Long bone fractures,
- Head/neck bruising,
- Apnea, and
- Seizures.

When 3 or more of these factors were present in children less than 3 years old, the positive predictive value for abuse approached 100%. Specifically concerning is the combination of intracranial hemorrhage and either retinal hemorrhages or rib fractures. For this reason, a thorough physical examination may still not be enough in younger children. Nearly 20% to 50% of children with AHT were found to have axial or appendicular fracture as well, so a skeletal survey and dilated retinal examination performed by an ophthalmologist is recommended by the American Academy of Pediatrics for all such patients.[4,87–91] Management of these patients is similar to that of accidental trauma with life-threatening issues addressed first and prevention of secondary injury second. Law enforcement and state, county, or tribal protective service should be involved early, although medical management must supersede forensic evidence collection for the sake of the child.

SUMMARY

Recognition and management of ciTBI is crucial to provide the best possible outcome for injured pediatric patients. The ED evaluation and initial resuscitation can have a profound impact on the patient's eventual outcome. Presenting GCS and hyperglycemia can be early clues to the degree of ciTBI suffered by the patient. Likely the most important interventions the emergency physician can make are the most basic interventions, including:

- Expeditious airway management,
- Elevated and midline head position,
- Maintenance of normal O_2 and CO_2 parameters,
- Judicious volume resuscitation and prevention of hypotension,
- Rapid imaging to identify surgically managed lesions, and
- Normal temperature maintenance and adequate sedation.

ICP-directed therapy can be considered during ED resuscitation as the patient transitions to surgical or critical care management. Although still the usual care, several authors have debated whether ICP reduction should be the goal of therapy. Interventions such as decompressive craniotomy, therapeutic hypothermia, and other adjunctive therapies have not shown the desired outcomes, although this outcome may be related to timing, patient cohort, or a host of other factors. AHT should be considered in light of the patient's age, the history obtained, and the degree of injury sustained. If suspected, a skeletal survey and dilated retinal examination should be performed to evaluate for occult or old injuries. Ultimately, the role of the ED should be to resuscitate and stabilize the critically injured child. Future research should focus on treatment regimens that show favorable patient-centered outcomes.

REFERENCES

1. Taylor CA. Traumatic brain injury–related emergency department visits, hospitalizations, and deaths—United States, 2007 and 2013. MMWR Surveill Summ 2017;66:1–16.

2. Schneier AJ, Shields BJ, Hostetler SG, et al. Incidence of pediatric traumatic brain injury and associated hospital resource utilization in the United States. Pediatrics 2006;118(2):483–92.
3. Thurman DJ. The epidemiology of traumatic brain injury in children and youths: a review of research since 1990. J Child Neurol 2016;31(1):20–7.
4. Keenan HT, Runyan DK, Marshall SW, et al. A population-based study of inflicted traumatic brain injury in young children. JAMA 2003;290(5):621–6.
5. Agran PF, Anderson C, Winn D, et al. Rates of pediatric injuries by 3-month intervals for children 0 to 3 years of age. Pediatrics 2003;111(6):e683–92.
6. Dunning J, Daly JP, Lomas J, et al. Derivation of the children's head injury algorithm for the prediction of important clinical events decision rule for head injury in children. Arch Dis Child 2006;91(11):885–91.
7. Oman JA, Cooper RJ, Holmes JF, et al. Performance of a decision rule to predict need for computed tomography among children with blunt head trauma. Pediatrics 2006;117(2):e238–46.
8. Kuppermann N, Holmes JF, Dayan PS, et al. Identification of children at very low risk of clinically-important brain injuries after head trauma: a prospective cohort study. Lancet 2009;374(9696):1160–70.
9. Osmond MH, Klassen TP, Wells GA, et al. CATCH: a clinical decision rule for the use of computed tomography in children with minor head injury. Can Med Assoc J 2010;182(4):341–8.
10. Stiell I, Lesiuk H, Vandemheen K, et al. Obtaining consensus for the definition of "clinically important" brain injury in the CCC study. Acad Emerg Med 2000;7(5):572.
11. Atzema C, Mower WR, Hoffman JR, et al. Defining "clinically unimportant" CT findings in patients with blunt head trauma. Acad Emerg Med 2002;9(5):451.
12. Chang W-TW, Badjatia N. Neurotrauma. Emerg Med Clin North Am 2014;32(4):889–905.
13. Wing R, James C. Pediatric head injury and concussion. Emerg Med Clin North Am 2013;31(3):653–75.
14. Blyth BJ, Bazarian JJ. Traumatic alterations in consciousness: traumatic brain injury. Emerg Med Clin North Am 2010;28(3):571–94.
15. McHugh GS, Engel DC, Butcher I, et al. Prognostic value of secondary insults in traumatic brain injury: results from the IMPACT study. J Neurotrauma 2007;24(2):287–93.
16. Adelson P. Guidelines for the acute medical management of severe traumatic brain injury in infants, children, and adolescents. Pediatr Crit Care Med 2003;4(3):1–75.
17. Spaite DW, Hu C, Bobrow BJ, et al. The effect of combined out-of-hospital hypotension and hypoxia on mortality in major traumatic brain injury. Ann Emerg Med 2017;69(1):62–72.
18. Chesnut RM, Marshall LF, Klauber MR, et al. The role of secondary brain injury in determining outcome from severe head injury. J Trauma 1993;34(2):216–22.
19. Patel R, Lenczyk M, Hannallah RS, et al. Age and the onset of desaturation in apnoeic children. Can J Anaesth 1994;41(9):771–4.
20. Davis DP, Meade W Jr, Sise MJ, et al. Both hypoxemia and extreme hyperoxemia may be detrimental in patients with severe traumatic brain injury. J Neurotrauma 2009;26(12):2217–23.
21. Smith RL, Lin JC, Adelson PD, et al. Relationship between hyperglycemia and outcome in children with severe traumatic brain injury. Pediatr Crit Care Med 2012;13(1):85.

22. Kochanek P, Carney N, Adelson P. Guidelines for the acute medical management of severe traumatic brain injury in infants, children, and adolescents. Pediatr Crit Care Med 2012;13(1 SUPPL):S1–82.

23. ATLS Subcommittee, American College of Surgeons' Committee on Trauma, International ATLS working group. Advanced trauma life support (ATLS®): the ninth edition. J Trauma Acute Care Surg 2013;74(5):1363.

24. American Academy of Pediatrics ACoEP. APLS - the pediatric emergency medicine resource. 5th edition. Dallas (TX): Jones & Bartlett Learning; 2012.

25. Kenefake ME, Swarm M, Walthall J. Nuances in pediatric trauma. Emerg Med Clin North Am 2013;31(3):627–52.

26. Dieckmann RA, Brownstein D, Gausche-Hill M. The pediatric assessment triangle: a novel approach for the rapid evaluation of children. Pediatr Emerg Care 2010;26(4):312–5.

27. Cicero MX, Cross KP. Predictive value of initial Glasgow coma scale score in pediatric trauma patients. Pediatr Emerg Care 2013;29(1):43–8.

28. Holmes JF, Palchak MJ, MacFarlane T, et al. Performance of the pediatric Glasgow Coma Scale in children with blunt head trauma. Acad Emerg Med 2005; 12(9):814–9.

29. Lieh-Lai MW, Theodorou AA, Sarnaik AP, et al. Limitations of the Glasgow Coma Scale in predicting outcome in children with traumatic brain injury. J Pediatr 1992; 120(2):195–9.

30. Murphy S, Thomas NJ, Gertz S, et al. Tripartite stratification of the Glasgow Coma Scale in children with severe traumatic brain injury and mortality: an analysis from a multi-center comparative effectiveness study. J Neurotrauma 2017. [Epub ahead of print].

31. Acker SN, Ross JT, Partrick DA, et al. Glasgow motor scale alone is equivalent to Glasgow Coma Scale at identifying children at risk for serious traumatic brain injury. J Trauma Acute Care Surg 2014;77(2):304–9.

32. American Heart Association. Pediatric advanced life support provider manual. Dallas (TX): American Heart Association; 2017.

33. Babbitt CJ, Halpern R, Liao E, et al. Hyperglycemia is associated with intracranial injury in children younger than 3 years of age. Pediatr Emerg Care 2013;29(3): 279–82.

34. Esposito T, Ingraham A, Luchette F, et al. Urogenital trauma. J Trauma 2005;59: 1314–9.

35. Stewart TC, Alharfi IM, Fraser DD. The role of serious concomitant injuries in the treatment and outcome of pediatric severe traumatic brain injury. J Trauma Acute Care Surg 2013;75(5):836–42.

36. Sakles JC, Mosier JM, Patanwala AE, et al. Apneic oxygenation is associated with a reduction in the incidence of hypoxemia during the RSI of patients with intracranial hemorrhage in the emergency department. Intern Emerg Med 2016;11(7): 983–92.

37. Cook T, Wolf A, Henderson A. Changes in blood-gas tensions during apnoeic oxygenation in paediatric patients. Br J Anaesth 1998;81(3):338–42.

38. Shein SL, Ferguson NM, Kochanek PM, et al. Effectiveness of pharmacological therapies for intracranial hypertension in children with severe traumatic brain injury—results from an automated data collection system time-synched to drug administration. Pediatr Crit Care Med 2016;17(3):236–45.

39. Welch TP, Wallendorf MJ, Kharasch ED, et al. Fentanyl and Midazolam are ineffective in reducing episodic intracranial hypertension in severe pediatric traumatic brain injury. Crit Care Med 2016;44(4):809–18.

40. Pouraghaei M, Moharamzadeh P, Soleimanpour H, et al. Comparison between the effects of alfentanil, fentanyl and sufentanil on hemodynamic indices during rapid sequence intubation in the emergency department. Anesth Pain Med 2014;4(1):e14618.

41. Shapiro H, Wyte S, Harris A. Ketamine anaesthesia in patients with intracranial pathology. Br J Anaesth 1972;44(11):1200–4.

42. Gibbs J. The effect of intravenous ketamine on cerebrospinal fluid pressure. Br J Anaesth 1972;44(12):1298–302.

43. Gardner A, Dannemiller F, Dean D. Intracranial cerebrospinal fluid pressure in man during ketamine anesthesia. Surv Anesthesiol 1973;17(4):320.

44. Jabre P, Combes X, Lapostolle F, et al. Etomidate versus ketamine for rapid sequence intubation in acutely ill patients: a multicentre randomised controlled trial. Lancet 2009;374(9686):293–300.

45. Cohen L, Athaide V, Wickham ME, et al. The effect of ketamine on intracranial and cerebral perfusion pressure and health outcomes: a systematic review. Ann Emerg Med 2015;65(1):43–51, e42.

46. Bar-Joseph G, Guilburd Y, Tamir A, et al. Effectiveness of ketamine in decreasing intracranial pressure in children with intracranial hypertension: clinical article. J Neurosurg Pediatr 2009;4(1):40–6.

47. Walls RM. Rapid-sequence intubation in head trauma. Ann Emerg Med 1993; 22(6):1008–13.

48. Bramwell KJ, Haizlip J, Pribble C, et al. The effect of etomidate on intracranial pressure and systemic blood pressure in pediatric patients with severe traumatic brain injury. Pediatr Emerg Care 2006;22(2):90–3.

49. Patanwala AE, Erstad BL, Roe DJ, et al. Succinylcholine is associated with increased mortality when used for rapid sequence intubation of severely brain injured patients in the emergency department. Pharmacotherapy 2016;36(1): 57–63.

50. Bruce DA, Raphael RC, Goldberg AI, et al. Pathophysiology, treatment and outcome following severe head injury in children. Pediatr Neurosurg 1979;5(3): 174–91.

51. Muizelaar JP, Marmarou A, Ward JD, et al. Adverse effects of prolonged hyperventilation in patients with severe head injury: a randomized clinical trial. J Neurosurg 1991;75(5):731–9.

52. Spaite DW, Hu C, Bobrow BJ, et al. Mortality and prehospital blood pressure in patients with major traumatic brain injury: implications for the hypotension threshold. JAMA Surg 2017;152(4):360–8.

53. Bell MJ, Adelson PD, Hutchison JS, et al. Differences in medical therapy goals for children with severe traumatic brain injury—an international study. Pediatr Crit Care Med 2013;14(8):811.

54. Clifton GL, Miller ER, Choi SC, et al. Fluid thresholds and outcome from severe brain injury. Crit Care Med 2002;30(4):739–45.

55. Vavilala MS, Bowen A, Lam AM, et al. Blood pressure and outcome after severe pediatric traumatic brain injury. J Trauma Acute Care Surg 2003;55(6):1039–44.

56. Wade CE, Grady J, Kramer G, et al. Individual patient cohort analysis of the efficacy of hypertonic saline/dextran in patients with traumatic brain injury and hypotension. J Trauma Acute Care Surg 1997;42(5S):61S–5S.

57. Agbeko RS, Pearson S, Peters MJ, et al. Intracranial pressure and cerebral perfusion pressure responses to head elevation changes in pediatric traumatic brain injury. Pediatr Crit Care Med 2012;13(1):e39–47.

58. Ng I, Lim J, Wong HB. Effects of head posture on cerebral hemodynamics: its influences on intracranial pressure, cerebral perfusion pressure, and cerebral oxygenation. Neurosurgery 2004;54(3):593–8.
59. Gaither JB, Chikani V, Stolz U, et al. Body temperature after EMS transport: association with traumatic brain injury outcomes. Prehosp Emerg Care 2017;21: 575–82.
60. Bao L, Chen D, Ding L, et al. Fever burden is an independent predictor for prognosis of traumatic brain injury. PLoS One 2014;9(3):e90956.
61. Maekawa T, Yamashita S, Nagao S, et al. Prolonged mild therapeutic hypothermia versus fever control with tight hemodynamic monitoring and slow rewarming in patients with severe traumatic brain injury: a randomized controlled trial. J Neurotrauma 2015;32(7):422–9.
62. Adelson PD, Wisniewski SR, Beca J, et al. Comparison of hypothermia and normothermia after severe traumatic brain injury in children (cool kids): a phase 3, randomised controlled trial. Lancet Neurol 2013;12(6):546–53.
63. Crompton EM, Lubomirova I, Cotlarciuc I, et al. Meta-analysis of therapeutic hypothermia for traumatic brain injury in adult and pediatric patients. Crit Care Med 2017;45(4):575–83.
64. Adams H, Kolias AG, Hutchinson PJ. The role of surgical intervention in traumatic brain injury. Neurosurg Clin N Am 2016;27(4):519–28.
65. Cooper DJ, Rosenfeld JV, Murray L, et al. Decompressive craniectomy in diffuse traumatic brain injury. N Engl J Med 2011;364(16):1493–502.
66. Hutchinson PJ, Kolias AG, Timofeev IS, et al. Trial of decompressive craniectomy for traumatic intracranial hypertension. N Engl J Med 2016;375(12):1119–30.
67. Carney N, Totten AM, O'reilly C, et al. Guidelines for the management of severe traumatic brain injury. Neurosurgery 2017;80(1):6–15.
68. Bray R. Propofol infusion syndrome in children. Paediatr Anaesth 1998;8:491–9.
69. Liesemer K, Bratton SL, Zebrack CM, et al. Early post-traumatic seizures in moderate to severe pediatric traumatic brain injury: rates, risk factors, and clinical features. J Neurotrauma 2011;28(5):755–62.
70. Lewis RJ, Yee L, Inkelis SH, et al. Clinical predictors of post-traumatic seizures in children with head trauma. Ann Emerg Med 1993;22(7):1114–8.
71. Temkin NR, Dikmen SS, Wilensky AJ, et al. A randomized, double-blind study of phenytoin for the prevention of post-traumatic seizures. N Engl J Med 1990; 323(8):497–502.
72. Szaflarski JP, Sangha KS, Lindsell CJ, et al. Prospective, randomized, single-blinded comparative trial of intravenous levetiracetam versus phenytoin for seizure prophylaxis. Neurocrit Care 2010;12(2):165–72.
73. Ropper AH. Hyperosmolar therapy for raised intracranial pressure. N Engl J Med 2012;367(8):746–52.
74. Kamel H, Navi BB, Nakagawa K, et al. Hypertonic saline versus mannitol for the treatment of elevated intracranial pressure: a meta-analysis of randomized clinical trials. Crit Care Med 2011;39(3):554–9.
75. Rickard A, Smith J, Newell P, et al. Salt or sugar for your injured brain? A meta-analysis of randomised controlled trials of mannitol versus hypertonic sodium solutions to manage raised intracranial pressure in traumatic brain injury. Emerg Med J 2014;31(8):679–83.
76. Brenkert TE, Estrada CM, McMorrow SP, et al. Intravenous hypertonic saline use in the pediatric emergency department. Pediatr Emerg Care 2013;29(1):71–3.

77. Wright DW, Kellermann AL, Hertzberg VS, et al. ProTECT: a randomized clinical trial of progesterone for acute traumatic brain injury. Ann Emerg Med 2007; 49(4):391–402, e392.
78. Yutthakasemsunt S, Kittiwatanagul W, Piyavechvirat P, et al. Tranexamic acid for patients with traumatic brain injury: a randomized, double-blinded, placebo-controlled trial. BMC Emerg Med 2013;13(1):20.
79. Roberts I, Yates D, Sandercock P, et al. Effect of intravenous corticosteroids on death within 14 days in 10008 adults with clinically significant head injury (MRC CRASH trial): randomised placebo-controlled trial. Lancet 2004; 364(9442):1321–8.
80. Deans KJ, Minneci PC, Lowell W, et al. Increased morbidity and mortality of traumatic brain injury in victims of nonaccidental trauma. J Trauma Acute Care Surg 2013;75(1):157–60.
81. Duhaime A-C, Christian CW, Rorke LB, et al. Nonaccidental head injury in infants—the "shaken-baby syndrome". N Engl J Med 1998;338(25):1822–9.
82. Caffey J. The whiplash shaken infant syndrome: manual shaking by the extremities with whiplash-induced intracranial and intraocular bleedings, linked with residual permanent brain damage and mental retardation. Pediatrics 1974;54(4): 396–403.
83. Piteau SJ, Ward MG, Barrowman NJ, et al. Clinical and radiographic characteristics associated with abusive and nonabusive head trauma: a systematic review. Pediatrics 2012;130(2):315–23.
84. Hettler J, Greenes DS. Can the initial history predict whether a child with a head injury has been abused? Pediatrics 2003;111(3):602–7.
85. Maguire SA, Kemp AM, Lumb RC, et al. Estimating the probability of abusive head trauma: a pooled analysis. Pediatrics 2011;128(3):e550–64.
86. Maguire S, Pickerd N, Farewell D, et al. Which clinical features distinguish inflicted from non-inflicted brain injury? A systematic review. Arch Dis Child 2009; 94(11):860–7.
87. King WJ, MacKay M, Sirnick A, Canadian Shaken Baby Study Group. Shaken baby syndrome in Canada: clinical characteristics and outcomes of hospital cases. CMAJ 2003;168(2):155–9.
88. Alexander R, Sato Y, Smith W, et al. Incidence of impact trauma with cranial injuries ascribed to shaking. Am J Dis Child 1990;144(6):724–6.
89. Atwal G, Rutty G, Carter N, et al. Bruising in non-accidental head injured children; a retrospective study of the prevalence, distribution and pathological associations in 24 cases. Forensic Sci Int 1998;96(2):215–30.
90. Merten D, Osborne D, Radkowski M, et al. Craniocerebral trauma in the child abuse syndrome: radiological observations. Pediatr Radiol 1984;14(5):272–7.
91. Lazoritz S, Baldwin S, Kini N. The Whiplash Shaken infant syndrome: has Caffey's syndrome changed or have we changed his syndrome? Child Abuse Negl 1997; 21(10):1009–14.

Pediatric Thoracic Trauma
Recognition and Management

Stacy L. Reynolds, MD

KEYWORDS

- Pediatric • Thoracic trauma • Chest • Child

KEY POINTS

- Pulmonary contusions, pneumothoraces, hemothoraces, and rib fractures occur most commonly when children sustain thoracic trauma.
- The narrow trachea, compliant chest wall, lower functional residual capacity, and higher oxygen demand of children pose specific challenges in treating the unique injury patterns of thoracic trauma in children.
- Rib fractures occur less commonly in children even in association with cardiopulmonary resuscitation and should prompt consideration of nonaccidental trauma.
- Blunt cardiac injury should not increase the chance of arrhythmia or shock in children unless shock or arrhythmia are present at or before the emergency department presentation.
- Chest computed tomography may increase the detection of occult chest injuries but infrequently detects clinically significant occult injury, and chest radiograph provides a reasonable screening tool for most chest injuries in children.

INTRODUCTION

Thoracic injuries account for less than one-tenth of all pediatric trauma-related injuries but comprise 14% of pediatric trauma-related deaths.[1] Many affected patients die at the scene when injuries do occur. Thoracic trauma includes injuries to the lungs, heart, aorta and great vessels, tracheobronchial tree, and structures of the chest wall. Pulmonary contusions, pneumothoraces, hemothoraces, and rib fractures occur most commonly.[2]

During the first decade of life, most chest injuries result from falls or motor vehicle accidents.[1] Penetrating trauma occurs rarely. More than half of pediatric blunt thoracic trauma occurs in association with head, abdominal, and limb injuries.[1] The case-specific mortality for patients with thoracic trauma increases to 20% for patients with concomitant abdominal injuries and exceeds 30% for patients with associated head injuries. Isolated chest trauma occurs less frequently and with lower mortality rates.

Disclosure Statement: None.
Division of Pediatric Emergency Medicine, Department of Emergency Medicine, Carolinas Medical Center, 1000 Blythe Boulevard, 3rd Floor Medical Education Building, Charlotte, NC 28203, USA
E-mail address: Stacy.Reynolds@carolinas.org

Emerg Med Clin N Am 36 (2018) 473–483
https://doi.org/10.1016/j.emc.2017.12.013   emed.theclinics.com

Certain unique anatomic features of the developing child provide a rationale for thoracic injury patterns. The trachea is narrow and easily compressed, and small changes in airway diameter produce respiratory distress.[3] Children less than 10 years of age have a lower functional residual capacity and a higher oxygen demand; thus, hypoxemia develops more quickly than in adults.[3] The mediastinum is not fixed in children, and there is more opportunity for visceral displacement leading to loss of preload and hypotension.[3] A child's short stature increases the incidence of improper restraint placement.[1] The pediatric chest wall is compliant, and the flexible ribs are unlikely to fracture; this can foster direct transmission of force to the lung parenchyma.[4] As a result, pulmonary contusions occur more commonly in the pediatric population. Rib fractures, when they do occur, herald more significant internal injuries in children. The chest wall seems to be fully developed by 13 years of age and responds to injury like the adult chest wall.[5]

The compliant chest wall of a child can also make the evaluation of patients more challenging, as there can be significant injury with little or no external signs of trauma. A thorough examination being mindful of risk factors for intrathoracic injury is imperative. These risk factors for thoracic trauma include a low systolic blood pressure, elevated age-adjusted respiratory rate, abnormal results on thoracic examination, abnormal chest auscultation, femur fracture, and Glasgow Coma Scale less than 15.[6] Clinicians should consider thoracic injury in pediatric patients with such risk factors, a suggestive examination, or radiographic findings of injury.

PNEUMOTHORAX AND HEMOTHORAX
Clinical Recognition

Tachypnea, decreased breath sounds, chest wall crepitus, and chest wall injury increase suspicion for pneumothoraces.[1] Decreased breath sounds on the left side may also occur in a right main stem intubation, and this should be considered when evaluating intubated patients with chest trauma.[3] Severe gastric distention from prolonged bagging can distort the left-sided lung examination as well.[3] An abnormal chest examination or work of breathing warrants further investigation for injury in pediatric trauma patients.

Tension pneumothorax occurs when air overfills the pleural space and causes displacement of the lung parenchyma and mediastinal structures. Diastolic filling of the heart is reduced by obstructed return of blood from the vena cava. This condition will progress to shock and cardiac arrest without decompression. Tension pneumothorax should be suspected with jugular venous distention, a displaced cardiac apex beat suggesting mediastinal shift, loss of breath sounds to one side, or contralateral tracheal deviation.[1] Decreasing end-tidal carbon dioxide levels and hyperresonance of the chest may also indicate tension pneumothoraces. These findings suggest potentially life-threatening injury, and the tension pneumothorax should be decompressed as quickly as possible.

Pneumomediastinum occurs in up to 10% of patients with blunt thoracic trauma.[7] Because pneumomediastinum may indicate aerodigestive injury, many patients received extended workups on this finding alone historically. However, in the absence of clinical symptoms, the workup of pneumomediastinum rarely yields findings of other injuries.[7] It has been postulated that benign pneumomediastinum may result from subclinical alveolar rupture.[7] Injuries of the tracheobronchial tree or esophagus warrant consideration with pneumomediastinum but are rarely present without other examination findings.

Open pneumothorax and lung lacerations occur rarely except in cases of penetrating trauma.[1] Open pneumothoraces occur when air fills the pleural space from an external wound along the chest wall. Failure to recognize the wound can rapidly produce tension physiology. Fortunately, these injuries are rare. Lung lacerations can predispose to air leaks, pneumothoraces, and hemothoraces.[1] Most lung lacerations will heal without surgical intervention and can be treated with tube thoracostomy alone. Hemothorax results from injury to the intrathoracic vessels, injury to the lung parenchyma, or from rib fractures that damage the intercostal vessels.[3] Blunt trauma causes shear forces and increased pressure that puts the mediastinal vessels at risk for tearing.[3] Hemothoraces and pneumothoraces often occur together. Penetrating injuries may cause hemorrhage from direct injury to a vessel.

Diagnostic Testing

Chest radiographs are used to screen for thoracic injury. Chest radiographs demonstrating air in the pleural space with or without displacement of the trachea and the mediastinal structures indicate a pneumothorax. Radiographs in patients with pneumothoraces may demonstrate any of the following: hyperlucency at the apex or lung borders, hyperlucency tracing the mediastinal structures, a deep sulcus sign, hyperlucency along the diaphragm, or loss of lung markings.[8] Hemothorax may be indicated by pleural effusions on chest radiographs. A chest radiograph demonstrates high sensitivity for clinically significant chest trauma and serves as an adequate screening tool to limit computed tomography (CT) imaging of the chest.[9]

Chest CT does increase the sensitivity of occult pneumothoraces and hemothoraces, but the clinical significance of these additional findings over chest radiography is limited. CT chest was shown to increase the diagnosis of pneumothorax from 7.2% to 18.7% in a large retrospective study of 1035 pediatric blunt trauma activations; however, only one patient required a change in management with chest tube placement before going to the operating room for an exploratory laparotomy.[10] Other studies have demonstrated similar findings.[11] The largest prospective study was a planned secondary analysis of a large cohort of pediatric patients with blunt trauma, including more than 8000 undergoing chest radiograph (CXR).[12] CT identified an additional 2.8% of patients with occult pneumothoraces, but most patients were managed with observation alone.[12] The investigators concluded that observational management of occult pneumothoraces should be strongly encouraged.[12] Although CT has a higher sensitivity for pneumothoraces and hemothoraces, it seems that CXR may be a better predictor of clinically significant injuries and outcomes.

Ultrasound also has a high sensitivity for detecting pneumothoraces. In adult studies, the sensitivity of ultrasound for clinically significant pneumothoraces was around 80% with a specificity of 100%.[13] Studies of neonatal pneumothorax demonstrated a sensitivity of 100%.[14] Lung sliding appears on ultrasound if the visceral and parietal pleura are free to slide over each other with respiration. Additionally, comet tail artifacts require the parietal and visceral pleura to be aligned for visualization. Comet tail artifacts occur when water under the visceral pleura vibrates. Both lung sliding and comet tails will be interrupted and abolished by subcutaneous emphysema, pleural adhesions, or air or blood distending the pleural. Absence of lung sliding and comet tail artifacts suggest the presence of a pneumothorax.

Management Goals

The main goal of management is to decompress the chest and restore ventilation. When time allows, chest tube thoracostomy provides the most reliable means of treatment. A gloved finger acting as a unidirectional valve provides a life-saving alternative in the resuscitation of blunt traumatic arrest.[1] When a large air leak causes pneumo-thoraces with pneumomediastinum, consider placing multiple chest tubes to adequately decompress the chest.[1] Tension pneumothorax is fatal without interven-tion and warrants immediate chest tube placement. In cases of hemothorax, it is important to evacuate the blood, which can cause empyema or undergo fibrous scaring to entrap the lung.[3] Chest tube placement both decompresses the lung and provides a way to monitor for ongoing or rapid bleeding. Hemorrhage exceeding 20% to 25% of blood volume or losses of 4% of blood volume per hour should prompt surgical exploration.[1] Fortunately, vascular injuries of this severity are rare in children. Tube thoracostomy is often sufficient for management. Open pneumothoraces require an occlusive dressing to stop accumulation of air through the wound and immediate chest tube placement to decompress the pleural space. The chest tube should not be placed through the existing wound.

Pneumomediastinum often requires only observational management assuming the mediastinal air does not indicate a more serious injury, such as a tear in the tracheo-bronchial tree.[2] Pneumomediastinum in a patient with a persisting air leak, as in tracheobronchial injury, may require multiple chest tubes and surgical intervention to correct the injury. Esophageal injury should also be considered in such severe cases.

Antibiotic use is controversial but often done routinely in patients with chest tube placement or substantial tissue destruction from injury.[3] There is considerable varia-tion in this practice by region. Practitioners should consult with their local trauma ser-vices for current recommendations.

LUNG PARENCHYMAL INJURY
Clinical Recognition

Pulmonary contusions may be diagnosed clinically by respiratory distress, abnormal breath sounds in the consolidated area, resting tachypnea, and, less commonly, he-moptysis.[4] Pulmonary contusions often occur without external indictors of chest wall injury or rib fractures.[3] High-energy forces damage the alveolar spaces leading to edema, hemorrhage, and subsequent inflammation.[1] Lung contusions and lacera-tions are the predominant injuries with or without rib fractures, pneumothoraces, or hemothoraces.[4]

Two main mechanisms damage the lung: direct compression or tearing of the lung or severe displacement of the lung as with decelerating injuries.[4] With rapid deceler-ation, the lung is displaced and the lung, tracheobronchial tree, or mediastinal struc-tures may tear.[4] The damaged lung suffers hemorrhage, edema, and consolidation that impairs ventilation leading to ventilation/perfusion mismatch and hypoxia.[4] If the pleura is torn, pneumothorax with or without hemothorax will also occur.[4] Small contusions begin to heal over the course of a week.[2] Lung contusions, however, can lead to acute respiratory distress syndrome and respiratory failure.[3] Furthermore, 20% of patients with lung contusions will develop pneumonia.[4]

Diagnostic Testing

Plain films will demonstrate nonanatomic areas of consolidation.[4] Lung contusions often spare the periphery of the lung and are poorly defined.[8] The initial radiograph will underestimate the size of the contusion, and radiographs should be repeated 24 hours later.[2] It takes hours for the hemorrhage, edema, and inflammation of the injured lung tissue to manifest by radiograph. Ultrasound has the potential to diagnose a pulmonary contusion more rapidly than radiographs because B lines from edema and alveolar disruption show up rapidly on ultrasound. Alveolar bleeding pushes air out of the lung making it appear like hepatic tissue, referred to as hepatization. When hepatization is present, pulmonary contusion should be apparent by both ultrasound and radiograph. High-resolution CT scans detect the most minor lung contusions with high sensitivity. However, CT may overestimate the significance of an injury and may diagnose small contusions of limited clinical significance.[4]

Management Goals

The main goal of therapy is to restore adequate oxygenation.[4] Adequate pain management and normovolemia will promote respiratory function.[2] In up to 30% of cases, respiratory failure occurs requiring intubation with mechanical ventilation and positive end-expiratory pressure.[4] Although there is no evidence to support broad-spectrum antibiotic use with large pulmonary contusions, the practice is widely accepted.[1] Pneumatocoeles and posttraumatic pseudocysts are rare complications of lung injury and usually resolve without lung resection over several months.[2]

RIB FRACTURES
Clinical Recognition

Rib fractures occur less frequently in children than in adult patients. The chest wall of a child is extremely compliant resulting in fewer rib fractures and more direct lung injury. The incidence of hemothorax increases with increasing rib fractures.[15] In a large pediatric study, mortality increased from 1.8% among children without rib fractures to 5.0% for children with one rib fracture and exceeded 8.0% when 7 ribs were fractured.[15] A study of 328 children and 6627 adult patients compared the rates of associated injuries for pediatric and adult patients with rib fractures.[16] Pediatric patients with rib fractures sustained more brain injuries, abdominal solid organ injuries, and lung injuries than adult patients, though the overall mortality rates were similar at 5%.[16] Rib fractures are a signal of high transmission of force and potential for severe injury. The absence of rib fractures, however, does not rule out significant internal injury.

Flail chest involves a segment of fractured ribs that move freely but opposite to the chest wall during respiration.[1] These injuries occur very rarely in children and are almost uniformly associated with underlying pulmonary injuries.[1] This injury should be considered for patients with respiratory distress or paradoxic motion of the chest wall.

Rib fractures warrant consideration of nonaccidental trauma in infants and toddlers.[3] A large study of children found the rate of abuse for children less than 24 months of age with rib fractures to be 56%.[17] A retrospective study of children less than 3 years of age demonstrated that 72% of the patients with rib fractures were abused.[18] For children less than 1 year of age, 82% of rib fractures indicated child abuse.[19] Interestingly, abused children with rib fractures sustained fewer lung injuries.[18] Rib fractures from abuse most often occur in the posterior ribs and result from squeezing.[18] However, squeezing of the chest in cardiopulmonary resuscitation (CPR) does not seem to cause rib fractures. A retrospective study of children less than 1 year of age requiring CPR found that 2-finger CPR rarely caused rib fractures.[20] The investigators concluded that posterior rib fractures after CPR require investigation for nonaccidental trauma.[20]

Diagnostic Testing

Nondisplaced rib fractures are often difficult to detect. Posterior rib fractures secondary to nonaccidental trauma are especially challenging to diagnose. Repeat radiographs at 10 days may be required to look for the callous formation of healing fractures.[20] Displaced rib fractures are easier to visualize but not in all cases. Chest CT offers greater sensitivity for detecting rib fractures. However, rib fractures should not be the only indication for chest CT, as isolated rib fractures heal well and are benign injuries. Ultrasound will detect rib fractures, but the utility of ultrasound for rib fractures is operator dependent.

Management Goals

Pain relief minimizes the atelectasis and risk of pneumonia following rib fractures. Aggressive management of pain should be the standard of care for children and adults.[2] Epidural anesthesia and regional blocks may be used to manage fracture pain in selected cases. Patients with rib fractures should be assessed carefully for consideration of associated severe injuries.[3] Children may rarely require intubation and positive pressure ventilation depending on the extent of injury.

BLUNT CARDIAC INJURY
Clinical Recognition

Blunt cardiac injuries are rare in the emergency department (ED) because many victims die before hospital presentation.[1] Lung contusions and rib fractures are commonly associated with these injuries.[1] Cardiac contusions warrant consideration when cardiac output is low in trauma.[1] Patients with a cardiac contusion present with arrhythmia, low cardiac output, or abnormal cardiac serum enzymes.[2]

Stable, asymptomatic patients with a possible cardiac contusion rarely develop cardiac arrhythmias or cardiac arrest. In a multicenter, retrospective study of patients less than 18 years of age diagnosed with blunt cardiac injury, hemodynamically stable patients who presented with a normal sinus rhythm did not develop cardiac arrhythmias or cardiac failure.[21] All patients who did develop an arrhythmia or pump failure displayed a serious arrhythmia or shock in the ED.[21] Among admitted pediatric patients with a diagnosis of blunt cardiac injury, 5% developed cardiac sequela, including mitral or tricuspid insufficiency or a traumatic ventricular septal defect.[21] Although these injuries are rare, not all cardiac sequelae were detected during the hospital evaluation and follow-up was strongly recommended.[21]

Commotio cordis is a unique entity that deserves specific attention. It is a phenomenon of sudden death after chest trauma without evidence of cardiac contusion, coronary arterial abnormalities, or a lesion in the conduction system.[3] The postulated mechanism is cardiac arrest following a disorganized rhythm initiated by blunt force to the chest.[3] Preventative measures, such as midchest protective gear, are recommended by some sports leagues to mitigate potential injuries.[3]

Diagnostic Testing

The Eastern Association for the Surgery of Trauma's (EAST) guidelines recommend an electrocardiogram (EKG) for all patients in whom a blunt cardiac injury is suspected.[22] Troponin I testing is supported in adult patients, and the combination of a negative EKG and negative troponin I level rules out blunt cardiac injury in adult patients.[22] The evidence for pediatric patients does not support or refute the use of troponin I to diagnose blunt cardiac injury, and the EAST's guidelines do not make a recommendation for the pediatric population.[22]

Management Goals

The goals of management are adequate analgesia, monitoring for arrhythmia, and inotropic support if needed.[2] Supportive management includes cardiac monitoring, and frequent blood pressure monitoring. Inotropes are required in rare circumstances to support cardiac function.[3] Patients with unstable hemodynamics should undergo echocardiography to look for structural disruption in the heart.[3] All patients with suspected blunt cardiac injury require outpatient follow-up.

INJURIES OF THE AORTA AND GREAT VESSELS
Clinical Recognition

The mobility of the pediatric mediastinum makes traumatic aortic injury very rare in a child. It occurs in only 0.06% to 0.1% of pediatric trauma patients and accounts for only 2.1% of pediatric deaths from trauma.[8] High-energy mechanisms with rapid deceleration, such as motor vehicle accidents and falls, most commonly result in such injuries.[2] These injuries can also occur with penetrating trauma but are less common.

Aortic injuries most commonly occur at the aortic isthmus at the ligamentum arteriosum distal to the left subclavian artery where the aorta is tethered. Shearing forces twist the mobile ascending aorta at its point of fixation to produce pseudoaneurysms or focal aortic dissections.[8] Injury at this anatomic site leads to widening of the aorta and blurring of the mediastinal contour. This subtle finding on a chest radiograph may be the only indication of injury.

Diagnostic Testing

Suggestive features on chest radiography include mediastinal widening, loss of a defined aortic knob, pleural effusion, deviation of the esophagus or main stem bronchus, apical cap, or first or second rib fractures.[3] The size of the thymus in young children can mask traditional diagnostic features, and CT may be required to make the diagnosis.[3] The injury should be strongly considered in any child with a severe deceleration mechanism.

CT angiography of the chest is the study of choice for diagnosis. Thoracic CT has a negative predictive value approaching 100%.[8] Chest CT may reveal a pseudoaneurysm, focal dissection, thrombus, intimal irregularity, or hidden mediastinal hematoma.[8] Some investigators have suggested thoracic CT should be reserved for patients with a high clinical suspicion of vascular injury or an abnormal mediastinal silhouette on a radiograph.[10]

Management Goals

Surgical management provides definitive treatment. Temporizing measures to reduce shear forces to the aorta includes pain control and may include beta-blocker therapy to decrease the heart rate and blood pressure.[2] However, most of these patients will present with multiple injuries; beta-blocker therapy will be largely impractical for ED management in most cases. The injuries are often fatal. The emergency physician reduces mortality most effectively through early recognition.

PENETRATING TRAUMA

Penetrating trauma occurs nearly 6-fold less often than blunt trauma in children.[8] However, penetrating trauma accounts for 20% of all deaths among children less than 19 years of age.[5] Penetrating thoracic wounds occur by stabbing, firearms, or impalement injuries and impose a mortality rate of about 14%.[5] About one-third of injuries will be managed with tube thoracostomy alone, and an additional 35% of patients will require operative intervention.[5] Although penetrating trauma remains less common in children, violent injuries by stabbing and firearms are increasing.[5]

Management Goals

The main goal of management is to resuscitate patients with hemorrhagic shock and surgically correct ongoing hemorrhage. Immediate surgery is indicated for patients with shock and among patients with chest tube output exceeding 20% of blood volume or a persistent output exceeding 2 mL/kg/h based on body weight.[23] Blood is the resuscitation fluid of choice for such patients. Delayed resuscitation strategies have not been supported with data in the pediatric population.[23] Similarly, ED thoracotomy has limited indications for children with penetrating trauma and should be reserved for patients who lose signs of life in the ED.[23]

ESOPHAGEAL INJURIES
Clinical Recognition

Esophageal injury is rare but can occur with extreme increases in intra-abdominal or gastric pressure from blunt trauma.[1] The esophagus is one of the best protected structures of the thorax.[3] Blunt thoracic trauma causes esophageal injury in less than 0.1% of patients.[8] Chest pain or epigastric pain with mediastinal air, fever or sepsis, or pleural effusion should prompt consideration of esophageal disruption.[3]

Diagnostic Testing

Both water-soluble contrast esophagram and esophagoscopy are required to fully evaluate esophageal injuries.[3] Chest radiographs may increase suspicion of esophageal injury if infiltrates, pleural effusion, or pneumomediastinum is present in patients with clinical symptoms. Fluid accumulation in the mediastinum will cause widening. Perforation may appear as focal extraluminal air at the site of esophageal injury on a CT scan. CT has increased sensitivity over radiographs to detect esophageal injury.

Management Goals

The main goal of ED management is early recognition. Fluids and broad-spectrum antibiotics should be administered to avoid sepsis.[3] Surgical closure is common in adults, but most children can be managed with supportive care and drainage of any infectious fluid collections.[1] Antibiotics and parenteral nutrition are required to allow the injury to heal.[2] Surgical repair should be undertaken in patients with complications or failure to improve.

DIAPHRAGMATIC INJURIES
Clinical Recognition

Most diaphragmatic injuries occur when the abdomen is forcibly compressed and the diaphragm is stressed by high pressures.[1] The timing of impact in the respiratory cycle plays an important role.[24] The left hemidiaphragm ruptures in two-thirds of cases and most often in the posterolateral area.[3] Liver and spleen injuries accompany most diaphragmatic injuries.[3] Penetrating trauma can directly injure the muscle of the diaphragm, but this is rare.[1]

Diaphragmatic injuries may be asymptomatic early in care and are often missed initially. Bowel sounds in the chest suggest this injury. In severe defects, the bowel will compress the lung parenchyma and cause respiratory distress mandating emergent surgical repair. Diaphragmatic injuries will present in a delayed fashion if visceral herniation does not occur initially. Delayed presentations include vague chest pain, difficulty breathing, vomiting, or bowel obstruction.[24]

Diagnostic Testing

The subtle radiographic findings in these injuries include opacifications in the lung bases, air above the diaphragm, pleural effusions, displacement of the stomach bubble into the thoracic cavity, or a nasogastric tube in the chest.[8] CT imaging may reveal diaphragmatic injuries missed on a radiograph. Features suggestive of diaphragmatic disruption include an abnormal diaphragmatic line or high-riding diaphragm. The presence of intestinal loops in the chest with or without pleural effusion also strongly suggests diaphragmatic injury.[3]

Management Goals

The main goal of ED management is to recognize the injury and support the patients' respiratory function in severe cases. This injury should be considered in all patients requiring a chest tube to avoid bowel perforation. Surgical repair is required in most patients and highly successful.[24] Pulmonary hypertension and permanent lung parenchymal damage may complicate delayed presentations of injury.

TRAUMATIC ASPHYXIA
Clinical Recognition

Traumatic asphyxia occurs rarely. The injury occurs in high-speed motor vehicle accidents from improperly placed restraint devices or as a complication of crush injuries to the head or torso.[25] The mechanism for traumatic asphyxia is similar between trauma and nontrauma patients. Intrathoracic and mediastinal pressure increase with compressive force to the abdomen against a closed glottis.[25] As intrathoracic pressure increases, right atrial blood is pushed into the innominate and jugular veins and capillaries break in the cervicofacial region in response.[25]

Patients may present with facial and bulbar conjunctival petechiae as early as 2 to 3 hours after the injury.[25] Oral mucosal petechiae, facial edema, and facial cyanosis may occur. Neurologic symptoms are less common and include agitation, loss of consciousness, confusion, seizures, anoxic injury, cerebral edema, or ischemia.[25]

Management Goals

Most cases of traumatic asphyxia resolve spontaneously and carry a good prognosis. Adequate oxygenation and adequate cerebral perfusion are the goals of management to promote healing and avoid secondary neurologic injury.[25] Mild symptoms usually reverse in 1 to 2 days.[25] The prognosis is good for patients who survive the initial hours of management.

TRACHEOBRONCHIAL INJURIES
Clinical Recognition

The most common clinical presentation of a tracheobronchial injury is mediastinal air tracking into the neck with subcutaneous emphysema.[4] A persistent, large air leak or respiratory collapse may also indicate an airway injury.[3] Stridor, hoarse voice, and difficulty swallowing additionally warrant consideration. Tracheobronchial injuries are often subtle and may be unrecognized in the trauma bay during the initial resuscitation.

Tracheobronchial injuries, although rare, are lethal in up to one-third of cases in the first hour.[2] Force to the chest against a closed glottis, rapid deceleration, or direct disruption from a crush injury predispose patients to injuries of the tracheobronchial tree.[1] The airways may be directly obstructed by blood, vomit, or foreign bodies.

Airway obstruction will present with stridor, respiratory distress or failure, or hypoxia and cyanosis but usually without subcutaneous emphysema.

Diagnostic Testing

Chest radiographs may demonstrate pneumothoraces and subcutaneous emphysema but will not localize tracheobronchial injuries. CT imaging identifies most but not all tracheobronchial injuries. Bronchoscopy is often required to diagnose tracheobronchial disruption and to identify the location of injury.[3] A high clinical suspicion is required to pursue the diagnosis.

Management Goals

Most tracheobronchial injuries will be recognized after the ED stabilization of patients. When tracheal injury is suspected, intubation in the operating room with bronchoscopy should be considered. Partial tears may become complete tracheal disruption during direct laryngoscopy in the ED. Tracheostomy or cricothyroidotomy may be emergently required. Intubation past the injured area may serve as a temporizing measure if the air leak of a tracheal injury is difficult to manage.[4] This measure may allow a tear to heal with conservative management, though most injuries will require surgical repair.[4]

REFERENCES

1. Tovar JA, Vazquez JJ. Management of chest trauma in children. Paediatr Respir Rev 2013;14:86–91.
2. Van As AB, Manganyi R, Brooks A. Treatment of thoracic trauma in children: literature review, Red Cross War Memorial Children's Hospital data analysis, and guidelines for management. Eur J Pediatr Surg 2013;23:434–43.
3. Bliss D, Silen M. Pediatric thoracic trauma. Crit Care Med 2002;30(11):S409–15.
4. Tovar JA. The lung and pediatric trauma. Semin Pediatr Surg 2008;17:53–9.
5. Mollberg NM, Tabachnick D, Lin FJ, et al. Age-associated impact on presentation and outcome for penetrating thoracic trauma in the adult and pediatric patient populations. J Trauma Acute Care Surg 2013;76(2):273–8.
6. Holmes JF, Sokolove PE, Brant WE, et al. A clinical decision rule for identifying children with thoracic injuries after blunt torso trauma. Ann Emerg Med 2002; 39(5):492–9.
7. Neal MD, Sippey M, Gaines BA, et al. Presence of pneumomediastinum after blunt trauma in children: what does it really mean? J Pediatr Surg 2009;44: 1322–7.
8. Hammer MR, Dillman JR, Chong ST, et al. Imaging of pediatric thoracic trauma. Semin Roentgenol 2012;47(2):135–46.
9. Yanchar NL, Woo K, Brennan M, et al. Chest x-ray as a screening tool for blunt thoracic trauma in children. J Trauma Acute Care Surg 2013;75(4):613–9.
10. Golden J, Isani M, Bowling J, et al. Limiting chest computed tomography in the evaluation of pediatric thoracic trauma. J Trauma Acute Care Surg 2016;81(2): 271–7.
11. Holscher CM, Faulk LW, Moore EE, et al. Chest computed tomography imaging for blunt pediatric trauma: not worth the radiation risk. J Surg Res 2013;184(1): 352–7.
12. Lee LK, Rogers AJ, Ehrlich PF, et al. Occult pneumothoraces in children with blunt torso trauma. Acad Emerg Med 2014;21(4):440–8.

13. Helland G, Gaspari R, Licciardo S, et al. Comparison of four views to single-view ultrasound protocols to identify clinically significant pneumothorax. Acad Emerg Med 2016;23(10):1170–5.
14. Cattarossi L, Copetti R, Brusa G, et al. Lung ultrasound diagnostic accuracy in neonatal pneumothorax. Can Respir J 2016;2016:6515069.
15. Rosenberg G, Bryant AK, Davis KA, et al. No breakpoint for mortality in pediatric rib fractures. J Trauma Acute Care Surg 2015;80(3):427–32.
16. Kessel B, Dagan J, Swaid F, et al, Israel Trauma Group. Rib fractures: comparison of associated injuries between pediatric and adult population. Am J Surg 2014; 208:831–4.
17. Lindberg DM, Beaty B, Juarez-Colunga E, et al. Testing for abuse in children with sentinel injuries. Pediatrics 2015;136(5):831–8.
18. Darling SE, Done SL, Friedman SD, et al. Frequency of intrathoracic injuries in children younger than 3 years with rib fractures. Pediatr Radiol 2014;44:1230–6.
19. Bulloch B, Schubert CJ, Brophy PD, et al. Cause and clinical characteristics of rib fractures in infants. Pediatrics 2000;105(4):E48.
20. Franke I, Pingen A, Schiffman H, et al. Cardiopulmonary resuscitation (CPR)-related posterior rib fractures in neonates and infants following recommended changes in CPR techniques. Child Abuse Negl 2014;38:1267–74.
21. Denise D, Krug S. Pediatric blunt cardiac injury: epidemiology, clinical features, and diagnosis. J Trauma 1996;40(1):61–7.
22. Clancy K, Velopulos C, Bilaniuk JW, et al. Screening for blunt cardiac injury: an Eastern Association for the Surgery of Trauma practice management guideline. J Trauma Acute Care Surg 2012;73(5):S301–6.
23. Cotton BA, Nance ML. Penetrating trauma in children. Semin Pediatr Surg 2004; 13(2):87–97.
24. Khan TR, Rawat J, Maletha M, et al. Traumatic diaphragmatic injuries in children: do they really mark the severity of injury? Our experience. Pediatr Surg Int 2009; 25:595–9.
25. Montes-Tapia F, Arroyo IB, Cura-Esquivel I, et al. Traumatic asphyxia. Pediatr Emerg Care 2014;30(2):114–6.

Printed and bound by CPI Group (UK) Ltd, Croydon, CR0 4YY

08/05/2025

01864711-0003